To

Melissa Lorton

Hope to get your back

Skiing.

Regards,

Richard Sanders MD

15 October 2013

Thoracic Outlet Syndrome

Thoracic Outlet Syndrome

A common sequela of neck injuries

Richard J. Sanders, M.D.
Department of Surgery
Rose Medical Center
School of Medicine
University of Colorado
Health Science Center
Denver, Colorado

Craig E. Haug, M.D.
School of Medicine
University of Colorado
Health Science Center
Denver, Colorado
Department of Surgery
Massachusetts General Hospital
Harvard Medical School
Boston, Massachusetts

Illustrations by
Susan Raymer, B.A.

With seven additional contributors

RICHARD J. SANDERS, M.D.
4545 E. 9th Avenue, Suite 240
Denver, Colorado 80220-3950

Acquisitions Editor: Lisa McAllister
Developmental Editor: Paula Callaghan
Project Coordinator: Susan Clarey
Production: McLaurine & Co.
Compositor: Circle Graphics
Printer/Binder: The Maple-Vail Book Manufacturing Group

Supported in part by a grant from the Rose Foundation,
Rose Medical Center, Denver, Colorado

3 5 6 4

Library of Congress Cataloging-in-Publication Data

Sanders, Richard J
    Thoracic outlet syndrome : a common sequela of neck injuries/
Richard J. Sanders, Craig E. Haug, with seven additional
contributors; illustrated by Susan Raymer.
     p.   cm.
    Includes bibliographical references and index.
    ISBN 0-397-51097-7
    1. Thoracic outlet syndrome –Surgery.   I. Haug, Craig E.
II. Title.
    [DNLM: 1. Neck---injuries. 2. Neck Muscles---pathology.
3. Thoracic Outlet Syndrome   WL 500 S215t]
RD531.S26   1991
617.5'3044—dc20
DNLM/DLC   91-14160
for Library of Congress   CIF

The authors and publisher have exerted every effort to ensure that drug selection and dosage set forth in this text are in accord with current recommendations and practice at the time of publication. However, in view of ongoing research, changes in government regulations, and the constant flow of information relating to drug therapy and drug reactions, the reader is urged to check the package insert for each drug for any change in indications and dosage and for added warnings and precautions. This is particularly important when the recommended agent is a new or infrequently employed drug.

This book is dedicated to
Charles Joseph Phillips
(1903–1990)
and
Kevin Martin Carlton
(1990–   )
The cycle is complete

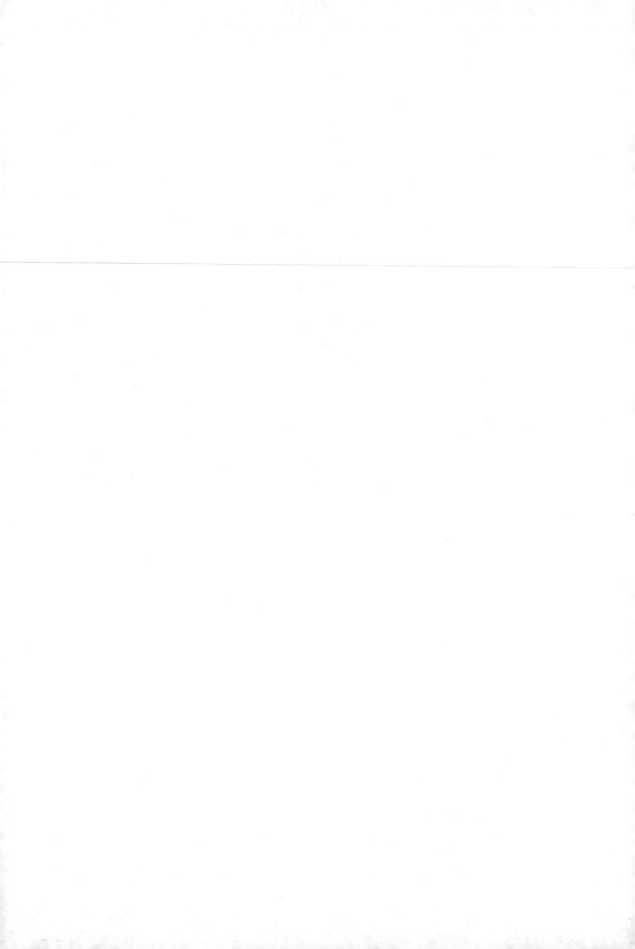

Contributors

Natalio Banchero, M.D.
> Professor of Physiology, School of Medicine, University of Colorado Health Science Center, Denver, Colorado

Craig E. Haug, M.D.
> Instructor in Surgery, School of Medicine, University of Colorado Health Science Center, Denver, Colorado; Department of Surgery, Massachusetts General Hospital, Harvard Medical School, Boston, Massachusetts

Catherine G.R. Jackson, Ph.D.
> Associate Professor of Kinesiology, and Department Chair, University of Northern Colorado, Greeley, Colorado

Roger F. Johnson, M.D., LL.B.
> Clinical Assistant Professor of Psychiatry, School of Medicine, University of Colorado Health Science Center; Adjunct Professor of Law, University of Denver College of Law, Denver, Colorado

Mary B. Mockus, M.D., Ph.D.
> Instructor in Surgery, School of Medicine, University of Colorado Health Science Center, Denver, Colorado

Susan L. Raymer, B.A.
> Medical Illustrator, Denver, Colorado

Richard J. Sanders, M.D.
> Attending Vascular Surgeon, Rose Medical Center; Clinical Professor of Surgery, School of Medicine, University of Colorado Health Science Center; Consulting Surgeon, Fitzsimons Army Hospital, Denver, Colorado

Stephen H. Shogan, M.D.
> Attending Surgeon, Rose Medical Center; Clinical Assistant Professor of Neurosurgery, School of Medicine, University of Colorado Health Science Center, Denver, Colorado

Richard Smith, M.D.
> Attending Neurologist, Rose Medical Center, Denver, Colorado

Angelika Voelkel, M.D.
> Attending Physician, Presbyterian Medical Center and Rose Medical Center; Clinical Assistant Professor of Physiatry, School of Medicine, University of Colorado Health Science Center, Denver, Colorado

Foreword

It is a privilege to write a foreword to this book. Dr. Sanders has integrated his years of interest and experience in the care of this syndrome into a volume that is complete, well organized, and easy to read. It is a further pleasure for me to read because it so very nearly represents my own thoughts concerning the thoracic outlet syndrome.

Dr. Sanders has presented the historical material effectively, going back to concise descriptions by Sir Astley Cooper. He brings before the reader conflicting arguments regarding many of the aspects of this often-controversial syndrome dispassionately and with a high degree of objectivity. Where there exist possibly confusing subjective material and ideas, he has taken great pains to identify them as such and to quantify some of the concepts that muddy the waters. Material regarding the clinical presentation is matched in completeness by careful attention to the details of treatment. The surgeon is even advised when to change his position at the operating table! There is some well justified repetition in the text, but it serves Dr. Sanders well in that he can present critical arguments at the point upon which they bear rather than making reference to a different or distant page. Such "repetition" makes it much easier to follow his train of thought. In the discussion of results, the many parameters that do relate to outcome are carefully sorted, delineated, and appraised. Throughout the book the text is supplemented by extensive clarification in the form of tabular material that brings forth the details of many other publications.

The final sections present Dr. Sanders' personal opinions in distinction to the more objective arguments offered earlier. And last, the detailed and extensive annotated bibliography goes so far as to offer titles still "in press": it would be hard to ask for more!

The publishers and editors have further done justice to the excellence of the subject material by printing it in highly legible type, and by providing us with many subheadings that enable one to focus on specific aspects quickly. This volume should stand for many years as the definitive work on an often ill-defined topic.

Wiley F. Barker, M.D.

Foreword

Most clinicians are uncomfortable with the concept of the Thoracic Outlet Syndrome (TOS). They occasionally see patients with some of the characteristics of the syndrome, but there are usually distracting factors and they find no objective evidence of disease. The diagnostic tests that clinicians find described in textbooks seem to lack sensitivity or specificity. Worst of all, the suggested treatment for the very real complaints are not universally successful. The result is a mixture of skepticism and confusion in the minds of most clinicians concerning the problem.

Given this gloomy background, Dr. Sanders has attacked the problem by summarizing his long-standing concern for and study of both his many patients and the recorded experience of others in this scholarly monograph. His objective is to throw some light on this still-confusing clinical syndrome.

The subtitle of this book indicates that Dr. Sanders has concentrated his studies on a still more controversial aspect of an already confusing topic—namely, the relation of Thoracic Outlet Syndrome to neck injury. "Whiplash" injury has acquired a sinister medico legal connotation as the last resort of the scoundrel. In this litigious age, whiplash injuries become the concern of physicians, attorneys, and insurers, who must manage those who complain of neck and arm pain following even slight injury to the neck, but who show no evidence of organic disease.

Such a suspect description of the syndrome paints the somber backdrop for this volume, which systematically examines essentially every aspect of the problem. Dr. Sanders not only draws heavily on his own experience with over 800 patients evaluated and treated by him over a period of 25 years, but it also presents one of the most thorough and scholarly analyses of the pertinent literature that now exists. It is from such a consistent and objective approach to confusing clinical problems that progress occurs. I know from personal experience that Dr. Sanders has had a persistent concern for the problem of TOS, whether it be in the operating room, in teaching conferences, or on the ski slopes. Like a backache, it is always with him.

In typically orderly fashion, the author serially examines the normal and abnormal anatomy of the neck region associated with the syndrome. Of particular importance is the summary of the original work Dr. Sanders and his colleagues have performed in trying to find microscopic evidence of muscle injury following various types of closed neck injury as associated clinically with the symptoms of TOS. The data are presented with admirable objectivity and self criticism.

The author is a surgeon, and he leads us gently by the hand along the rocky road he has trod in trying to treat patients operatively. Being a computer buff, he has kept meticulous records of his clinical experience, which he summarizes frequently. In this book, Dr. Sanders provides us with the logic that underlies why he has modified his operative approach to the problem. He is not one to jump frivolously from one operation to another in the operative approach to these patients.

Being a practicing clinical surgeon, the author provides details and good illustrations of precisely how to carry out the various procedures that he advocates. Surgeons of whatever specialty will find this book an excellent source for the details of technique that only one who has performed the procedure many times can provide.

The subject holds wide appeal for clinical specialists, be they neurosurgeons, neurologists, orthopedists, vascular surgeons, or physiotherapists, who become involved in the management of such patients.

Dr. Sanders is the first to admit that neither he nor anyone else has solved the still vexous problems associated with the syndrome, but his very persistence and dedication to the subject as documented in this book will hereafter serve as a milestone in progress toward an ultimate solution.

B. Eiseman, M.D.

Preface

Thoracic Outlet Syndrome (TOS) has been the subject of considerable debate for several decades, primarily because of its lack of objective diagnostic criteria. In the absence of facts, controversy abounds. When experts and specialists disagree, who should the rest of us believe?

This book provides the data currently available on TOS to help the reader decide how best to manage patients with symptoms of TOS. The diagnostic criteria are set forth and the treatment options described. Surgeons, physiologists, plus a neurologist, neurosurgeon, physiatrist, and physician/attorney have each contributed to this volume to present comprehensive coverage of this challenging subject.

One of the primary questions asked is whether a diagnosis can be made from subjective evidence alone or whether objective data must be present. The apparent absence of pathology in excised first ribs and scalene muscles adds further to the controversy over the existence of TOS without objective findings. Although a few objective tests are available for diagnosis, their results are often normal. In most patients, the diagnosis of TOS is based solely on clinical signs and symptoms.

Some of the confusion arises from thinking of TOS as a single disease rather than as a spectrum of abnormalities located in the same anatomical region and eliciting similar symptoms. This book defines the spectrum, classifies its various entities, and focuses on etiology and histopathology as the starting point to resolve the controversy. Also included are chapters on other aspects of TOS: anatomy, signs and symptoms, diagnosis, treatment, results, and recurrence. New to the TOS arena is the subject of histology. There is now microscopic evidence of structural changes in the scalene muscles of patients with TOS following neck injuries. Because trauma has assumed increasing importance in TOS, disability evaluation and the influence of litigation on symptoms and results is discussed.

Presented here are personal observations regarding patients who have undergone over 850 operations for TOS. The results are compared using life-table methods with follow-ups to 15 years. An attempt is made to present a perspective that emphasizes clinical observations and data; speculation and theory are clearly labelled. It is understood that clinical data that are not always pure and objective. For example, the success of an operation requires subjective evaluation by the patient. Nevertheless, until objective methods of assessment become available, subjective appraisal must suffice.

The book will be of help to vascular, general, thoracic, hand, orthopedic, and neurosurgeons, as well as physiatrists, generalists, internists, and neurologists. Practitioners who deal with neck and muscle trauma will also find this volume useful.

Acknowledgments

The authors express their thanks to several people for their assistance in preparing this volume: from the staff of Rose Medical Center, medical librarian Nancy Simon; physical therapists Peggy O'Reilly and Diana Nichols; photographers Larry Bartz and Peggy Randall; medical artist Sara Gustafson; Diane Yacovetta and Linda Schoening; from my office staff, Connie Rauzi, Yvonne Blush, Nelda Brown, and Gretchen Alson, R.N.; from the University of Colorado Health Science Center, Darryl Jones, Ph.D.; and to David Sanders for his review and comments.

Richard J. Sanders, M.D.
Craig E. Haug, M.D.

Introduction

Several friends have asked how I became involved with Thoracic Outlet Syndrome (TOS) and why I was writing a book on this somewhat controversial subject. It happened by serendipity. Apparently, because my interest in the subject was just slightly greater than that of many of my surgical colleagues, I began seeing increasing numbers of patients with TOS symptoms, probably because few other surgeons were interested in them. When I became fascinated with computers and the way they store information, I decided to enter my TOS patients into a database to make it possible to analyze the various clinical features.

Since the introduction of transaxillary first rib resection in 1966, increasing attention and controversy have developed around TOS as evidenced by the growing number of articles in the medical literature on this subject. By 1990, more than 400 articles had been written about different aspects of TOS, and there seemed to be a need for a single volume that would summarize them. The idea for this book then became twofold: to summarize the literature on TOS and to present the data from our several hundred TOS patients.

My interest in TOS began in 1964 when I observed Dr. David Roos perform his first transaxillary first rib resection. A short time before this operation, Dr. Roos had used this approach on someone else for a different reason and was impressed with how easily he could visualize the first rib. When he then encountered a patient with symptoms of TOS, he boldly decided to try this innovative new idea of transaxillary first rib resection. The exposure in that case was quite good and I was impressed with how relatively simple the procedure appeared.

Over the next three years, from 1965 to 1968, Dr. Sylvan Baer, Dr. James Monsour, and I accumulated 69 cases of transaxillary first rib resection for TOS and were gratified to find a 90% improvement rate. At the time of that publication,[1] we were aware of only one recurrence. Other interesting and unexpected findings in that study included a history of trauma in half of the patients; neck pain in 24%; occipital headaches in 14%; and improvement in these symptoms following rib resection.

Following the analysis of our first series of cases, we began questioning patients more thoroughly, asking them specifically whether or not they had experienced trauma or had complaints of pain in their neck or head. The incidence of positive answers increased dramatically. At the same time, more patients who had undergone successful first rib resection were developing recurrent symptoms many months postoperatively; the incidence of recurrence eventually exceeded 15%.

The patients with recurrent symptoms had a common pattern: tenderness over the scalene muscles of their neck; improvement in findings following a scalene muscle block with xylocaine; and the majority experienced good relief of symptoms following reoperation with scalenectomy. The findings at the second operation were always the same: The scalene muscles were taut and adherent to the nerves of the plexus and the subclavian artery.

The increasing number of failures raised an important question: If a significant number of patients undergoing first rib resection were requiring scalenectomy at a second operation, why not do scalenectomy as the first operation? It was also realized that scalenotomy had been a part of rib resection, and that scalenotomy included not only the anterior scalene muscle but also the middle scalene. Therefore, in 1972 we changed our operation for TOS from rib resection to supraclavicular scalenectomy, removing both anterior and middle scalene muscles as completely as possible to avoid the postoperative muscle adherence we had observed following first rib resection.

In 1978, we again analyzed our results. Dr. James Monsour, Dr. William Gerber, and I pooled our experiences with both rib resection and scalenectomy, keeping the statistics of each surgeon separately. It was interesting to see three different surgeons, doing independent data analysis of their separate experiences, coming up with slightly different early results (10–15% apart), but much closer late results (2–8% apart) for each operation.[2] The long term good-to-excellent results were 68% and 70%, respectively; for the two operations with fair and poor results, 30% and 32%, respectively. About 15% of the patients in each group were reoperated upon, the second operation performing what had not been done at the first. Reoperations led to improvement in the majority of patients.

In 1980, this analysis led to another change in operations. Because either rib resection or scalenectomy led to performance of the other operation at a later date in 15% of the patients, it was decided to perform the two operations simultaneously in an attempt to improve the success rate. Between 1980 and 1988, the third of our series of TOS operations was performed, combining anterior and middle scalenectomy with first rib resection through a supraclavicular approach. To our disappointment, the results of this combined operation have been identical to the results of each operation alone.[3]

The data from these 25 years of TOS surgery, along with the data from the medical literature between 1927 and 1989, are presented in the chapters that follow.

Richard J. Sanders, M.D.

References

1. Sanders RJ, Monsour JW, Baer SB. Transaxillary first rib resection for the thoracic outlet syndrome. Arch Surg 1968;97:1014–1023.
2. Sanders RJ, Monsour JW, Gerber FG, Adams WRA, Thompson N. Scalenectomy versus first rib resection for treatment of the thoracic outlet syndrome. Surgery 1979;85:109–121.
3. Sanders RJ, Pearce WH. The treatment of thoracic outlet syndrome: A comparison of different operations. J Vasc Surg 1989;10:626–634.

Contents

1
The Controversies Regarding Thoracic Outlet Syndrome

Richard J. Sanders
Stephen H. Shogan

Neurogenic TOS Without Objective Data
Overdiagnosis vs. Underdiagnosis

Diagnostic Criteria
Symptoms
Physical Findings
Adson Test
Neurophysiologic Diagnostic Tests

Indications for Surgery
Completion of Treatment for All Associated or Differential Conditions
Timing
Disabling Symptoms
Objective Diagnostic Criteria
Surgery as the "Last Resort"

Choice of Operation
First Rib Resection, Scalenectomy, or Both

Neurogenic TOS—Just Another Point for Nerve Compression

Geographic Location—Endemic Condition

Few subjects in medicine are as controversial as thoracic outlet syndrome (TOS). Although there is general recognition of arterial and venous TOS as specific types of vascular compression—conditions that are easily confirmed by arteriograms and venograms—neurogenic TOS is not so generally recognized. In dispute are those cases of neurogenic TOS that are associated with no osseous abnormalities and have either normal or nonspecific abnormal patterns on neuro-electric studies. Those cases, labeled "disputed TOS" by Wilbourn,[1] involve several areas of disagreement:

1. The existence of neurogenic TOS without objective data
2. Diagnostic criteria
3. Indications for surgery
4. Choice of operation

Neurogenic TOS Without Objective Data

Proponents of neurogenic TOS as a specific entity, even without positive objective electrical abnormalities, base their belief on two factors: 1) There is a group of clinical signs and symptoms, documented in large numbers of patients, that can be recognized as TOS; and 2) When conservative treatment fails, several surgical procedures have provided significant symptomatic relief to the majority of patients operated upon.

Those who believe that symptomatic nerve compression in the thoracic outlet area cannot exist when all objective tests are normal, do so on the basis of sound medical principles: When diagnoses are made without the backing of objective data, the numbers of diagnostic errors can be high. Although this statement may be true generally, it does not mean that brachial plexus compression cannot occur when neurophysiologic diagnostic tests are normal. In fact, in the experience of several surgeons, many successful results were observed in patients with normal neurophysiological studies.[2-4]

Arguments used to deny the existence of neurogenic TOS include these: the citation of case histories of nerve injuries during TOS surgery that made patients worse;[5,6] the detection of inaccuracies in reporting of patients classified as improved who later were found still to have symptoms;[7,8] the reliance on ulnar nerve conduction velocities (UNCV) as promoted by Urschel[9] was based upon falsified data;[10,11] and finally, the improvement rate from surgery is simply a placebo effect.

Even though each of these criticisms has validity, they are not, either individually or collectively, evidence that neurogenic TOS without objective findings is nonexistent. There is a recognized failure rate—nerve injuries are complications of surgery and a few patients are worse after surgery, but that does not mean that the diagnosis was incorrect; and errors in recording results have been made, although some of those could represent patients in whom symptoms that recurred caused late failure after initial improvement. The discrepancies in Urschel's studies are a moot point because few investigators have duplicated or confirmed his results and most diagnoses of neurogenic TOS are made on the basis of clinical data alone.[2, 4, 12–15]

The placebo effect of an operation is recognized for relief of pain.[15, 16] However, it is difficult to accept as a placebo effect the consistent early improvement rate of 80% to 90% in operated TOS patients noted by more than 20 investigators (see Chapter 12). The type of improvement most patients describe is relief of hand paresthesia within 24 hours while pain in neck and shoulders still remains for some time after surgery. Furthermore, many operated TOS patients are able to comb their hair, drive a car, and sleep through the night without their hands falling asleep; those are not typical placebo effects.

Proponents of the position that neurogenic TOS is nonexistent do not look at the whole spectrum of cases. Their opinions have been formed primarily on the basis of experiences with patients whose operations were unsuccessful or resulted in complications. Patients with good results do not seek doctors because they are no longer in need of medical attention. Thus, when made without viewing the entire group of patients operated upon for TOS, statements that the condition rarely exists and is overdiagnosed are subjective, based on impressions rather than fact.

Lack of a positive objective test to diagnose neurogenic TOS is sometimes used to deny its existence. However, this argument is a poor one. Neurogenic TOS is no different from many other conditions in medicine where there is a need for more precise diagnostic tests. Appendicitis is a good example of a diagnosis that is made on the basis of clinical criteria in the absence of objective tests for confirmation. Physicians acknowledge and accept a significant number of diagnostic errors in dealing with appendicitis because the risks of not operating are greater than the risks of surgery. In experienced hands, the risks of TOS surgery are small—less than 1% of patients are made worse when operations fail to relieve symptoms (see Chapter 11). In fact, most patients who have been operated upon for TOS feel their surgery was worthwhile (see Chapter 12). It is this significant improvement rate that supports the view that there is a neurogenic form of TOS which can be recognized clinically, even in the absence of objective findings.

Overdiagnosis vs. Underdiagnosis

There are two schools of thought regarding the frequency of TOS. Those who feel the diagnosis of TOS is made too often point out that some surgeons perform operations on patients with incomplete evaluations, no neuroelectric tests, only one or two positive nonspecifc findings, and inadequate conservative treatment prior to considering surgery. They strengthen their argument by noting the rarity of true neurogenic TOS as indicated by how seldom this condition is mentioned in the neurological literature.[17]

The other school of thought includes proponents of neurogenic TOS who feel the diagnosis is often missed for several reasons. Some physicians do inadequate clinical evaluations and rely too heavily on neurophysiologic, vascular laboratory, and angiographic studies that are usually normal in neurogenic TOS. Many patients are sent from doctor to doctor, treated with physical therapy for prolonged periods of time with no improvement, and a diagnosis of TOS is never considered.

When the patient finally sees someone who makes a diagnosis of TOS, surgery frequently produces dramatic relief.[18]

In fact, the criticisms of both sides have many elements of truth, and patients can best be served by heeding the guidelines of each side. A patient should have a thorough history and physical examination, neck x-rays, and appropriate studies to rule out other conditions that, if present, should be treated first. When that has been done, if several months of conservative therapy have been unsuccessful, if the symptoms are significantly interfering with the patient's life, and if clinical diagnostic criteria are present, the physician should inform the patient of the options available.[19] Those options include surgery, with its limitations and risks.

Diagnostic Criteria

Symptoms

There probably is more agreement regarding symptoms than regarding other diagnostic criteria. The history of paresthesia and pain in the upper extremity is fairly well accepted as the main symptom complex of TOS. In a few patients, only one of these is present. Although there may be other symptoms and often a history of neck trauma, the essentials of paresthesia and pain are not disputed. However, those are nonspecific complaints and can be due to a variety of causes, of which TOS is only one.

Physical Findings

Regarding physical examination, there are two areas of general agreement: supraclavicular tenderness and duplication of symptoms in the 90-degree abduction, external rotation position (90-degree AER position) are present in the vast majority of TOS patients. Although those are nonspecific, subjective findings, most physicians agree that they are significant diagnostic criteria for TOS. Their absence makes the diagnosis less likely. In some TOS patients, mild weakness in biceps or triceps muscles is present and a reduction in sensation to light touch may be found in specific fingers. However, those also are subjective findings and are demonstrable in less than half of the patients.

Adson Test

A positive Adson test (reduced radial pulse on rotating the head and deep breathing or upon abducting the arms to 90 degrees AER) is not present in the majority of patients undergoing operations for TOS. Nevertheless, some physicians still regard this as a necessary sign to establish a diagnosis.

Neurophysiologic Diagnostic Tests

There is general agreement that the more important function of neurophysiologic testing is to diagnose compression of more distal nerves (carpal tunnel syndrome, ulnar tunnel syndrome, ulnar nerve entrapment at the elbow) rather than compression at the thoracic outlet area. One reason for this might be the technical limitations of stimulating the nerve roots proximal to the brachial plexus (see Chapter 7).

However, there is disagreement regarding the indications for neurophysiologic tests to specifically diagnose TOS. To date, no specific changes characteristic of TOS have been recognized, except in those few cases with atrophy and wasting of the hand muscles. The abnormalities associated with TOS are nonspecific changes in electromyography (EMG), sensory evoked potentials (SEP), and delayed ulnar nerve conduction velocities (UNCV). There is disagreement among neurologists themselves as to the significance and meaning of these neurophysiologic abnormalities. While many studies demonstrate a positive correlation between abnormal electrical studies and good responses to TOS surgery, there is also just as good a correlation between normal electrical studies and improvement following TOS surgery.

Indications for Surgery

Completion of Treatment for All Associated or Differential Conditions

Everyone agrees that other causes of nonspecific symptoms should be sought and treated first. Cervical spine x-rays should be obtained in all patients. The indications for special imaging studies of the neck, such as CAT scans, MRI, or myelograms, are not an area of general agreement. Some physicians feel those should be performed on all patients before surgical treatment is considered while others recommend them only when there are clinical features suggesting cervical spine disease. The reasons for not ordering them routinely are that they are expensive and are rarely abnormal when there are no suggestive clinical features.

Timing

Most physicians agree that surgery for TOS should not be performed until the patient has failed to improve while on conservative management for at least a few months, but there is no consensus as to how long "a few" is. Physical therapy is prescribed for the majority of TOS patients, but precisely how physical therapy relieves symptoms is unknown. Perhaps the primary role of physical therapy is to gain time to permit the body's healing powers to do their work.

Disabling Symptoms

Disabling symptoms are accepted by most physicians as criteria for considering surgery, but the definition of "disabling" varies widely. In general it indicates interference with work, recreation, and/or the activities of daily living. This is a very subjective criterion because what is disabling to one patient may be easy to live with for another.

Objective Diagnostic Criteria

The presence of at least one positive objective test is required by some as an indication for surgery. This is the opinion of those who do not accept a diagnosis based solely upon subjective criteria.

Surgery as the "Last Resort"

If all diagnostic tests have been performed, all other treatable conditions have been treated, conservative management has been unsuccessful, and the patient still has the clinical picture of TOS with disabling symptoms, then only two options remain: The patient can live with the symptoms or undergo surgical decompression of the thoracic outlet area, realizing that there is no guarantee of success. At this point, opponents of neurogenic TOS would argue that the patient should not be offered the choice if there have been no abnormal objective tests; proponents would explain the options and let the patient make the decision.

Choice of Operation

First rib resection, scalenectomy, or both: No operation has proved superior to any other, although each procedure has its strong proponents (see Chapter 12). There are proponents for each of the five procedures listed below. The circumstances for selecting or not selecting each one vary among investigators. Each procedure, or combination of procedures, has enjoyed early success in the large majority of patients; each has seen the success rate deteriorate over time:

1. First rib resection
2. Cervical rib resection
3. Anterior scalenotomy
4. Anterior scalenectomy
5. Middle scalenectomy

Neurogenic TOS—Just Another Point for Nerve Compression

Throughout the body, peripheral nerves leave the spine and pass through small holes, long tunnels, and narrow spaces to reach their end points. Along the way, they are subject to irritation and compression by the numerous structures that they pass. The results of thoracic outlet decompression surgery should be viewed alongside the results of other forms of peripheral nerve decompression.

Results of surgery for nerve compression at the levels of the wrist, elbow, and cervical spine are presented in Table 1–1. In almost all of these cases at least one objective test was positive prior to surgery. In spite of this, the results of surgery are far from 100% cure. The majority of patients in each series experienced improvement in symptoms, not total relief; the average follow-up period tended to be short, seldom beyond two years and often less.

Table 1-1.   Results of Decompression Operations in Upper Extremities

Author	Year	No. Operations	Symptoms Present	Good	Fair	Failed	Length of Follow-up
Carpal Tunnel Decompression							
Semple, Cargill[20]	1969	37	<12 Mon.	97%		3%	not stated
		113	>12 Mon.	71%		29%	not stated
Gainer, Nugent[21]	1977	430		82%	10%	8%	not stated
Sakellarides[22]	1981	500[a]	<6 mon.	75%	25%		not stated
			>6 mon.	30%		70%[b]	not stated
Kulick et al.[23]	1986	130		81%		19%[c]	mean = 48 mon.
Ulnar Nerve Decompression at Elbow							
Craven, Green[24]	1980	30		81%		19%[c]	mean = 22 mon.
Chan et al.[25]	1980	235		82%		18%	mean = 24 mon.
Benoit et al.[26]	1987	70		66%		34%	mean = 13 mon.
Goldberg et al.[27]	1989	48		94%		6%	mean = 15 mon.
Cervical Root Decompression							
Andrews et al.[28]	1971	41		56%	21%	23%	not stated
Fager[29]	1983	49		100%			not stated
Manabe et al.[30]	1988	35		97%		3%	not stated

[a] = 500 total operations. The author did not subdivide the numbers in each group.
[b] = defined by author as "slight recovery."
[c] = combined fair and failed.

The results of both Semple and Cargill[20] and Sakellarides[21] were divided into two groups of patients: those with symptoms for less than a year prior to surgery and those with symptoms for more than a year prior to surgery. Both studies noted that better results were achieved in patients operated upon earlier in the course of their disease, before prolonged motor impairment had developed.

Goldberg et al. pointed out that the extent of postoperative improvement depended upon the grade of the neurologic deficit preoperatively. The best results were in patients with milder symptoms. In their patients with no objective neurologic findings preoperatively, 92% noted complete relief of symptoms following ulnar nerve release. The improvement rate fell in patients with intrinsic muscle weakness and muscle wasting and was proportional to the degree of these deficits. In patients with some motor weakness, symptomatic improvement dropped to 72% while complete motor recovery was less than 50%. In patients with severe motor deficits, although symptomatic improvement was common, functional recovery was unusual.[27]

Observations in TOS patients are similar. Gilliatt[31] and Wilbourn[1] have reported that following surgical decompression of the brachial plexus in patients with severe muscle wasting, there is usually improvement in symptoms but little return of function. In our own TOS patients, the best results are in those with sensory losses but few motor deficits. This raises an important issue: Are patients best served by withholding surgical treatment until objective signs are present or should surgery by considered earlier, on the basis of a clinical picture? While there are risks associated with operations, there are also risks in not operating soon enough.

Geographic Location—Endemic Condition

It has been suggested that TOS occurs only in certain areas of the country. Some physicians wonder why they see so few patients with TOS while other physicians in the same specialty, in specific locales, see them almost daily. This apparent geographic maldistribution is easy to explain. TOS is a more common condition than was once thought. The reason some physicians see large numbers of these patients is that they live in medical communities that have been educated to recognize TOS as a possible diagnosis in patients with paresthesia in their hands, particularly following neck injuries. The patients are referred from many sources, including neurologists, neurosurgeons, orthopedic surgeons, internists, family practitioners, physiatrists, general and thoracic surgeons, occupational and physical therapists, chiropractors, and attorneys, to mention a few.

In our practice, fewer than 25% of the patients seen for TOS are operated upon, as the majority are managed conservatively.

References

1. Wilbourn AJ. Thoracic outlet syndrome surgery causing severe brachial plexopathy. Muscle Nerve 1988; 11:66–84.
2. Dale WA. Management of thoracic outlet syndrome. Ann Surg 1975; 181:575–585.
3. McGough EC, Pearce MB, Byrne JP. Management of thoracic outlet syndrome. J Ther Card Med 1979; 77:169–174.
4. Sanders RJ, Monsour JW, Gerber FG, Adams WRA, Thompson N. Scalenectomy versus first rib resection for treatment of the thoracic outlet syndrome. Surgery 1979; 85:109–121.
5. Wilbourn AJ. Thoracic outlet syndrome: a reply (editorial). Muscle Nerve 1988; 11:1092.
6. Cherington M, Machanic B, Harper I, Parry L: Surgery for thoracic outlet syndrome may be hazardous to your health. Muscle Nerve 1986; 9:632–634.
7. Cherington M. A conservative point of view of the thoracic outlet syndrome. Am J Surg 1989; 158:394–395.
8. White BE. Diagnosis of thoracic outlet syndrome. Del Med J 1988; 60:606–607.
9. Urschel HC, Razzuk MA, Wood RE, Parekh M, Paulson DL. Objective diagnosis (ulnar nerve conduction velocity) and current therapy of the thoracic outlet syndrome. Ann Thorac Surg 1971; 12:608–620.
10. Wilbourn AJ. Evidence for conduction delay in thoracic outlet syndrome is challenged. N Engl J Med 1984; 310:1052–1053.
11. Urschel HC. Evidence for conduction delay in thoracic outlet syndrome is challenged. N Engl J Med 1984; 310:1052–1053.
12. Roos DB. Congenital anomalies associated with thoracic outlet syndrome. Anatomy, symptoms, diagnosis and treatment. Am J Surg 1976; 132:771–778.
13. Kelly TR. Thoracic outlet syndrome: current concepts of treatment. Ann Surg 1979; 190:657–662.
14. Qvarfordt PG, Ehrenfeld WK, Stoney RJ: Supraclavicular radical scalenectomy and

transaxillary first rib resection for the thoracic outlet syndrome. A combined approach. Am J Surg 1984; 148:111–116.

15. Dimond EG, Kittle CF, Crockett JE. Comparison of internal mammary artery ligation and sham operation for angina pectoris. Am J Cardiol 1960; 5:483–486.

16. Cobb LA, Thomas GI, Dillard DH, Merendino KA, Bruce RA. An evaluation of internal mammary artery ligation by a double-blind technic. N Engl J Med 1959; 260:1115–1118.

17. Wilbourn AJ. The thoracic outlet syndrome is overdiagnosed. Arch Neurol 1990; 47:228–230.

18. Roos D. The thoracic outlet syndrome is underrated. Arch Neurol 1990; 47: 327–328.

19. Mandel S. Thoracic outlet syndrome (editorial). Muscle Nerve 1988; 11: 1090–1091.

20. Semple JC, Cargill AO. Carpal-tunnel syndrome: results of surgical decompression. Lancet 1969; 1:918–919.

21. Gainer JB, Nugent GR. Carpal tunnel syndrome: report of 430 operations. South Med J 1977; 70:325–328.

22. Sakellarides HT. The management of carpal tunnel compression syndrome: follow-up of 500 cases over a 25 year period. Orthop Rev 1983; 12:77–81.

23. Kulick MI, Gordillo G, Javidi T, Kilgore ES Jr, Newmeyer WL. Long-term analysis of patients having surgical treatment for carpal tunnel syndrome. J Hand Surg 1986; 11A:59–66.

24. Craven PR Jr, Green DP. Cubital tunnel syndrome: treatment by medial epicondylectomy. J Bone Joint Surg 1980; 62A:986–989.

25. Chan RC, Paine KWE, Varughese G. Ulnar neuropathy at the elbow: comparison of simple decompression and anterior transposition. Neurosurgery 1980; 7:545–550.

26. Benoit BG, Preston DN, Atack DM, DaSilva VF. Neurolysis combined with the application of a silastic envelope for ulnar nerve entrapment at the elbow. Neurosurgery 1987; 20:594–598.

27. Goldberg BJ, Light TR, Blair SJ. Ulnar neuropathy at the elbow: results of medial epicondylectomy. J Hand Surg 1989; 14A:182–188.

28. Andrews ET, Gentchos EJ, Beller ML. Results of anterior cervical spine fusions done at the hospital of the University of Pennsylvania: a nine year follow up. Clin Orthop 1971; 81:15–20.

29. Fager CA. Evaluation of cervical spine surgery by postoperative myelography. Neurosurgery 1983; 12:416–421.

30. Manabe S, Tateishi A, Ohno T. Anterolateral uncoforaminotomy for cervical spondylotic myeloradiculopathy. Acta Orthop Scand 1988; 59:669–674.

31. Gilliatt RW, Willison RG, Dietz V, Williams IR: Peripheral nerve condition in patients with cervical rib and band. Ann Neurol 1978; 4:124–129.

2
History

Richard J. Sanders

Period I—The Cervical Rib: 1740–1927

Period II—The Cervical Rib Syndrome Without Cervical Rib: 1920–1956

Congenital Bands and Ligaments
Scalene Anticus Syndrome
Costoclavicular Syndrome
Normal First Rib
Rudimentary or Deformed First Rib
Scalene Medius and Minimus Muscles
Hyperabduction (Pectoralis Minor) Syndrome

Period III—Modern Era of Thoracic Outlet Syndrome: 1956–Present

New Surgical Approaches to Rib Resection
New Diagnostic Tests
Beginning of Disenchantment With First Rib Resection
Histology

The history of the thoracic outlet syndrome can be divided into three periods: 1) that of the cervical rib, its anatomy and its symptoms; 2) that of the cervical rib syndrome in the absence of a cervical rib—this is the period of the scalenus anticus syndrome, the costoclavicular syndrome, and the normal first rib; and 3) the current era of thoracic outlet syndrome as a group of symptoms that have several different anatomical causes. This era includes the introduction of objective diagnostic tests, such as arteriography and electrophysiologic studies, and the description of new surgical approaches to first rib resection.

Period I—The Cervical Rib: 1740–1927

The earliest history of what today is called thoracic outlet syndrome (TOS) began with the anatomical recognition of cervical ribs (Table 2–1). Although, there are very early references to cervical ribs by Galen and Vaselius, the first scientific study of cervical ribs was in 1740 by the German anatomist Hunauld.[1] A century later, in 1842, Gruber separated cervical ribs into four groups, a classification still used today.[2] Postmortem dissection was the primary method of diagnosing cervical ribs until 1894, when "skiagrams," or x-rays, became available. In that year, Pilling found 139 cases of cervical ribs that had been reported, nine of which were recognized during the patients' life.[3]

Sir Astley Cooper, in 1821, was the first to describe the symptoms of vascular compression from a cervical rib.[4] Although he did not treat the patient, his description is classic:

> "The subject . . . was a woman who was admitted to Guy's Hospital having no pulse at the wrist or elbow. Her hand was of a venous redness, always cold, generally denuded, yet seemed painful. There were small gangrenous spots upon it. . . . These appearances were found to be the consequence of a projection of the lower cervical vertebra towards the clavicle, and consequent pressure upon the subclavian artery."

Table 2-1.   **Period I—The Cervical Rib: 1740–1927**

A. Anatomical Descriptions
    Galen, Vesalius
    Hunauld, 1740—First description of extra ribs[1]
    Gruber, 1842—Classified cervical ribs into 4 groups[2]

B. Embryology
    Todd, 1912—Descent of limb theory[7]
    Jones, 1913—Elongation of vertebrae theory[8]

C. Clinical Description
    Cooper, 1821[4]

D. Surgical Resection
    Coote, 1861[6]

E. Physiology of Subclavian Aneurysms
    Halsted, 1916—Explanation: poststenotic dilitation[10]

Forty years after Cooper's recognition of the cervical rib syndrome, Wellshire wrote a brief clinical note in the Lancet describing a woman with a supraclavicular pulsation thought to be the subclavain artery being tented up by a cervical rib.[5] In 1861, Coote performed the first resection of a cervical rib for that condition.[6] During the next 35 years, only eight more operations were recorded. However, after 1895, when x-rays became available, the number of cervical rib resections increased. By 1907, Keen had found 42 reported cases and evaluated their clinical presentations;[3] 31 of the 42 were women. Neurologic symptoms of pain and paraesthesia were present in two-thirds, vascular symptoms in less than one-half. The medical therapy for cervical rib symptoms—massage, liniments, electricity, and douches—was seldom effective. Keen noted that trauma, even in the presence of a cervical rib, was the probable cause of symptoms in some cases.

Todd, in 1912,[7] and Jones, in 1913,[8] performed extensive studies of the embryology of the skeleton, including cervical ribs. Todd introduced the theory of the descent of the limb bud and Jones the theory of elongation of the vertebrae.

By 1916, Murphy could report that 112 articles had been written on the subject.[9] He is one of the first to point out the most serious complication from cervical rib excision: paralysis of the extremity. He describes that paralysis as occurring without obvious nerve injury and lasting two weeks to four months. Murphy points out that at operation the cervical rib is sometimes hard to find, and many first ribs had been removed when mistaken for cervical ribs.

While occlusion of the subclavian artery was recognized in the nineteenth century as the presenting problem in the early ones of cervical syndrome, it was Halsted, in 1916, who explained how cervical ribs caused aneurysms that subsequently thrombosed.[10] He reviewed 716 cases with cervical ribs and found mention of at least 27 aneurysms (4%); the aneurysms were always distal to the rib. Halsted postulated that the artery was narrowed by the rib and that the aneurysm was due to prolonged diastolic pressure elevation in the poststenoic segment. Halsted, in collaboration with Reid, went on to prove the theory by producing similar aneurysms in animals by partially ligating the aorta and observing poststenotic dilatation a few months later.[10] Although direct arterial pressure measurements subsequently disproved Halsted's hypothesis, his careful studies and precise observations have been confirmed by later researchers. Even today, his experimental approach serves as a model for scientific investigators.

Period II—The Cervical Rib Syndrome Without Cervical Rib: 1920–1956

Congenital Bands and Ligaments (Table 2–2)

Law, in 1920, described ligaments arising from tips of cervical ribs and inserting on the first rib or sternum.[11] He also noted "adventitious ligaments arising from normal seventh cervical transverse processes" inserting at various places on the first rib or adjacent ligaments. He operated upon four cases in which "the ligament was taut as a bowstring, and stretched over it and sharply angulated,

Table 2-2.   **Period II—Cervical Rib Syndrome Without Cervical Rib: 1920–1956**

A. Congenital Ligaments and Bands
  Law, 1920—First description[11]

B. Scalenus Anticus Syndrome
  Adson and Coffey, 1927—Decided that scalene was cause of symptoms with or without cervical rib[16]
  Ochsner, Gage, and DeBakey, 1935—Suggested trauma and muscle hypertrophy[18]
  Naffziger and Grant, 1938—Named Scalenus Anticus Syndrome[19]

C. Costoclavicular Syndrome
  Eden, 1939—Described the syndrome[20]
  Falconer and Wendell, 1943—Named the syndrome[21]

D. Normal First Rib
  Bramwell, 1903—First mentioned it as cause of symptoms[24]
  Tom Murphy, 1910—Credited with first resection[25]
  Stopford, 1919—Reported 10 cases and noted trauma as a cause[15]

E. Abnormal of Rudimentary First Rib
  Keen, 1907—First clinical description[3]
  Thorburn, 1908—First resection (uncertain of 1st rib vs. cervical rib)[27]
  Brickner and Milch, 1925—Noted that either normal or abnormal first ribs can produce the same clinical picture[26]

F. Middle Scalene Muscle Variations
  Stiles, 1929—First pointed out middle scalene as cause of symptoms[19]
  Kirgis and Reed, 1948—Recommended both anterior and middle scalenotomy in symptomatic patients[32]

G. Pectoralis Minor Syndrome (Hyperabduction Syndrome)
  Wright, 1945[37]

were the two lower cords of the brachial plexus." Division of both the anterior scalene muscle and congenital band gave relief of symptoms in all four cases. No patient had a cervical rib. More than 50 years later, Roos elaborated upon the bands and ligaments described by Law, dividing them into nine types.[12, 13]

Scalene Anticus Syndrome

As early as 1905 the role of the anterior scalene muscle in the "cervical rib syndrome" was recognized. In that year, Murphy described the anterior scalene muscle as the counteracting force in compressing the artery and nerves against a cervical rib.[14] During the next 20 years, other surgeons divided the anterior scalene muscle as part of operations designed to remove other structures, such as the first rib[15] or congenital bands.[11] However, Adson appears to be the first to plan an operation exclusively for anterior scalenotomy.[16]

Adson's classic article of 1927 includes several significant items: The now famous "Adson test" is described as obliteration of the radial pulse with rotation of the neck and deep inspiration. Thirty-six cases are reported of cervical rib resection with complications of postoperative numbness in eight and slight palsies in four.

These procedures were done via a transverse or posterior neck incision through which the cervical rib was removed without cutting the scalene muscles. Adson then described a new anterior neck approach in which the anterior scalene muscle is divided first. When he first used that technique, he noted that the subclavian artery was released from pressure by the muscle. He therefore, left the cervical rib unresected and was pleasantly surprised when the patient's symptoms improved. By eliminating rib resection, the neurologic complications of rib resection disappeared.[16]

Scalenotomy changed Adson's approach to the cervical rib syndrome. During the next 20 years, he operated on 89 patients with cervical ribs, removing the rib in only 26 (29%), usually those with complete cervical ribs. The rest (71%) were treated by scalenectomy alone. Good results occurred in 81% of those with cervical rib resection and in 90% of those receiving scalenectomy only. Fifty-three patients without cervical ribs were also part of the series. Their improvement rate was 81%.[17]

The first article to deal exclusively with scalenotomy in the absence of cervical ribs was by Ochsner, Gage, and DeBakey in 1935.[18] They called the condition the "Scalene Anticus Syndrome," or the "Naffziger Syndrome," recognizing Howard Naffziger of San Francisco as the originator of the name. In 1938, Naffziger published his own series of 18 patients with the condition.[19] However, enthusiasm for scalenotomy and the scalene anticus syndrome was short-lived because several patients failed to improve following surgery. Other explanations for pain, paraesthesia, and weakness of the upper extremity were sought.

Costoclavicular Syndrome

The costoclavicular syndrome was first described by Eden in 1939[20] and named by Falconer and Weddell in 1943.[21] The abnormality is a narrow space between clavicle and first rib at the point where the neurovascular bundle passes. Like scalenus anticus syndrome, the theory of costoclavicular compression was developed to explain the symptoms of patients with cervical rib syndrome who had no cervical rib. For treatment of this condition, these authors recommended resection of the normal first rib.

A more radical treatment for costoclavicular syndrome was introduced in 1953 by Lord[22]: claviculectomy. In 1961, he and Rosati reported 31 claviculectomies among the 61 extremities treated surgically by neurovascular compression.[23] Few surgeons ever adopted such an extensive procedure for neurologic symptoms in TOS, although many use it for subclavian vein thrombectomy or repair, or when subclavian artery resection and grafting is required, particularly in large people.

Normal First Rib

As early as 1903, Bramwell talked of neurovascular compression resulting from a normal first rib rather than from a cervical rib.[24] In 1910, Tom Murphy of Australia is credited with describing the first excision of a normal first rib for "cervical rib syndrome."[25] In 1916, J.B. Murphy of Chicago reported the removal of several normal first ribs to relieve neurovascular symptoms.[9] Stopford, in 1919, pointed out that the first rib, rather than the cervical rib or the anterior scalene muscle, could be the cause of neurovascular compression.[15] In 1925, Brickner and Milch noted two distinct types of symptomatic first rib cases: those with normal first ribs and those with rudimentary or deformed ribs.[26] The symptoms produced by the two types are the same.

Rudimentary or Deformed First Rib

As long ago as 1740, Hunauld described abnormal first ribs in anatomical dissections.[1] Keen, in 1907, was first to recognize and describe symptoms from an abnormal first rib,[3] and in the following year, Thorburn was first to resect a deformed first rib.[27] White, in 1945, reviewed the subject extensively and reported 10 cases of his own.[28] Abnormal first ribs are at least as common as cervical ribs. The combined incidence in the general population of cervical and abnormal first ribs is approximately 1%. The distinction between them is academic because the symptoms and treatment for these abnormalities is identical.

Scalene Medius and Minimus Muscles

Middle scalene muscle abnormalities as a cause of neurovascular symptoms were first suggested by Stiles in 1929.[19] In 1947, Telford and Mottershead described a frequent anatomical finding on the first rib: fusion of the fibers of insertion of the anterior and middle scalene muscles, creating a sling of fibrous tissue over which the lowest cords of the brachial plexus must pass.[29] In the same year, Gage made several observations of anatomical variations and anomalies of the middle scalene muscle.[30] In 1948, based on anatomical dissections, Telford and Mottershead,[31] as well as Kirgis and Reed,[32] independently described the scalene minimus muscle as being present in 34% and 55%, respectively, of their specimens.

In 1959, Daseler and Anson recorded a variation of 0.1 to 2.0 cm in the normal space between the points of insertions on the first rib of the anterior and middle scalene muscles.[33] Since then, while performing scalenectomies, several surgeons have observed a large incidence of middle scalene muscle variation.[34-36]

Hyperabduction (Pectoralis Minor) Syndrome

Subclavian artery occlusion caused by raising the arm over the head was studied in depth by Wright in 1945.[37] His interest in this subject began when he saw a 37-year-old man with superficial gangrene of two fingertips, followed by four more symptomatic patients without gangrene. All five had in common the obliteration of their radial pulses by hyperabduction of their arms to 180 degrees. Wright then studied 150 normal subjects and found 83% obliterated their pulses at 180 degrees too. He labeled those people who developed symptoms of numbness and tingling with their arms raised, particularly in bed at night, as having "Hyperabduction Syndrome." Most people required no treatment for this, but for severe discomfort, pectoralis minor tenotomy could be offered.

Period III—Modern Era of Thoracic Outlet Syndrome: 1956–Present

The term "thoracic outlet syndrome" was first used in 1956 by Peet;[38] independently, Rob and Standeven, in 1958,[39] used the term "thoracic outlet compression syndrome." Their purpose was to categorize the various anatomical abnormalities in the supraclavicular area under a single term, since they all produced similar symptoms. The term "thoracic outlet syndrome," or "TOS," is now widely accepted (Table 2–3).

New Surgical Approaches to Rib Resection

In the 1960s, three new approaches for removing the first rib for TOS were described. Clagett, in 1962, introduced the posterior route in his presidential address to the American Association for Thoracic Surgery.[40] It was this article that rekindled interest in the topic of neurovascular compression in the upper extremity. Four years later, in 1966, Roos described the transaxillary approach,[41] and in 1968, Gol reported using an infraclavicular incision for the same procedure.[42] A combination of a supraclavicular and infraclavicular incision has not been formally described, but we have used it successfully and describe it in Chapter 10 of this volume. The rationale for first rib resection was that the first rib was the common

Table 2-3.   **Period III—Current Era of TOS: 1956–Present**

A. The Name: Thoracic Outlet Syndrome
    Peet, 1956[39]
    Rob and Standeven, 1958[40]

B. Approaches to First Rib Resection
    Clagett, 1962—Posterior[41]
    Roos, 1966—Transaxillary[42]
    Gol, 1968—Infraclavicular[43]

C. Objective Diagnostic Tests
    1. Vascular
        Adson, 1927—"Adson maneuver"[16]
        Lange, 1962—arteriography[44]
        Winsor, 1966—plethysmography[45]
    2. Electrophysiology
        Caldwell, 1971—Ulnar nerve conduction velocity[48]
        Hongladaron, 1976—F-wave abnormalities[49]
        Glover, 1981—Somatosensory evoked potentials[50]

D. Histochemical Microscopy
    Machleder, 1986[52]
    Sanders, 1990[53]

denominator for all of the specific causes of TOS. Determining a specific etiology was not essential because first rib resection relieved all causes.[43]

New Diagnostic Tests

Since 1960, a variety of objective tests have been developed to aid in establishing diagnoses of arterial or neurological abnormalities. These tests have been used in patients with a wide variety of symptoms, including patients with TOS.

Lang, in 1962, first described the use of arteriography in TOS.[44] For patients with arterial insufficiency, diminished pulses, or suspected aneurysms, arteriography is of prime importance. Noninvasive arterial evaluation (plethysmography) in TOS patients was introduced in 1966.[45] However, since very few TOS patients have vascular compression, this test was abandoned for routine use.[47]

Neurophysiologic testing has been tried in TOS patients in many forms. Urschel et al., in 1968,[47] and Caldwell et al., in 1971,[48] introduced ulnar nerve conduction velocities; Hongladaron, in 1976, studied F-wave conduction velocity in TOS;[49] and Glover et al. reported experiences with sensory evoked potential responses in diagnosis TOS in 1981.[50] Each of these has added a little more to the knowledge of TOS.

Beginning of Disenchantment With First Rib Resection

In the 1970s, transaxillary first rib resection was the "state of the art" for treating TOS. However, by 1979, routine first rib resection was questioned when a comparison made between patients treated with anterior and middle scalenectomy and those treated with transaxillary first rib resection revealed identical results in each group but the morbidity of rib resection was higher.[46] In 1982, Dale reported the findings of a national survey in the United States of complications from transaxillary rib resection among 259 surgeons.[51] The number of nerve injuries was significant, and led to a recommendation of caution when advising rib resection.

Histology

The most recent event in the story of TOS has been the introduction of histochemical and morphometric evaluation of the anterior scalene muscles by Machleder et al. in 1986.[52] Further histochemical studies by Sanders et al. have demonstrated fiber changes as well as scar tissue in both anterior and middle scalene muscles of TOS patients.[53] These studies, which are more fully described in Chapter 5, should lead to more knowledge regarding the precise pathology of TOS.

References

1. Hunauld. Sur le nombre des cotes, moindre ou plus grand qu a l'ordinaire. Hist Acad Roy d Sc de Paris, 1740.
2. Gruber W. Ueber die halsrippen des menschen mit vergleichend-anatomischen. Bemerkungen, St. Petersburg, 1869.

3. Keen WW. The symptomatology, diagnosis, and surgical treatment of cervical ribs. Am J Med Sci 1907; 133:173–218.
4. Cooper A. On exostosis. In: Cooper, Cooper, and Travers. Surgical essays, London, 3rd Ed: 1821; 128.
5. Willshire. Lancet 1860; 2:633.
6. Coote H. Exostosis of the left transverse process of the seventh cervical vertebra, surrounded by blood vessels and nerves; successful removal. Lancet 1861; 1: 360–361.
7. Todd TW. The descent of the shoulder after birth: its significance in the production of pressure-symptoms on the lowest brachial trunk. Anat Anz 1912; 41:385–397.
8. Jones FW. Discussion on cervical ribs: the anatomy of cervical ribs. Proc R Soc Med 1913; 6:95–112.
9. Murphy JB. Cervical rib excision. Collective review on surgery of cervical rib. Clin John B Murphy 1916; 5:227–240.
10. Halsted WH. An experimental study of circumscribed dilation of an artery immediately distal to a partially occluded band, and its bearing on certain cases of cervical rib. J Exp Med 1916; 24:271–286.
11. Law AA. Adventitious ligaments simulating cervical ribs. Ann Surg 1920; 72:497–499.
12. Roos DB. Congenital anomalies associated with thoracic outlet syndrome. Anatomy, symptoms, diagnosis and treatment. Am J Surg 1976; 132:771–778.
13. Roos DB. New concepts of thoracic outlet syndrome that explain etiology, symptoms, diagnosis, and treatment. Vasc Surg 1979; 13:313–321.
14. Murphy JB. A case of cervical rib with symptoms resembling subclavian aneurism. Ann Surg 1905; 41:399–406.
15. Stopford JS, Telford ED. Compression of the lower trunk of the brachial plexus by a first dorsal rib: with a note on the surgical treatment. Br J Surg 1919; 7:168–177.
16. Adson AW, Coffey JR. Cervical rib: a method of anterior approach for relief of symptoms by division of the scalenus anticus. Ann Surg 1927; 85:839–857.
17. Adson AW. Surgical treatment for symptoms produced by cervical ribs and the scalenus anticus muscle. Surg Gynecol Obstet 1947; 85:687–700.
18. Ochsner A, Gage M, Debakey M. Scalenus Anticus (Naffziger) syndrome. Am J Surg 1935; 28:669–695.
19. Naffziger HC, Grant WT. Neuritis of the brachial plexus mechanical in origin: the scalenus origin. Surg Gynecol Obstet 1938; 67:722.
20. Eden KC. Complications of cervical rib. Vascular complications of cervical ribs and first thoracic rib abnormalities. Br J Surg 1939–40; 27:111–139.
21. Falconer MA, Weddell G. Costoclavicular compression of the subclavian artery and vein. Lancet 1943; 2:539–543.
22. Lord JW Jr. Surgical management of shoulder girdle syndromes: New operative procedure for hyperabduction, costoclavicular, cervical rib, and scalenus syndromes. Arch Surg 1953; 60:69–83.
23. Rosati LM, Lord JW Jr. Neurovascular compression of the shoulder. Modern Surgery Monographs. New York: Grune & Stratton, 1961.
24. Bramwell E. Lesion of the first dorsal nerve root. Rev Neurol Psychiatr 1903; 1:236–239.
25. Murphy T. Brachial neuritis caused by pressure of first rib. Aust Med J 1910; 15:582.
26. Brickner WM, Milch H. First dorsal, simulating cervical rib—by maldevelopment or by pressure symptoms. Surg Gynecol Obstet 1925; 40:38–44.
27. Thorburn W. The symptoms due to cervical ribs. Dreschfeld Memorial 1908: 85–111.
28. White JC, Poppel MH, Adams R. Congenital malformations of the first thoracic rib: a cause of brachial neuralgia which simulates the cervical rib syndrome. Surg Gynecol Obstet 1945; 81:643–659.

29. Telford ED, Mottershead S. The costoclavicular syndrome. Br Med J 1947; 1:325–328.
30. Gage M, Parnell H. Scalenus anticus syndrome. Am J Surg 1947; 73:252–268.
31. Telford ED, Mottershead S. Pressure at the cervico-brachial junction: an operative and anatomical study. J Bone Joint Surg 1948; 30:249–265.
32. Kirgis HD, Reed AF. Significant anatomic relations in the syndrome of the scalene muscles. Ann Surg 1948; 127:1182–1201.
33. Daseler EH, Anson BJ. Surgical anatomy of the subclavian artery and its branches. Surg Gynecol Obstet 1959; 108:149–174.
34. Grayson P. Thoracic outlet syndrome. J Bone Joint Surg (Br) 1975; 57:11.
35. Thomas GI, Jones TW, Stavney LS, Manhas DR. The middle scalene muscle and its contribution to the TOS. Am J Surg 1983; 145:589–592.
36. Reilly LM, Stoney RJ. Supraclavicular approach for thoracic outlet decompression. J Vasc Surg 1988; 8:329–334.
37. Wright IS. The neurovascular syndrome produced by hyperabduction of the arms. Am Heart J 1945; 29:1–19.
38. Peet RM, Hendriksen JD, Anderson TP, Martin GM. Thoracic outlet syndrome: Evaluation of a theraputic exercise program: Proc Mayo Clin 1956; 31:281–287.
39. Rob CG, Standeven A. Arterial occlusion complicating thoracic outlet compression syndrome. Brit Med J 1958; 2:709–712.
40. Clagett OT. Presidential address: research and prosearch. J Thorac Cardiovasc Surg 1962; 44:153–166.
41. Roos DB. Transaxillary approach for first rib resection to relieve thoracic outlet syndrome. Ann Surg 1966; 163:354–358.
42. Gol A, Patrick DW, McNeel DP. Relief of costoclavicular syndrome by infraclavicular removal of first rib. J Neurosurg 1968; 28:81–94.
43. Sanders RJ, Monsour JW, Baer SB. Transaxillary first rib resection for the thoracic outlet syndrome. Arch Surg 1968; 97:1014–1023.
44. Lang EK. Roentgenographic diagnosis of the neurovascular compression syndromes. Radiology 1962; 79:58–63.
45. Winsor T, Brow R. Costoclavicular syndrome. Its diagnosis and treatment. JAMA 1966; 196:109–111.
46. Sanders RJ, Monsour JW, Gerber FG, Adams WRA, Thompson N. Scalenectomy versus first rib resection for treatment of the thoracic outlet syndrome. Surgery 1979; 85:109–121.
47. Urschel HC, Paulson DL, McNamara JJ. Thoracic outlet syndrome. Ann Thorac Surg 1968; 6:1–10.
48. Caldwell JW, Crane CR, Krusen EM. Nerve conduction studies. An aid in the diagnosis of the thoracic outlet syndrome. South Med J 1971; 64:210–212.
49. Hongladarom T. "F"-Wave conduction velocity in thoracic outlet syndrome. N Engl J Med 1976; 295:1382–1383.
50. Glover JL, Worth RM, Bendick PJ, Hall PV, Markand OM. Evoked responses in the diagnosis of thoracic outlet syndrome. Surgery 1981; 89:86–93.
51. Dale A. Thoracic outlet compression syndrome: critique in 1982. Arch Surg 1982; 117:1437–1145.
52. Machleder HI, Moll F, Verity A. The anterior scalene muscle in thoracic outlet compression syndrome: histochemical and morphometric studies. Arch Surg 1986; 121:1141–1144.
53. Sanders RJ, Jackson CGR, Banchero N, Pearce WH. Scalene muscle abnormalities in traumatic thoracic outlet syndrome. Am J Surg 1990; 159:231–236.

3
Etiology

Richard J. Sanders

Definition

Etiology
Osseous Causes
Soft Tissue Causes

Pathophysiology

Classification
By Etiology
By Anatomy
By Symptoms
By Clinical Presentation

Definition

The simplest definition of thoracic outlet syndrome (TOS) is: *neurovascular symptoms in the upper extremity due to pressure on the nerves and vessels in the thoracic outlet area.* The specific structures compressed are usually the nerves of the brachial plexus and occasionally the subclavian artery or subclavian vein.

The term thoracic outlet syndrome includes all of the specific anatomical syndromes that occur in the thoracic area—cervical rib syndrome, first rib syndrome, scalenus anticus syndrome, and many others. Clinically, each of those conditions elicits symptoms that are indistinguishable from those of the other. From a diagnostic and therapeutic point of view, it is helpful to localize the site of pathology to the supraclavicular area even though the specific abnormality is yet unidentified. The diagnosis of TOS is useful in ruling out other sites of pathology, such as the cervical spine, elbow, or wrist. Once the diagnosis of TOS is established, the pathology should be defined as accurately as possible, because the different entities that comprise TOS are not all treated in the same way.

Etiology

A large number of conditions are included under the heading of thoracic outlet syndrome (Table 3–1). Some of these entities are not specific diseases; like the term "thoracic outlet syndrome," they are labels that define the area of pathology without specifying a cause. They are synonyms for TOS and include such names as *brachiocephalic syndrome*, *cervicobrachial syndrome*, and *cervicothoracic syndrome*. Any of those terms could be used instead of thoracic outlet syndrome. The term cervicobrachial syndrome was introduced by Aynesworth in 1940[1] for the same reasons that Peet in 1956 suggested the term thoracic outlet syndrome.[2] Perhaps the medical community was not ready for a such a comprehensive term in 1940 because the name cervicobrachial syndrome never became popular. By 1956, times had changed and "thoracic outlet syndrome" became the accepted name.

All causes of TOS can be divided into osseous and soft tissue types, which are described separately.

Osseous Causes

Bony Abnormalities Recognizable on X-ray

Osseous causes of TOS may be abnormalities recognizable on x-ray or may be soft tissue abnormalities compressing the neurovascular bundle against a normal first rib. *Cervical ribs*, *rudimentary first ribs*, and callus from *fractures of the first rib or*

Table 3–1.   **Synonyms for Thoracic Outlet Syndrome**

1. Brachiocephalic Syndrome
2. Cervicobrachial Neurovascular Syndrome
3. Cervicothoracic Syndrome

clavicle can easily be seen on chest and neck x-rays. These bony abnormalities press against the lower or upper nerves of the brachial plexus. They account for almost all subclavian artery aneurysms and occlusions associated with TOS and sometimes are the cause of venous compression as well.

Normal First Rib

A normal first rib can be passively responsible for neurovascular compression in a variety of circumstances. The cords of the plexus are usually draped over the first rib as they pass to the arm. *Weak shoulder muscles* and *drooping or sagging shoulders* have the potential of weighing the arms downward, stretching the cords of the plexus over the rib and eliciting neurological symptoms. *Rucksack or backpack paralysis* implies the same mechanism of downward traction on the plexus by heavy loads on the shoulders.

The combination of a bony abnormality and TOS symptoms does not mean the symptoms are always caused by the obvious abnormality. In their classical article of 1927, Adson and Coffey noted that patients with cervical ribs often obtained symptomatic relief by scalenotomy alone, without cervical rib removal, suggesting that the cervical rib is a predisposing cause.[3] However, symptoms develop only when something else occurs to the scalene muscles, such as an injury or muscle disease.

The Costoclavicular Syndrome

First described in 1939 by Eden,[4] and named in 1943 by Falconer and Weddell,[5] costoclavicular syndrome is neurovascular compression between clavicle and first rib. These bones usually appear normal on x-ray, but they apparently curve enough toward each other that structures passing between them can be squeezed. Neurologic and/or vascular symptoms can be produced. The vascular symptoms are more often arterial than venous, but either can occur.

Neurovascular compression by either sagging shoulders or a tight costoclavicular space is difficult to prove. Although some surgeons claim costoclavicular narrowing can be confirmed at operation by manipulating the arm with a finger in the costoclavicular space to feel the "pinching" action, these criteria are very subjective and can also be demonstrated in asymptomatic patients.

Soft Tissue Causes

The soft tissue causes of TOS can be traumatic, congenital, inflammatory, or even neoplastic. Any entity that causes swelling and/or fibrosis of the scalene muscles can elicit symptoms of TOS.

Scalene Muscle Trauma

The association of trauma and TOS was first discussed by Ochsner, Gage, and DeBakey in 1935.[6] They reported six patients, three of whom developed their symptoms after neck injuries. They theorized that scalene muscle spasm caused elevation of the first rib which, in turn, irritated the nerves of the brachial plexus. Nerve irritation stimulated more muscle spasm, thereby establishing a vicious cycle. The concept of elevation of the first rib was questioned in 1948 by Telford and Mottershead, who stated that in 470 scalenotomies they had yet to see the first rib fall following tenotomy.[7]

Friedberg, in 1938, reported 20 cases of scalenus anticus syndrome associated with rotator cuff tendinitis or cervical spine strain.[8] In 1940, Aynesworth described another 20 cases of Scalenus Anticus Syndrome, many of which had cervical ribs and 80% of which had histories of trauma.[1] Scalenotomy was performed in all cases, usually without resection of the cervical rib. Interestingly, most patients enjoyed symptomatic improvement, including relief of their headaches, even though their cervical ribs remained. This led Aynesworth to postulate that trauma caused fibrosis and contracture of the anterior scalene muscle, which in turn compressed the brachial plexus and subclavian artery to produce symptoms. Almost 50 years were to pass before microscopic evidence of muscle injury would be available to support Aynesworth's theory.[9]

Holden et al., in 1951, observed that trauma was the cause of acute scalenus anticus syndrome and that the trauma "need not be of great severity."[10] They noted that other muscles were also in spasm—the trapezius, rhomboid, pectoralis major, and deltoid muscles—and that scalenotomy obviously would not relieve the symptoms from myositis arising in these areas.

Stowell, in 1956, divided scalenus anticus syndrome into "post-traumatic and non-traumatic groups."[11] Whiplash injuries were especially common in the post-traumatic group and many of these patients were erroneously labeled as having "cervical disc pathology." Unilateral occipital headaches were a common complaint and were noted to be "invariably relieved by scalenus anticus division."[11]

Observations of the association of thoracic outlet syndrome with trauma continued in the 1960s and 1970s as they had with the scalenus anticus syndrome decades earlier. Several authors recorded a significant incidence of trauma in their TOS patients.[12–17] In 1978 Woods found that among 1,958 patients with soft tissue neck injuries, 23% had TOS.[15] While the majority improved with conservative therapy, 41% required scalenectomy. Similarly, in 1986 Capistrant noted that among 111 patients with cervical strains and whiplash injuries, 36% had TOS and 20% of these received first rib resections.[18]

Precisely how trauma produces TOS is still open to speculation, but several observations made over the past few decades offer some clues. The demonstration of consistent microscopic changes in the muscles of people who have experienced neck trauma just prior to the onset of symptoms, suggests that the anterior and/or middle scalene muscles may be the source of pathology. Anatomical dissections in the operating room and laboratory have revealed that the nerves of the brachial plexus usually pass through the narrowest part of the scalene triangle, where there is no space;[19] the nerves normally touch these muscles. Elevation of the arms tends to push the plexus even higher in the scalene triangle, forcing the nerves against the scalene muscles. Following trauma, if these muscles have been tightened or hardened by an inflammatory process, it is easy to envision how these nerves could be irritated and produce neurologic symptoms.

Tight scalene muscles also explain some of the non-neurologic symptoms seen in traumatic TOS patients, such as neck pain, neck stiffness, and occipital headache. In a few patients, headaches are the predominant complaint.[20] These symptoms are most likely muscular in origin and are consistently relieved by scalenotomy or scalenectomy, with or without rib resection. Scalene muscle injury, secondary to trauma, is emerging as the commonest etiology of TOS.

Evidence of the important role of trauma is seen in a list of etiologies from 668 operated cases of TOS (Table 3–2).[21] In 86% trauma was the cause. Automobile accidents were the commonest type of injury—56%; job related trauma accounted for 22%. Although the incidence of osseous abnormalities was close to 5%, most of these patients had histories of trauma immediately preceding the onset of their symptoms; they are classified under trauma. The 2% incidence of bony abnormalities recorded in Table 3–3 represent patients without histories of trauma.

Congenital Bands and Ligaments

Congenital bands and ligaments are frequently found attached to the first rib. The costovertebral ligament is probably the commonest band, running from the transverse process of C-7 to insert on the first rib with the middle scalene muscle.

Table 3–2.   **Etiologies and Abnormalities Included in Term "Thoracic Outlet Syndrome"**

Osseous
    A. Abnormal x-ray
        1. Cervical rib
        2. Abnormal, anomalous, or rudimentary first rib
        3. Fractured clavicle
        4. Fractured first rib
    B. Normal x-ray
        1. Normal first rib syndrome
        2. Sagging shoulder syndrome
        3. Rucksack paralysis
        4. Costoclavicular syndrome
        5. Effort thrombosis (this might be traumatic)
        6. Nonthrombotic subclavian obstruction

Soft Tissue
    A. Traumatic
        1. Scalenus anticus syndrome
        2. Scalenus medius syndrome
    B. Congenital
        1. Cervical ligaments and bands
        2. Anomalous scalene muscle insertions
        3. Scalenus minimus muscle
        4. Nonthrombotic subclavian vein obstruction
        5. Hyperabduction (pectoralis minor) syndrome
    C. Inflammatory
        1. Infections—acute, chronic, viral
        2. Connective tissue diseases
    D. Neoplasm

Table 3–3.   Etiology—668 Operated Cases of TOS

Trauma		86%
Rear end auto accident	32%	
Side or front auto	24	
Work injury	20	
Work related, no injury	2	
Other trauma	8	
Cervical or rudimentary first rib (without trauma)		2%
Axillary vein occlusion		1%
Arterial insufficiency		1%
Soft tissue/unknown (no history of trauma)		10%
		100%

(From Sanders RJ, Pearce WH. The treatment of thoracic outlet syndrome: A comparison of different operations. J Vasc Surg 1989; 10:626–634. With permission.)

Telford and Mottershead observed such a tight muscle band in 34% of their anatomical dissections.[7] Roos has described a large number of variations among these bands and has observed them in the majority of transaxillary rib resections.[22] The ligaments narrow the scalene triangle, making it easier for adjacent structures to compress the neurovascular bundle.

Because those bands and ligaments are present in more than half of the normal population, and since less than 1% of the population ever develop TOS, it appears that these congenital bands provide a predisposition to develop symptoms, but are seldom the primary cause. While the ligaments have been present since birth, it usually requires a neck injury to elicit symptoms. The injury, rather than the congenital band, is the immediate cause of TOS. The same statement applies to most cervical and abnormal first ribs.

Inflammation

Acute or chronic infections, connective tissue diseases, degenerative diseases, and tumors are all capable of establishing inflammatory reactions in the scalene muscles, which, in turn, can elicit symptoms of TOS. Many of those conditions are self-limiting or subject to remission and the symptoms subside spontaneously. Examples of them, in the authors' experiences, include muscular dystrophy and sarcoidosis, diagnoses that were confirmed microscopically.

Pathophysiology

The pathophysiology of venous TOS begins with venous obstruction. The symptoms of pain and swelling are those of venous hypertension. Improvement in symptoms is associated with either recanalization of the occluded vein or development of collateral veins around the venous block. The mechanism of venous obstruction may be a combination of anatomical narrowing at the subclavian innominate junction plus one or more episodes of shoulder trauma causing intimal injury to the subclavian vein. This is further discussed in Chapter 15.

The pathophysiology of arterial TOS is based upon the effects of arterial compression by bony abnormalities. The changes in fluid hemodynamics that are produced by subclavian artery stenosis are responsible for the subsequent changes of poststenotic dilatation, mural thrombosis, and peripheral embolization. These are more fully discussed in Chapter 14.

Neurologic symptoms of paresthesia, weakness, and pain are due to brachial plexus irritation and compression caused by the structures forming the scalene triangle or costoclavicular space. Cervical ribs act as a fulcrum beneath the plexus; because they push up against the nerves, symptoms may be aggravated when the arms hang down and be relieved when the arms are elevated. In contrast, scalene muscles that are taut or scarred by injury or disease will have symptoms elicited by elevating the arms and relieved by hanging them down. The scalene muscles normally touch the nerves of the brachial plexus. As the arm is abducted and elevated, the nerves are raised upwards, into the narrower portion of the scalene triangle. If the muscles are soft, no symptoms are elicited; but if they are scarred and tight, plexus irritation and paresthesia occur.

It is easy to appreciate how nerves can be stretched or compressed by bony abnormalities. However, it is more difficult to understand how neck trauma elicits the symptoms of nerve compression. The pathophysiology of traumatic TOS is probably a combination of an anatomic predisposition to plexus pressure plus an injury to the scalene muscles. The predisposition can be a congenital band, ligament, or cervical rib that narrows the scalene triangle, or it can be a variation in anatomical relationships whereby the cords of the brachial plexus emerge at a point high in the scalene triangle where the anterior and middle scalene muscles are very close together.[19] Injury to the scalenes results in muscle fibrosis and mild plexus compression by tightened or spastic anterior and middle scalene muscles.

Even though objective data is difficult to accumulate, this theory of the etiology of traumatic TOS is supported by several isolated observations. Anatomic predisposition is suggested by the observation that 83% of patients operated upon for TOS had a high emergence of the nerves of the brachial plexus from the scalene triangle, where there was no space, compared to an incidence of only 40% in cadaver controls[19] (see also Chapter 4). Histologic abnormalities have now been identified in the scalene muscles of traumatic TOS patients[9] (see also Chapter 5). The positive correlation between improvement following scalene muscle block and improvement following scalenectomy or rib resection gives validity to implicating the scalene muscles as the site of pathology (Chapter 7). Finally, support for this hypothesis comes from the clinical improvement noted in the large majority of patients with a diagnosis of traumatic TOS following surgery in which the scalene muscles were divided or removed[21] (see also Chapter 12).

In a clinical study of over 600 patients operated upon for TOS, the incidence of bony abnormalities, primarily cervical ribs, was 4.5%, six to nine times greater than the incidence of 0.5% to 0.7% in the general population. However, in over 70% of these patients with cervical ribs, neck trauma precipitated the onset of symptoms.[21] This supports the thesis that most cervical ribs are predisposing factors for TOS rather than the primary cause.

Classification

To better understand the spectrum of abnormalities that can produce thoracic outlet syndrome, some type of classification is needed. There are several ways TOS can be classified: by etiology, anatomy, symptoms, or clinical presentation.

By Etiology

All conditions are either congenital or acquired. Each group can be further subdivided into osseous and soft tissue abnormalities.

A. Congenital
   1. Osseous—Cervical ribs and rudimentary first ribs
   2. Soft tissue—Congenital bands and ligaments, scalene minimus muscle
B. Acquired
   1. Osseous—Fractures of clavicle and first rib
   2. Soft tissue—Scalene trauma, inflammation, infection

By Anatomy

All conditions are either osseous or soft tissue abnormalities. These can be further differentiated into congenital and acquired groups.

A. Osseous
   1. Congenital—Cervical ribs and rudimentary first ribs
   2. Acquired—Fractures of clavicle and first rib
B. Soft Tissue
   1. Congenital—Congenital bands and ligaments, scalene minimus muscle, scalene muscle/plexus anatomical relationships
   2. Acquired—Scalene trauma, inflammation, infection

By Symptoms

Arterial, venous, or neurologic symptoms are another way to classify TOS. Arterial problems are usually associated with osseous abnormalities like cervical ribs, abnormal first ribs, or fractures of the first rib or clavicle. Venous obstruction is usually congenital and due to an enlarged costoclavicular ligament or subclavius muscle. Neurologic symptoms are usually present in all cases, including those with arterial and venous compression.

Wilbourn subdivides neurogenic TOS into two groups: true or disputed TOS.[23] True neurogenic TOS has abnormalities by x-ray or abnormal neurophysiologic tests. Disputed neurogenic TOS includes all of the other cases that lack objective criteria.

A. Arterial TOS

   1. Ischemic changes in fingers—Pain, coldness, color changes, digital gangrene

   2. Arterial cut-off—Pulse loss and bruit on physical exam

   3. Arterial damage—as seen on arteriography

B. Venous TOS

   1. Swelling and cyanosis

   2. Venous obstruction—As seen on positional venography

C. Neurogenic TOS

   1. True—Abnormal X-ray, or abnormal neurophysiologic tests

   2. Disputed—Neurologic symptoms, but normal x-rays and neurophysiologic tests

By Clinical Presentation

Presenting symptoms are used to first divide patients into vascular or neurogenic groups. The vascular patients, comprising less than 5% of all TOS patients, are either arterial or venous. Next, because a history of trauma is easy to determine, trauma is used to subdivide patients with neurogenic TOS into traumatic or nontraumatic groups. Finally, chest x-rays further separate patients into groups with osseous or soft tissue abnormalities.

A classification based on symptoms, a history of trauma, and chest x-rays is as follows:

   I. Arterial TOS

  II. Venous TOS

III. Neurogenic TOS

   A. Traumatic TOS

     1. Soft tissue—Scalene muscle injury

     2. Osseous—Rare cases of fractured clavicle or first rib

   B. Nontraumatic TOS

     1. Osseous

       a. Cervical rib

       b. Abnormal or rudimentary first rib

       c. Sagging shoulders (stretching plexus over rib)

       d. Costoclavicular syndrome

     2. Soft Tissue

       a. Inflammation

         1) Viral

         2) Connective tissue diseases

　　　　3) Sarcoidosis

　　　　4) Irradiation

　　　　5) Other infections

　　b. Congenital bands or ligaments

　　c. Pectoralis minor (Hyperabduction) syndrome

　　d. Large costoclavicular ligament

　　e. Large subclavius muscle

　　f. Postoperative scalene scarring

　　g. Tumor, Hodgkins, others

　　h. Variations in scalene muscle/brachial plexus relationships

　　　　A simpler version of the clinical classification of neurogenic TOS is presented in Table 3–4. Using the categories of traumatic, osseous, and nontraumatic TOS, it is interesting to review the etiologies of three groups of patients who were operated on for TOS over a period of 22 years (Table 3–5). In the earliest series, 1964–67, trauma was listed as the etiological factor in 54% of the patients. It was in reviewing this group of cases that the relatively high incidence of trauma in TOS patients became apparent. In the next series, 1972–79 and 1980–85, every patient was specifically asked if an accident or injury to the neck had preceded the onset of symptoms. The incidence of trauma increased to 89% and 91%, respectively.

　　　　Today, few patients with TOS have osseous abnormalities or vascular symptoms. TOS has evolved from a vascular disease, due to osseous abnormalities and with objective vascular signs, to a nerve compression syndrome, due to costoclavicular narrowing or scalene muscle pathology but with no objective findings.

Table 3–4.   **Clinical Classification of Neurogenic TOS**

Class	Etiology	History	X-ray	Treatment
Traumatic TOS	Scalene injury	Pos.	Neg.	Scalenectomy and/or rib resection
Osseous TOS (Abnormal x-ray)	Cervical rib, abnormal first rib, fractures of clavicle or first rib	Neg.	Pos.	Excise bone
Nontraumatic TOS	All other causes with normal x-rays and no history of trauma	Neg.	Neg.	Variable— depends on cause

Table 3–5.   **Etiology**

	1965–71	1972–79	1980–86	1965–86
Number of operations	76	281	223	580
Traumatic TOS	54%	89%	91%	85%
Osseous TOS	2%	1%	1%	2%
Nontraumatic TOS	44%	10%	8%	13%

There are still a few cases of vascular and nerve compression that produce ischemic or muscle wasted hands, but they comprise less than 5% of the TOS cases seen by most physicians.

References

1. Aynesworth KH. The cervicobrachial syndrome. A discussion of the etiology with report of twenty cases. Ann Surg 1940; 111:724–742.
2. Peet RM, Hendriksen JD, Anderson TP, Martin GM. Thoracic outlet syndrome: evaluation of a therapeutic exercise program. Proc Mayo Clin 1956; 31:281–287.
3. Adson AW, Coffey JR. Cervical rib: a method of anterior approach for relief of symptoms by division of the scalenus anticus. Ann Surg 1927; 85:839–857.
4. Eden KC. Complications of cervical rib. Vascular complications of cervical ribs and first thoracic rib abnormalities. Br J Surg 1939–40; 27:111–139.
5. Falconer MA, Weddell G. Costoclavicular compression of the subclavian artery and vein. Lancet 1943; 2:539–543.
6. Ochsner A, Gage M, DeBakey M. Scalenus anticus (Naffziger) syndrome. Am J Surg 1935; 28:669–695.
7. Telford ED, Mottershead S. Pressure at the cervico-brachial junction: an operative and anatomical study. J Bone Joint Surg 1948; 30:249–265.
8. Freiberg JA. The scalenus anterior muscle in relation to shoulder and arm pain. J Bone Joint Surg 1938; 20:860–861.
9. Sanders RJ, Jackson CGR, Banchero N, Pearce WH. Scalene muscle abnormalities in traumatic thoracic outlet syndrome. Am J Surg 1990; 159:231–236.
10. Holden WD, Murphy JA, Portmann AF. Scalene anticus syndrome: unusual diagnostic and therapeutic aspects. Am J Surg 1951; 81:411–416.
11. Stowell A. The scalenus anticus syndrome. J Int Coll Surg 1956; 26:711–717.
12. Woods WW. Personal experiences with surgical treatment of 250 cases of cervicobrachial neurovascular compression syndrome. J Int Coll Surg 1965; 44:273–283.
13. Timmis H. Discussion in Dale WA: Management of thoracic outlet syndrome. Ann Surg 1975; 181:585.
14. Capistrant TD. Thoracic outlet syndrome in whiplash injury. Ann Surg 1977; 185:175–178.
15. Woods WW. Thoracic outlet syndrome. West J Med 1978; 128:9–12.
16. Sanders RJ, Monsour JW, Gerber FG, Adams WRA, Thompson N. Scalenectomy versus first rib resection for treatment of the thoracic outlet syndrome. Surgery 1979; 85:109–121.
17. Qvarfordt PG, Ehrenfeld WK, Stoney RJ. Supraclavicular radical scalenectomy and transaxillary first rib resection for the thoracic outlet syndrome. A combined approach. Am J Surg 1984; 148:111–116.
18. Capistrant TD. Thoracic outlet syndrome in cervical strain injury. Minn Med 1986; 69:13–17.
19. Sanders RJ, Roos DB. The surgical anatomy of the scalene triangle. Contemporary Surg 1989; 35:11–16.
20. Raskin NH, Howard MW, Ehrenfeld WK. Headache as the leading symptom of the thoracic outlet syndrome. Headache 1985; 25:208–210.
21. Sanders RJ, Pearce WH. The treatment of thoracic outlet syndrome: a comparison of different operations. J Vasc Surg 1989; 10:626–634.
22. Roos DB. New Concepts of thoracic outlet syndrome that explain etiology, symptoms, diagnosis, and treatment. Vasc Surg 1979; 13:313–321.
23. Wilbourn AJ. Thoracic outlet syndrome surgery causing severe brachial plexopathy. Muscle Nerve 1988; 11:66–74.

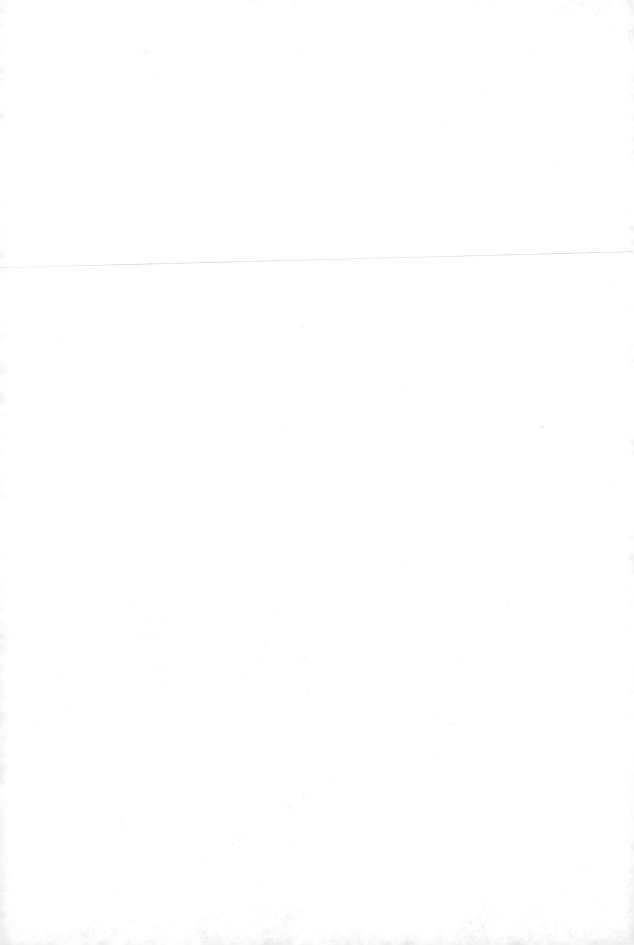

4
Anatomy

Mary B. Mockus
Craig E. Haug
Richard J. Sanders

The Four Anatomical Spaces

Cervical Ribs

Ligaments and Bands
Nerves

Subclavian Vessels

Thoracic Duct

The Four Anatomical Spaces

The thoracic outlet area is located just above the first rib where the subclavian vessels enter and exit the chest. Because many vital nerves and vessels travel through this relatively small area, mechanical pressure against them is not unusual. Appreciation of the normal anatomy and its variations is essential in understanding the various etiologies of TOS and the approaches to surgical repair.

The thoracocervical region has been described by Pollak[1] as a long tunnel through which the neurovascular structures of the region must pass. Usually these structures coexist harmoniously. However, when the delicate equilibrium between contents and container is disturbed, the neurovascular bundle yields to the firmer osseous and fibromuscular components, resulting in symptomatic compression. The goal of surgery for TOS is to widen the tunnel by removing the various structures, such as the first rib, scalene muscles, or pectoralis minor tendon, that form the sides of the tunnel.

The tunnel has four sections: the sternocostovertebral space, the scalene triangle, costoclavicular space, and the pectoralis minor (coracopectoral) space, which lies laterally. These are described below and shown in Figure 4-1.

Sternocostovertebral Space

The sternocostovertebral space is the largest and most proximal portion of the tunnel. It is bounded anteriorly by the sternum, posteriorly by the spine, and laterally by the first rib. The subclavian artery and vein traverse the space, as do the

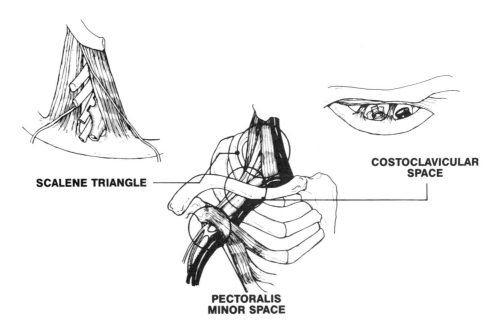

SCALENE TRIANGLE

COSTOCLAVICULAR SPACE

PECTORALIS MINOR SPACE

Fig. 4-1.   Three major spaces in the thoracic outlet area.

five roots of the brachial plexus. In this area the nerve roots have just left the spine and have not yet formed trunks. The space includes the apex of the lung, the pleura, the sympathetic trunk, jugular vein, and lymphatics of the neck. Compression of nerves or vessels is rare in this area and when it occurs, is usually the result of enlargement or tumors of the thyroid, thymus, parathyroid, lymph nodes, or lung. Pancoast tumors present here.

Scalene Triangle

This area is bounded by the anterior scalene muscle anteriorly, the middle scalene muscle posteriorly, and the first rib at its base. Any one of these three structures can cause compression of the neurovascular bundle and the clinical picture of TOS.

Anterior Scalene Muscle

The anterior scalene muscle has a constant site of origin from the third through the sixth cervical vertebrae but its point of insertion, generally on the scalene tubercle of the first rib, can vary. The insertion on the tubercle is between the subclavian artery and vein, with an expansion to the pleural dome. Variants include insertion behind the artery, between the artery and the brachial plexus, or an extended area of insertion that includes the entire base of the scalene triangle. The latter variant may result in the anterior and middle scalene muscles forming a vise around the neurovascular bundle.[2] The insertion of the anterior scalene muscle merges with the middle scalene muscle in 20% of individuals. In half of all individuals, the insertions are overlapping on the first rib, while in the other half they are joined in a common insertion. A complete fusion of the muscles has also been described.[2,3]

Deep to the anterior scalene muscle lie the subclavian artery and nerve trunks of the brachial plexus. Usually, the nerves pass through a slit formed by the anterior and middle scalene muscles (Fig. 4-2). In some cases, however, the fifth and sixth cervical roots actually pass between bundles of the anterior scalene muscle rather than the hiatus between the anterior and middle scalene muscles. In one study, this variant was seen in 45% of cadavers and 21% of TOS patients.[4]

The anterior scalene muscle, at its widest part, has a sharp falciform posterior border that overlies the transverse process of the seventh cervical vertebra. Hypertrophy of this transverse process, coupled with spasmodic contraction of the anterior scalene muscle, has been suggested as a mechanism for compression of the brachial plexus.

Middle Scalene Muscle

The middle scalene muscle originates from the transverse processes of the second through the seventh cervical vertebrae and inserts on the superior aspect of the first rib at Chassaignac's retroarterial tubercle. This insertion is broader and more posterior than that of the anterior scalene muscle. The middle scalene may also have an expansion that inserts on the fibrous septum of the pleural dome.

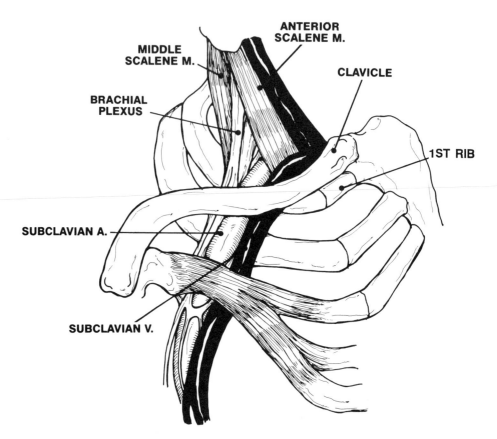

Fig. 4-2.   The scalene triangle contains the subclavian artery and the nerves of the brachial plexus. The subclavian vein lies anterior to the triangle.

Lateral fibers of the middle scalene descend below the first rib to insert on the second rib.

Insertion of the middle scalene muscle in a more forward or anterior position can cause compression of the trunks of the brachial plexus by contact with the sharp, anterior edge of the muscle. In a cadaver study published in 1948, the most frequently encountered anatomy was that of the lower trunk of the brachial plexus resting on the anterolateral margin of the middle scalene muscle.[3] Fibromuscular bands along this border of the muscle may be one of the pathogenic mechanisms for TOS in the absence of a cervical rib. Among 33 patients treated for TOS by Thomas et al., middle scalene muscle abnormalities were observed in 58%.[5]

First Rib

The first thoracic rib forms the floor of the scalene triangle. Its long axis forms a 45-degree angle with the horizontal. Thus, its anterior end projects at the level of the fourth or fifth thoracic vertebra, and the apex of the lung projects above the anterior end of the first rib. Muscles inserting on the first rib include the anterior and middle scalenes, the first digitation of the serratus anterior, and the intercostals. The neurovascular bundle runs across the first rib with the artery and T-1 being close to the rib. Fractures or congenital rib anomalies like bony ridges, hypoplasia, or abnormalities of curvature may compromise the integrity of the neurovascular bundle (Fig. 4-3).

Scalene Triangle Variations

Studies suggest that a narrow scalene triangle may contribute to the etiology of TOS.[4,5] The base of the triangle was reported by Daseler and Anson to average 1.1 cm in width, based upon measurements in 100 cadavers.[6] When studied at operation for TOS, Kirgis and Reed found the average base of the triangle to be 0.77 cm in men and 0.67 cm in women[3] (Fig. 4-4, A and B).

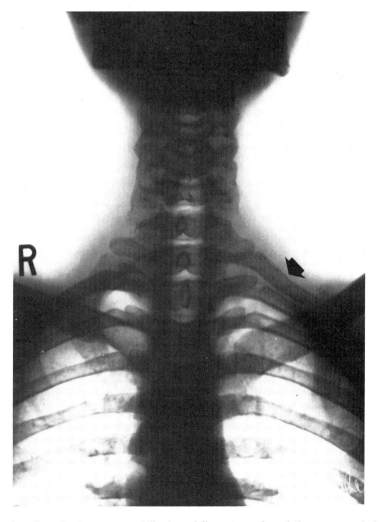

Fig. 4-3.   Left anomalous first rib. At times it is difficult to differentiate a first rib from a cervical rib. In this x-ray, the right first rib is normal. Its transverse process is T-1. The left first rib comes from a similar transverse process and, therefore, is a first, not cervical, rib.

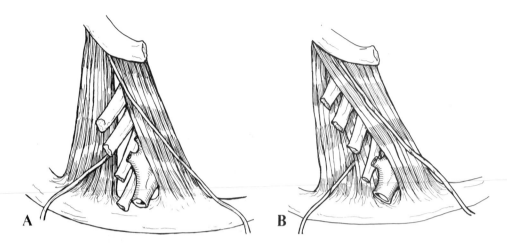

Fig. 4-4. Variations in the relationships within the scalene triangle. **A**—The usual relationships found in most cadavers. The triangle is wider and the nerves emerge a little lower than in most TOS patients. **B**—The narrow tight triangle noted in most TOS patients. The nerves emerge high in the triangle touching the scalene muscles as they emerge. *(From Sanders RJ, Roos DB. The surgical anatomy of the scalene triangle. Contemporary Surg 1989; 35:11–16. With Permission.)*

Little attention has been paid to the other end of the triangle, the apex. Here, the fibers of origin of the anterior and middle scalene muscles intermingle in a solid muscle mass with no opening for at least two to three cm below the apex. It is here that the upper nerves of the plexus, C-5, C-6, and often C-7, emerge from the scalene triangle. In an anatomical study of cadavers and TOS patients, one of the most significant findings was that the nerves of the plexus exited from the very apex of the triangle in 40% of cadavers (controls) compared to 83% of TOS patients.[4] The high emergence of the nerves in almost all of the TOS patients might be an important anatomic variation predisposing these people to TOS symptoms (Fig. 4-4, A and B).

Other variations in the triangle include the proximity of the muscles to each other and adherence of nerves to muscle. Interdigitating muscle fibers run between the two scalenes in 75% of TOS patients compared to 40% of cadavers.[6,7] Adherence of nerves to the anterior scalene is more common in TOS patients than in cadavers, 90% versus 29%, respectively.[4] Adherence to the middle scalene occurred in 61% of TOS patients compared to 32% of cadavers. In that study, it was pointed out that adherence in preserved cadavers was more difficult to assess than adherence in the living, which may have affected the results.[4]

Costoclavicular Space

The costoclavicular space is the area between clavicle and first rib. The anterior border is the costoclavicular ligament; the posterior border is not well-defined but is near the posterior edge of the middle scalene muscle. The space

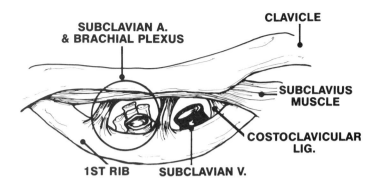

Fig. 4-5.   The costoclavicular space includes all of the structures of the scalene triangle plus the subclavian vein.

contains all of the contents of the scalene triangle and, in addition, the subclavian vein and subclavius muscle (Fig. 4-5).

Clavicle

The clavicle follows a curved path between its two joints, the medial sternoclavicular joint, which is relatively fixed, and the lateral acromioclavicular joint, which has a wide range of motion due to the extensive mobility of the scapula. Anything that affects the position of the scapula and changes the position of the acromioclavicular joint can influence the size of the costoclavicular space. Contraction of the pectoralis minor, serratus anterior, or lower fibers of the trapezius muscle can pull down the scapula and lateral end of the clavicle, thereby narrowing the costoclavicular space. Newborns have a large costoclavicular space because of their elevated scapulas. Subsequent body growth leads to progressive acromioclavicular descent, which may explain the rarity of costoclavicular compression in children. Poor posture and an asthenic habitus, theoretically, can also narrow the space.

Exostosis, tumors, fractures, and particularly the space occupying callus of healed fractures of the clavicle or first rib, are each capable of narrowing the costoclavicular space and compressing the neurovascular bundle.

First Rib

The first rib is fixed anteriorly at the sternum and posteriorly at the spine, leaving its lateral portion as the only part that is mobile. Both anterior and middle scalene muscles insert here and, theoretically, each can elevate the first rib and narrow the costoclavicular space. Because the middle scalene muscle is larger than the anterior scalene and because the middle scalene inserts more laterally on the first rib giving it a greater lever arm, it plays a larger role in rib elevation and narrowing of the costoclavicular passage. It should be stressed that movement of the first rib is probably minimal and that these anatomical differences are of questionable clinical significance.

Pectoralis Minor Space

The pectoralis minor space lies below the insertion of the pectoralis minor tendon into the coracoid process and superficial to the ribs of the chest wall (Fig. 4-1). It is traversed by the brachial plexus and subclavian artery and vein. During hyperabduction of the arm, angulation and compression of the nerves or vessels can occur.

Cervical Ribs

Embryology

Teleologically, lower animal forms, such as reptiles, have ribs articulating with their cervical vertebrae. Todd[8] and Jones[9] suggested that in higher animal forms there is a negative selection pressure that prevents development of ribs from cervical vertebrae. This lack of development is a result of the appearance of limb buds. The spinal column grows faster than the limb bud, causing the cervical nerve roots to angulate caudally and gather together into a plexus. Since the nervous system is further developed than the osseous system at this point in embryologic life, the segmental nerves, being pulled downward by the descent of the upper limb bud, physically block the ribs and arrest their growth. A cervical rib appears when this process is incomplete.

In man, evidence of rib rudiments are the anterior tubercles of the transverse processes of normal cervical vertebrae.[9] To further support the theory of the nerve roots inhibiting rib development, it is noted that cervical ribs are usually associated with an underdeveloped T-1 nerve, suggesting that it was too small to prevent growth of the cervical rib. Further, in cases where the T-2 nerve root contributed to the brachial plexus, the first rib was often seen to be rudimentary (Jones[9]). The incidence of such underdeveloped first ribs is 0.25–0.76% (Table 4–1).

Classification

Based upon extensive anatomical dissections, Gruber, in 1869, divided cervical ribs into four stages of development (Table 4–2).[15] Incomplete cervical ribs (types I and II), usually attach to the first rib by a tight band from the tip of the cervical rib to the first rib (Figs. 4-6 and 4-7). The rib and the band lie within or on the medial border of the middle scalene muscle. This narrows the space within the scalene triangle and can cause pressure against the neurovascular bundle, thereby producing neurologic or vascular symptoms. With complete ribs, the neurovascular bundle must arch over the rib, increasing the probability of compression symptoms, particularly when the shoulder girdle is lowered (Figs. 4-7 and 4-8).

Incidence and Sex Distribution

When the frequency of cervical ribs was determined by anatomical dissections, the incidence was quite small, 0.056%.[16] With the introduction of x-rays,

Table 4–1. **Incidence of Cervical and Rudimentary First Ribs**

Author	Year	No. x-rays	Cervical Ribs			Rudimentary First Ribs		
			Total	Female	Male	Total	Female	Male
Southham[10]	1924	2,000	13(0.45%)	10(77%)	3(23%)			
Haven[11]	1939	5,000	37(0.74%)	26(70%)	11(30%)	38(0.76%)	19(50%)	19(50%)
Etter[12]	1944	40,000	68(0.17%)	men only		114(0.29%)		
Sycamore[13]	1944	2,000	10(0.5%)	men only		10(0.5%)		
Eaton[14]	1946	7,706	45(0.58)	29(65%)	16(35%)			
TOTALS		56,700	173(0.3%)	65(68%)	30(32%)	162(0.34%)	19(50%)	19(50%)

Table 4–2. **Gruber Classification of Cervical Ribs**

Type I—<2.5 cm, barely beyond transverse process
Type II—Longer, >2.5 cm incomplete rib with free end
Type III—Complete rib with fibrous connection to first rib
Type IV—Complete rib with cartilaginous joint connecting to first rib

the ability to find incomplete cervical ribs improved enormously. In five reviews of over 50,000 chest films, the incidence of cervical ribs ranged from 0.17% to 0.74% and averaged 0.3% (Table 4–1). The incidence in women was twice that of men (68% versus 32%). These figures are of particular interest because they reveal approximately the same sex distribution as patients who develop TOS with cervical ribs (83% women)[17, 18] or without cervical ribs (71% women).[19]

TOS Symptoms

No more than 10% of people with cervical ribs ever develop symptoms. Those who do become symptomatic usually relate the onset of symptoms to some type of trauma[17] in which the neck could have been stretched.[19] Symptoms of arterial compression, enough to produce subclavian artery stenosis and aneurysmal dilatation, are almost always associated with an osseous abnormality, most commonly a cervical rib or rudimentary first rib. Arterial damage is rare without such bony abnormalities. Even though cervical ribs are capable of compressing the subclavian artery, most symptoms from cervical ribs are from nerve compression.

Ligaments and Bands

At least 12 different fibrous structures in the thoracic outlet area have been identified at operation or during cadaver dissection. Table 4–3 lists the nine types described by Roos.[20] Some of the most significant ligaments are those that run from either the transverse process of C-7 or from the tip of a cervical rib and attach to the first rib. These ligaments lie within the body or on the anterior surface of the

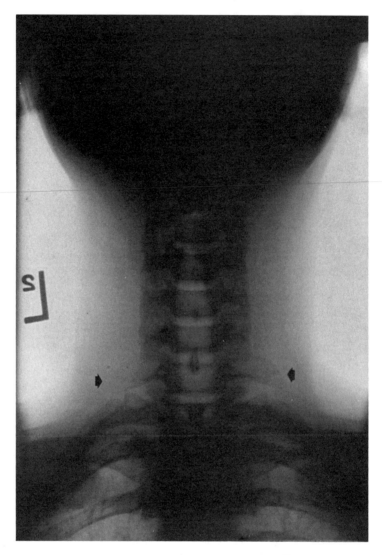

Fig. 4-6.   Bilateral, Type I cervical ribs (Gruber classification; see Table 4–2).[15] These ribs are short and easily missed. They frequently have a band running from their tip to the first rib.

middle scalene muscle where the lower cords of the brachial plexus can be pulled taut against the ligament and elicit TOS symptoms. In 1965, Bonney reported 13 such cases[21] and Gilliat et al., in 1970 and 1978, reported another 9 and 14 cases, respectively.[22, 23] In each series, a few patients had complete cervical ribs, but the majority did not; rather, the commonest finding was an incomplete cervical rib, or a long transverse process of C-7, with the tip of the bone pointing downward and a tight band running to the first rib. In each of these series, symptomatic relief usually was obtained by surgically dividing the ligaments and not removing the first rib.

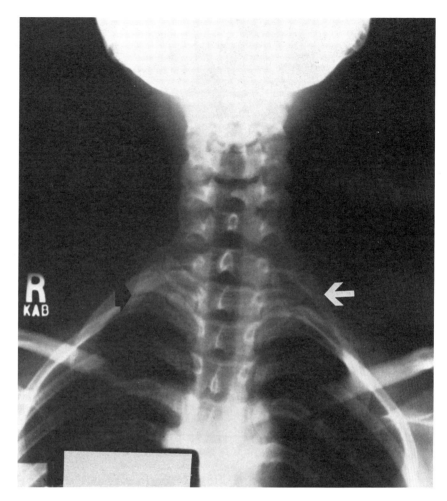

Fig. 4-7.   Cervical ribs: Gruber classification Type II (right) and Type III (left). Cervical ribs are frequently bilateral.

Nerves

Brachial Plexus

The brachial plexus takes origin from the spinal nerves as follows: At each vertebral level, the spinal cord gives rise to anterior and posterior roots that unite to form spinal nerves within the spinal canal. As the spinal nerve exits the intervertebral foramen, it divides into two small and two large branches or rami. The large anterior rami of C-5, C-6, C-7, C-8, and T-1 pass laterally between the anterior and middle scalene muscles and form the brachial plexus. T-1 exits below the neck of the first rib but will later pass above the lateral edge of the rib to soon fuse with C-8.

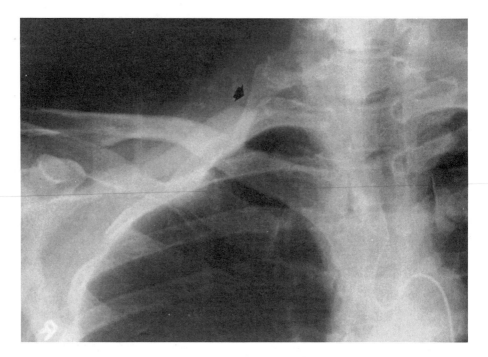

Fig. 4-8.   Complete cervical rib, Gruber classification Type III or Type IV.

Either within the scalene triangle or just lateral to it three trunks are formed: superior trunk, from fusion of C-5 and C-6; middle trunk, from C-7 alone; and inferior trunk, from fusion of C-8 and T-1. The three trunks separate into anterior and posterior divisions that in turn fuse to form the lateral, medial, and posterior cords. Clinically, only the formation of the trunks is visualized during scalenectomy; formation of cords occurs lateral to the operative field.

Phrenic Nerve

The position of the phrenic nerve, in relation to the anterior scalene muscle, is of major surgical importance. The phrenic arises chiefly from C-4 but usually receives a twig from C-3 and another from C-5. It travels near the lateral edge of the anterior scalene muscle cephalad and crosses the anterior scalene from lateral to medial as it moves caudad towards the chest (Fig. 4-9). By the time it crosses the subclavian artery, it is usually on the medial side of the anterior scalene and separated from the artery by the thickness of the muscle. The phrenic nerve is held in close contact with the anterior scalene muscle by a thin layer of connective tissue. The nerve does not lie in the scalene fat pad.

When the phrenic nerve receives a contribution from C-5, the junction of that branch with the phrenic is often visible at the upper end of the surgical field when performing scalenectomy. Because that junction lies near the lateral edge of the anterior scalene muscle, the phrenic nerve will then descend across the anterior scalene in the center of the operative field to reach the medial side. When

Table 4–3. **Congenital Bands and Ligaments Described by Roos[20]**

Type 1: Extending from the anterior tip of an incomplete cervical rib to the middle of the first thoracic rib, this band inserts just posterior to the scalene tubercle on the upper rib surface.

Type 2: This band arises from an elongated C-7 transverse process, in the absence of a cervical rib, and also attaches to the first rib just behind the scalene tubercle in the same place that a band from an incomplete cervical rib attaches. The presence of this band can be predicted by a transverse process of C-7 extending beyond the transverse process of T-1, as seen on AP cervical spine x-rays.

Type 3: The type 3 band both originates and inserts on the first rib. It starts posteriorly, near the neck of the rib and inserts more anteriorly, just behind the scalene tubercle. It is the smallest, deepest, and most difficult of the bands to visualize.

Type 4: Originating along with the middle scalene muscle from a transverse process, the fourth band runs on the anterior edge of the middle scalene muscle, inserting with it on the first rib. The lower nerves of the plexus may lie against it.

Type 5: The scalene minimus muscle is the fifth band. It arises with the lower fibers of the anterior scalene muscle, runs parallel to this muscle but passes deep to the muscle, behind the subclavian artery but in front of the plexus, to insert on the first rib. Normally, the entire anterior scalene muscle passes anterior to the artery. Any fibers that pass anterior to the plexus but posterior to the artery belong to the scalene minimus muscle.

Type 6: When the scalene minimus muscle inserts onto Sibson's fascia over the cupola of the pleura and lung instead of onto the first rib, it is labelled separately to distinguish its point of insertion.

Type 7: A fibrous cord running on the anterior surface of the anterior scalene muscle down to the first rib and attaching to the costochondral junction or sternum. In this position, the band lies immediately behind the subclavian vein, where it may indent the vein and be the cause of partial venous obstruction.

Type 8: This band arises from the middle scalene muscle and runs under the subclavian artery and vein to attach to the costochondral junction.

Type 9: The last band is a web of muscle and fascia filling the inside posterior curve of the first rib.

the phrenic does not receive a contribution from C-5, the path of the nerve is more medial, making scalenectomy easier.

The phrenic nerve is a single structure 87% of the time. In the other 13%, an accessory phrenic nerve is present and responsible for innervation of the lateral leaf of the diaphragm.[4] When single, the nerve usually lies in the medial position described above. When double, the usual positions for the nerves are one each on the medial edge and on the lateral edge of the anterior scalene muscle. The lateral nerve (accessary phrenic) often moves toward the medial side of the anterior scalene as it passes caudally towards the first rib. It may unite with the medial

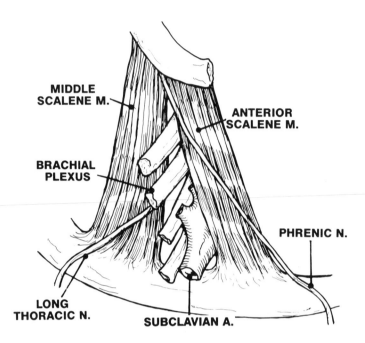

MIDDLE
SCALENE M.

ANTERIOR
SCALENE M.

BRACHIAL
PLEXUS

PHRENIC N.

LONG
THORACIC N.

SUBCLAVIAN A.

Fig. 4-9.   Scalene triangle demonstrating the usual positions of the phrenic and long thoracic nerves. The phrenic crosses from the lateral to medial side of the anterior scalene muscle as it descends. The long thoracic nerve emerges from the belly of the middle scalene and drops over the edge of the first rib.

branch in the neck, below the clavicle, or may remain as an independent nerve all the way to the lateral leaf of the diaphragm.

When a nerve remains on the lateral side of the anterior scalene muscle for most of its course, it is in danger of being stretched or cut during scalenectomy because it lies in the middle of the dissection. Extra care is required to avoid its injury. On the other hand, medial-lying phrenic nerves can remain undisturbed and often untouched during scalenectomy.

The phrenic nerve enters the chest superficial to the subclavian artery. It usually passes deep to the subclavian vein. However, one of the phrenic nerve anomalies is its passage superficial to the subclavian vein (prevenous), where it can obstruct the vein. Although there are only two reported cases of subclavian vein obstruction from *prevenous phrenic nerves* (see Chapter 15), three studies have shown the prevenous position of the phrenic nerve in 7%,[24] 5%,[25] and 4%[26] of cadaver dissections, respectively.

Long Thoracic Nerve

The long thoracic nerve is formed from branches of C-5, C-6, and C-7. The C-6 branch and occasionally the C-5 branch pass through the body of the middle scalene muscle, run over the lateral edge of the first rib, and unite with a branch from C-7 to form the long thoracic nerve (Fig. 4-9). The nerve has no consistent landmark inside the middle scalene muscle. When performing middle scalenectomy, a few muscle bundles at a time are grasped with a smooth forceps and squeezed. If the nerve is present in this bite, the shoulder jumps. If the shoulder remains quiet, it is safe to excise those muscle bundles. In performing transaxillary first rib resection, the long thoracic nerve can be injured if the scissors dividing the intercostal muscles strays too far away from the lateral edge of the first rib.

Suprascapular Nerve

This nerve arises as one of the first branches of C-5 or the superior trunk of the plexus and travels laterally, over the scapula and through the suprascapular notch, to innervate the supraspinatus muscle. It usually is seen when mobilizing C-5 and C-6 prior to middle scalenectomy.

Dorsal Scapular Nerve

The dorsal scapular nerve arises primarily from C-5 and passes across or through the middle scalene muscle on its path toward the rhomboid and levator muscles. Its path parallels that of the long thoracic nerve in the middle scalene muscle and the two nerves cannot be differentiated when a nerve segment is visualized during the course of middle scalenectomy. During surgery, it is common to identify one nerve in the belly of the middle scalene and occasionally two nerves are seen; but it is not possible to be certain whether it is the long thoracic or dorsal scapular nerve that is actually being visualized.

Subclavian Vessels

Subclavian Artery

The relationship of the subclavian artery to the clavicle varies considerably. The artery may lie anywhere from just below the clavicle to 4 cm above it. In TOS patients, the artery lies above the clavicle more often than in cadavers, 56% versus 22%, respectively.[4] When considering surgical approaches to the subclavian artery, the level of the artery is of great importance. A high-lying artery is often reached with ease through a short supraclavicular incision; exposure of a lower-lying artery requires a more extensive approach such as claviculectomy, dividing the clavicle, or splitting the sternum.

Two branches of the subclavian artery, the suprascapular and dorsal scapular, frequently cross above or below the anterior scalene muscle. When encountered, these branches can be ligated and divided with impunity as collaterals are rich in this area.

Subclavian Vein

The subclavian vein represents one of the situations in the body where a vein is separated from its companion artery by a muscle. The vein lies superficial to the anterior scalene muscle. It is usually single but can be double. It runs in the medial corner of the costoclavicular space, which is bounded medially by a tight ligament of the same name. Enlargement of that ligament can encroach on the subclavian vein and cause stenosis, intimal thickening, scarring, and eventual thrombosis.

Thoracic Duct

The thoracic duct lies in the anteromedial corner of the thoracic outlet area. It ascends from the chest, dorsal and medial to the left subclavian artery, rising about 3 to 4 cm above the clavicle. It then arches forward, passes ventral to the subclavian artery and descends to empty into the left subclavian vein near its junction with the internal jugular vein. The duct is seldom encountered during supraclavicular operations on the scalene muscles because it usually lies medial to the area of dissection. However, variations in the course of this duct are common and the duct may run laterally, in the scalene fat pad, where it can be entered in the course of scalenectomy. If that occurs, the thoracic duct should be ligated to prevent postoperative leakage.

References

1. Pollak EW. Thoracic outlet syndrome: diagnosis and treatment. Mount Kisco, NY: Futura Publishing Co, 1986.
2. Telford ED, Mottershead S. Pressure at the cervico-brachial junction: an operative and anatomical study. J Bone Joint Surg 1948; 30:249–265.
3. Kirgis HD, Reed AF. Significant anatomic relations in the syndrome of the scalene muscles. Ann Surg 1948; 127:1182–1201.
4. Sanders RJ, Roos DB. The surgical anatomy of the scalene triangle. Contemp Surg 1989; 35:11–16.
5. Thomas GI, Jones TW, Stavney LS, Manhas DR. The middle scalene muscle and its contribution to the TOS. Am J Surg 1983; 145:589–592.
6. Daseler EH, Anson BJ. Surgical anatomy of the subclavian artery and its branches. Surg Gynecol Obstet 1959; 108:149–174.
7. Roos DB. The place for scalenectomy and first rib resection in thoracic outlet syndrome. Surgery 1982; 92:1077–1085.
8. Todd TW. The descent of the shoulder after birth: its significance in the production of pressure-symptoms on the lowest brachial trunk. Anat Anz 1912; 41:385–397.
9. Jones FW. Discussion on cervical ribs: the anatomy of cervical ribs. Proc R Soc Med 1913; 6:95–112.
10. Southam AH, Bythell WJ. Cervical ribs in children. Br Med J 1924; 2:844–855.
11. Haven H. Neurocirculatory scalenus anticus syndrome in the presence of developmental defects of the first rib. Yale J Biol 1939; 11:443–448.
12. Etter LE. Osseous abnormalities of the thoracic cage seen in forty thousand consecutive chest photorentgenograms. Am J Roentg 1944; 51:359–363.
13. Sycamore LK. Common congenital anomalies of the bony thorax. Am J Roentg 1944; 51:593–599.
14. Eaton LM. Neurologic causes of pain in the upper extremities: with particular reference to syndromes of protruded intervertebral disk in the cervical region and mechanical compression of the brachial plexus. Surg Clin North Am 1946; 26:810–833.
15. Gruber W. Ueber die halsrippen des menschen mit vergleichend-anatomischen. Bemerkungen, St. Petersburg, 1869.

16. Adson AW, Coffey JR. Cervical rib: a method of anterior approach for relief of symptoms by division of the scalenus anticus. Ann Surg 1927; 85:839–857.
17. Scher LA, Veith FJ, Haimovici H, Samson RS, Ascer E, Sushil KG, Sprayregen S. Staging of arterial complications of cervical rib: guidelines for surgical management. Surgery 1984; 95:644–649.
18. Brown SC, Charlesworth D. Results of excision of a cervical rib in patients with the thoracic outlet syndrome. Br J Surg 1988; 75:431–433.
19. Sanders RJ, Pearce WH. The treatment of thoracic outlet syndrome: a comparison of different operations. J Vasc Surg 1989; 10:626–634.
20. Roos DB. New concepts of thoracic outlet syndrome that explain etiology, symptoms, diagnosis, and treatment. Vasc Surg 1979; 13:313–321.
21. Bonney G. The scalenus medius band. A contribution to the study of the thoracic outlet syndrome. J Bone J Surg 1965; 47B:268–272.
22. Gilliatt RW, Le Quesne PM, Logue V, Sumner AJ. Wasting of the hand associated with a cervical rib or band. J Neurol Neurosurg Psychiatry 1970; 33:615–624.
23. Gilliatt RW, Willison RG, Dietz V, Williams IR. Peripheral nerve conduction in patients with a cervical rib and band. Ann Neurol 1978; 4:124–129.
24. Hovelacque A, Monod O, Evrard H, Beuzart J. Etude anatomique du nerf phrenique pre-veineux. Ann D'Anatomie Path 1936; 13:518–522.
25. Hughes ESR. Venous obstruction in the upper extremity. Brit J Surg 1948; 36:155–163.
26. Schroeder WE, Green FR. Phrenic nerve injuries; report of a case. Anatomical and experimental researches, and critical review of the literature. Am J Med Sci 1902; 123:196–220.

5
Histology and Histochemistry of Scalene Muscles

Catherine G. R. Jackson
Natalio Banchero
Richard J. Sanders

Although scalene muscles have been incriminated as the site of pathology in traumatic thoracic outlet syndrome (TOS) for over 60 years,[1] few abnormalities have been described in these muscles. The first histologic studies of scalene muscles were from a few patients with scalenus anticus syndrome. Through routine histological methods, their scalene muscles demonstrated mild fibrosis.[2, 3] Later studies, using similar clinical laboratory procedures that included formalin fixation, found the same amount of connective tissue in the scalene muscles of TOS patients as was found in normal patients.[4]

It is now known that formalin fixation can mask subtle changes in muscular cytoarchitecture. Subsequent studies, utilizing more current freezing techniques and histochemical stains employed by muscle pathologists, have shown consistent histological abnormalities in the scalene muscles of patients with traumatic TOS.[5, 6] Unfortunately, the significance of these findings remains partially unknown because limited information on normal scalene muscle makes comparison with the muscle from TOS patients difficult. Nevertheless, there are enough histochemical differences between normal skeletal muscle and the scalene muscles of TOS patients to warrant a description of the observation to date. These findings, as well as the difficulties encountered in obtaining control tissue, are presented in this chapter.

Techniques

General Handling

Muscle tissue prepared by the routine procedures used in hospital clinical pathology laboratories does not show the anatomical features that are essential for studying the muscle pathology of thoracic outlet syndrome because it is difficult to assess information from longitudinal or tangential sectioning. Muscle tissue must be in good cross section in order to determine its normality or abnormality as has been established extensively by muscle pathologists.[7, 8] The tissue, once properly oriented, should be cut perpendicular to the longitudinal axis of the fibers. Careful processing of the tissue is both time-consuming and tedious but is mandatory. The muscle sample should not be handled excessively and any stretch or mechanical trauma should be avoided. The ends where the tissue may have been compressed by surgical instruments should be discarded from evaluation, and sample handling from the operating room to the site of processing should last less than 45 minutes.

Open Biopsy Technique

The fascia over the anterior scalene is incised in the longitudinal direction of the fibers with care to avoid the phrenic nerve. After exposure of the fascicles, the muscle should be handled with as little trauma as possible and should not be touched, stretched, or manipulated excessively by surgical instruments. The outer layers of the muscle that contain the epimysium should not be sampled; the piece should be taken deep to the muscle surface. The sample should come from the mid-belly of the muscle; tendinous origins and insertions should be avoided. Multiple muscle biopsies are preferred and will aid analysis.

A 2–3-cm-long and 0.5-cm diameter portion of muscle is isolated with a right angle forceps, which is used to pass ties around both ends of the muscle cylinder (Fig. 5-1A, B, and C). The muscle is then cut outside the two ties and is removed. We do not stretch the tissue at this point, although some investigators prefer to do so, particularly if electron microscopy is used.

Once collected, the tissue is placed on a gauze sponge barely moistened with saline; excessive fluid on the gauze should be avoided because it will produce artifacts that interfere with interpretation. The sample can then be subdivided and oriented in the operating room because the tissue is more flexible when freshly obtained. If that is not possible, then it is carefully oriented just before processing. The sample is taken immediately to the laboratory for freezing.

If electron microscopy is to be done, the tissue must be handled more carefully than for light microscopy and speed is more important. The tissue must be fixed immediately in the operating room, reducing ischemic time to as few seconds as possible.

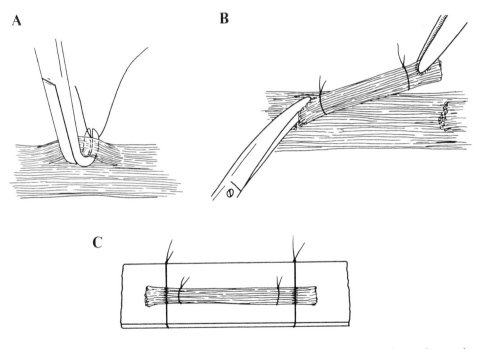

Fig. 5-1.   Technique of skeletal muscle biopsy. **A:** A right angle or curved hemostat is passed around a muscle bundle, 0.5 cm in diameter, and tied firmly enough to hold but not so tightly that it cuts through the muscle bundle. **B:** The bundle is excised, a few cm outside the two ties, which are 2–3 cm apart. **C:** The muscle is fixed to a short piece of wood (tongue blade) with two additional ties to preserve its length, without excessive tension.

Specimen Preparation

Rapid freezing preserves the features of muscle and is a superior technique to conventional fixation with formalin, which shrinks the tissue and produces artifacts (Fig. 5-2, A and B). The sample should be frozen as quickly as possible after it is obtained in order to preserve enzyme activity. Since muscle tissue must be cut perpendicular to the longitudinal axis of the fibers, a dissecting microscope may assist those who are unfamiliar with the orientation of muscle fibers prior to freezing.

Fixation and Storage

There are several choices for mounting and fast freezing the muscle.[8] We prefer to mount the tissue on a labeled cork block using a paste of gum tragacanth. The block is then immersed in a metal beaker filled with isopentane that has been cooled in liquid nitrogen to $-160°C$.[7] The isopentane is at the correct temperature when a second "boil" occurs and small ice crystals are observed. The mounted tissue sample is quickly immersed for approximately 10 seconds.

Once the tissue on the cork is frozen, it may be stored in a sealed container at $-80°C$ until the time of sectioning in a cryostat. Many investigators have kept tissue thus frozen for up to five years with insignificant loss of enzyme activity in the staining process. However, such a long wait is not recommended as unforeseen events, such as electrical outages, may lead to loss of the sample.

Histological and Histochemical Stains

The tissue is cut in a cryostat at approximately $-20°C$ and picked up on coverslips. At this point there are numerous choices for a battery of histochemical and histological stains. The choice of stains will vary among investigators and their familiarity with both technique and interpretation. Many muscle pathologists can obtain the information they need with an hematoxylin and eosin (H and E) and a modified Gomori trichrome stain, used to assess morphology, and a tetrazolium reductase such as a nicotinamide adenine dinucleotide hydrogenase-tetrazolium reductase (NADH-TR), used to assess oxidative enzymes. For TOS specimens, other stains can be added for specific purposes: the hydrolase myosin adenosine triphosphatase (myosin ATPase) at three different pH's (4.2, 4.6, and 9.4) for fiber type and size; Verhoeff van-Gieson (VVG) for connective tissue; and periodic acid Schiff (PAS) for glycogen content.[7]

Methods of Tissue Analysis

There are many acceptable ways to analyze muscle tissue. Described below is the methodology we used to obtain the histologic descriptions that follow. Samples were evaluated both visually and by computerized image analysis. Image analysis

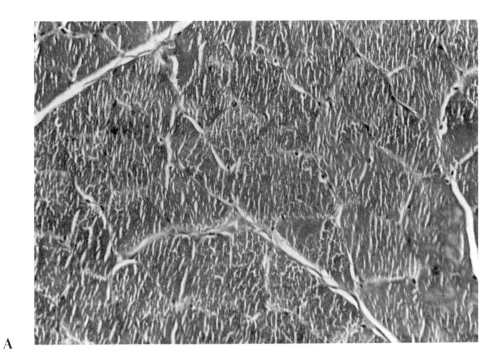

A

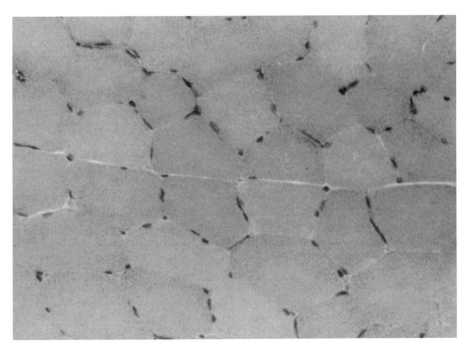

B

Fig. 5-2. Comparison of freeze fixation to formalin fixation in H and E at 120× (original magnification, 160×). **A:** Freeze fixation in normal muscle. Note the clearly defined cell borders and nuclei. **B:** Formalin fixation in muscle. Note the fractures and loss of cytoarchitecture.

was necessary because qualitative observations cannot detect small differences in the amount of connective tissue in muscle samples. Initial impressions and observations were noted in multiple samples taken from each muscle in each stain.

Type I and type II fibers were counted and measured in the myosin ATPases with three random fields per slide chosen for analysis using both a Data General Nova computer in line with an x-y digitizer and a Zeiss IBAS II image analysis system. The same slides were graded by trained observers for estimation of atrophy and fiber type percentage. A Joyce-Loeble Magiscan 2, Nikon, was used to evaluate the amount of connective tissue in VVG sections. Four fields were selected, two with heavy infiltration and two with minimal infiltration of connective tissue. The values obtained were averaged for each sample. The same slides were graded by trained observers as normal, borderline, or increased connective tissue; hypertrophy or atrophy of fibers; and normal or abnormal fiber percentage distribution.

Cytoarchitecture of Normal Muscle

Limb Skeletal Muscle

Fiber Types

Normal skeletal muscle contains two major fiber types distinguished by their reaction to the *myosin ATPase* stain. These have been called type I (slow-twitch) and type II (fast-twitch) fibers. The type II fibers can also be subdivided into type IIA (fast-twitch-oxidative-glycolytic) and IIB (fast-twitch-glycolytic).[9]

Fiber Size

The size of the type I and type II fibers in females is often similar but in males it is not uncommon for type II fibers to be slightly larger than type I's.[8]

Fiber Type Distribution

In normal human limb skeletal muscle, the ratio of type I to type II fibers is variable and in any individual may range from 60:40 to 40:60;[10] there are differences in individual muscles in the same person. While deep muscles have features different from superficial muscles, the majority of published studies present easily obtained superficial limb muscles.[10] The percentage of one type of fiber can also vary from superficial to deep so that sample sites in individual muscles must be consistent from subject to subject.[11]

Connective Tissue

Minimal amounts of connective tissue are visualized by VVG in the epimysium, perimysium, and endomysium. A study of body builders has shown that the approximate amount of connective tissue in skeletal muscle is 13%.[12]

General Morphology

H and E and *modified Gomori trichrome* can be used to determine general morphological features of muscle, and the trained histochemist or muscle pathologist can interpret most features seen in the other stains.

Oxidative Enzyme Distribution and Myofibrills

NADH-TR shows the oxidative enzyme distribution, the cytochemical architecture, and the ordered array of myofibrillar components of the muscle. The observation of disarray of the myofibrils in NADH-TR staining indicates a neuromuscular disorder, although it is a nonspecific finding.

Glycogen

PAS stains glycogen, among other components of the cell, and can be used to determine the presence or absence of this polysaccharide. Most normal cells show reactivity to PAS in varying amounts. Increased muscle activity preceding sampling can result in glycogen depletion, which is seen in PAS as a cell devoid of stain. A state of chronic muscle contracture can produce the same cellular reaction. Depletion can also be used to determine whether type I or type II fibers are recruited in a specific muscle. Glycogen stores are repleted in normal people within 48 hours of depletion.

Summary

Overall, normal skeletal limb muscle has a pattern of almost equal numbers of type I and type II fibers whose cross sectional size is similar. The type II fibers may be slightly larger than the type I fibers. Connective tissue is 12–15% of a cross sectional field. H and E and other general stains show that nuclei are peripheral and the pattern of other cellular components is very ordered. There is an ordered array of myofibrils seen in NADH-TR. Glycogen is seen in varying amounts in all fiber types and fibers are seen as depleted only if continuous, strenuous exercise or electrical stimulation preceded the tissue biopsy.

Electron Microscopy

Electron micrographs of normal muscle reveal that sarcomeres are ordered with respect to actins and myosins while the Z-lines in myofibrils are lined up with each other. Modest amounts of lipid are present and lipofuchsin granules are rarely seen.[8]

Scalene Muscle

Scalene muscle appears to be structurally similar to skeletal muscles throughout the body, and therefore it is assumed that the many general factors that are known to alter other muscles will affect the scalenes in a similar fashion. The physiologic aging process,[13–15] poor nutrition, metabolic illnesses, cancer, and starvation[16] can each cause type II fiber atrophy and a reduction in fiber cross sectional area (FCSA). General body trauma can also be expected to cause the same type of response in scalene muscles as it causes in other skeletal muscles.[17] Additionally, any generalized disease process that involves muscle can affect the scalenes[16] and therefore has the potential to produce TOS symptoms.

Normal Controls

A histological and histochemical profile of normal human scalene muscle proved to be a difficult task and is not yet complete. Initially, autopsy material was obtained but this proved to be an inadequate control source. There were few specimens available, which could not be obtained in a timely fashion before artifacts began to appear in the tissue, and little was known of the subjects' previous lifestyle and history of neck trauma. Most histochemical stains were nonreactive because the tissue enzymes upon which they depend were depleted. Furthermore, most of the autopsy specimens were from individuals who were much older or much younger than the TOS patients.

In collecting normal scalene muscles to compare to the muscles of traumatic TOS patients, it was known that many "normals" could have had neck injuries that they may or may not have recalled. The best tissue for a control is from an individual who has no disease of any kind and is undergoing neck surgery for reasons unrelated to neck muscle. Additionally, since muscle cytoarchitecture varies with age and gender, controls should match TOS patients in these parameters. Within such constraints a limited number of scalene muscles from individuals free of disease and remote trauma, within the age categories of the TOS patients, were deemed acceptable.

The scalene muscles of five nondiseased control patients exhibited the pattern of normal limb skeletal muscle described above. The indications for operations were: two patients for cervical ribs, arm and hand symptoms, and no history of neck trauma; two patients for causalgia following arm trauma without neck trauma; and one patient for a thyroid nodule on no medication. The histology and histochemistry in these control specimens revealed a normal distribution of fiber type averaging 50% of type I and type II, and sizes of type I and type II fibers that were within previously reported values for limb muscle (Table 5–1). They averaged 14.5% connective tissue in the field of muscle measured. Nuclei were in the periphery and PAS observations indicated that there was no apparent glycogen depletion. There was an ordered array of myofibrills in NADH-TR.

Diseased Controls

Samples from patients undergoing neck surgery for any cause other than TOS were obtained for control tissue after excluding those patients with histories of

Table 5–1.   Normal Controls

						Muscle Fibers	
Name	Sex	Age	Diagnosis[a]	Connective Tissue (%)	Type I (%)	Type II (μm^2)	Type I (μm^2)
Ba	M	33	TR	8	45	6,206	4,725
Me	M	22	TR	20	47	6,417	4,689
Pa	M	20	C	15	67	6,689	3,434
Mc	M	28	TH	<15	39	3,785	3,705
Av	M	25		14.5	50	5,774	4,138
Za	F	39	C	15	56	5,094	3,126

[a]TR = TOS with cervical rib; no neck trauma; C = causalgia; TH = thyroid nodule, euthyroid.
(*From Sanders RJ, Jackson CGR, Banchero N, Pearce WH. Scalene muscle abnormalities in traumatic thoracic outlet syndrome. Am J Surg 1990; 159:231–236. With Permission.*)

chronic neck pain. However, it was noted that these "controls" had some muscle changes similar to TOS patients. Thus, two categories of control patients were found: those whose muscles were within parameters of normal limb skeletal muscle and those whose muscles were significantly different. In the latter group of four patients, two had thyroid disease and were taking thyroid medication, one had parathyroidism, and one had causalgia. The histologic findings in these patients included type I fiber predominance and type II fiber atrophy, similar to TOS patients, but they had no increase in connective tissue (Table 5–2). All other histological and histochemical properties were similar to the undiseased control patients.

Cytoarchitecture of Scalene Muscle of TOS Patients

Subjects

Over 90% of the scalene muscles we have examined were from patients with histories of neck trauma. Therefore, the microscopic picture of their muscles is predominantly that of traumatic TOS. Forty-five anterior and 45 middle scalene muscles from 37 patients with TOS were analyzed. There were 31 females and 6 males; 8 patients had bilateral operations. Ages ranged from 19–42 years in twenty-eight patients and from 44–80 years in nine patients. Twenty-seven patients had symptoms for at least a year; ten had symptoms for 3–12 months. There were a few patients without histories of trauma.

Scalene Muscle of TOS Patients

Fiber Types, Size, and Distribution

The anterior and middle scalene muscles of TOS patients exhibited type I fiber predominance with an average of 78% type I fibers compared to 50% type I

Table 5–2. **Diseased Controls**

Name	Sex	Age	Diagnosis[a]	Muscle[b]	Connective Tissue (%)[*]	Type I (%)[*]	Type II Size, Visual Estimate
Sh	F	45	THS	SCM	<15	51	Normal
				AS	<15	84	Decreased
Ta	F	31	PT	AS	<15	70	Normal
Th	F	37	C	AS	<15	100	No fibers
				MS	<15	65	Decreased
Na	F	32	TH	SCM	<15	47	Normal
				AS	<15	70	Decreased

[a]PT = Hyperparathyroidism; THS = thyroiditis; TH = thyroid nodule, euthyroid; C = causalgia.
[b]SCM = Sternocleidomastoid muscle; AS = anterior scalene muscle; MS = middle scalene muscle.
[*] Values are means.
(*From Sanders RJ, Jackson CGR, Banchero N, Pearce WH. Scalene muscle abnormalities in traumatic thoracic outlet syndrome. Am J Surg 1990; 159:231–236. With Permission.*)

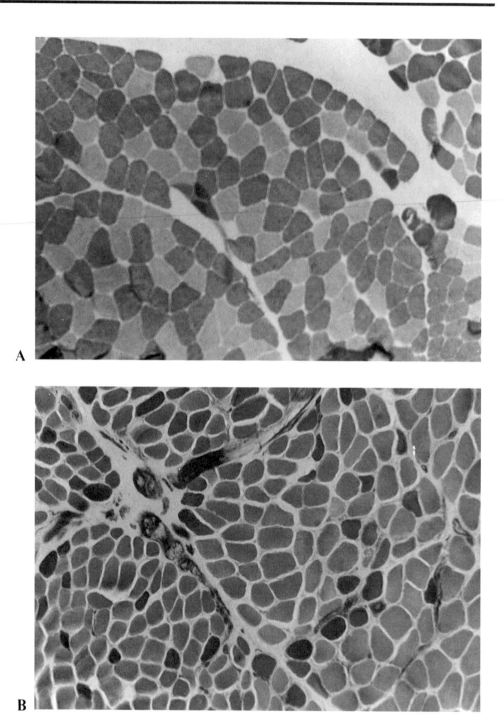

Fig. 5-3.   Fiber type distribution in scalene muscle control vs. TOS scalene muscle in myosin ATPase at pH 9.4 at 75× (original magnification, 100×). Type I fibers are light stain; type II fibers are dark stain. **A:** Control scalene muscle. Note the almost equal distribution of type I and type II fibers. **B:** TOS scalene muscle. Note the predominance of type I fibers, the connective tissue, and the atrophic type II fibers.

fibers in controls (Fig. 5-3, A and B). When a fiber type represented more than 70% of the total number of fibers it was classified as abnormal and predominant.[7, 8] The type II fibers were atrophic while the type I fibers were of normal size (Table 5–3 and Fig. 5-4, A and B). Additionally, type IIB fibers were rarely seen (Fig. 5-5, A and B).

Connective Tissue

The muscles of all TOS patients exhibited an increased amount of connective tissue in at least one of the two muscles, with many patients exhibiting it in both anterior and middle scalenes (Fig. 5-6, A and B). The amount of connective tissue in TOS patients averaged 36%, more than double the 14.5% average in control patients (Table 5–4 and Table 5–5). The visual estimates by trained observers was in good agreement with the increase measured by computerized image analysis, although it is recognized that all observers, regardless of experience, have some difficulty detecting modest increases in amounts.

General Morphology

H and E and *modified Gomori trichrome* stains disclosed the presence of internal nuclei and abnormal lipid deposits in the areas of focal fibrosis. *NADR-TR* revealed cores in the majority of TOS patients that were not present in either diseased or nondiseased controls, although the significance of this observation is currently unknown (Fig. 5-7). In *PAS*, glycogen depletion was noted in a small number of fibers but was not observed consistently in all samples. The overall picture was one of a subtle abnormality.

Table 5–3.   **Fiber Type Distribution and Size in Control and TOS Patients: Anterior and Middle Scalene Muscles Together[a]**

Subjects	No. Muscles	Type I Fiber (%)[b]	Type I Fiber Size (μm²)[b]	Type II Fiber Size (μm²)[b]
Control male	4	49.5 (±12.2)	4178 (±1370)	5774 (±2160)
Control female	1	56	3126	5094
TOS male	12	76 (±10.6)	3693 (±555)	2801 (±736)
TOS female	49	78.7 (±14.7)	2843 (±633)	1968 (±831)

[a]There was no statistically significant difference between anterior and middle scalene muscles in fiber distribution or size. The results of the two are therefore combined in this table.
[b]Values are means ± standard deviation.
(From Sanders RJ, Jackson CGR, Banchero N, Pearce WH. *Scalene muscle abnormalities in traumatic thoracic outlet syndrome. Am J Surg 1990; 159:231–236. With Permission.*)

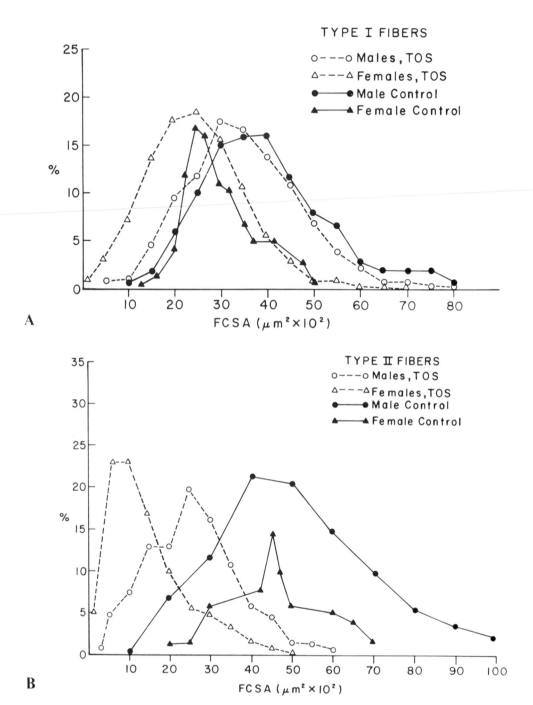

Fig. 5-4.   Histograms of type I and type II fiber cross-sectional areas in TOS vs. control scalene muscle. **A:** Type I fibers—6,145 fibers were measured; there is no significant difference between TOS and control patients ($P > 0.05$). **B:** Type II fibers—3,173 fibers were measured; fibers in TOS patients were significantly smaller than control fibers ($P < 0.001$).

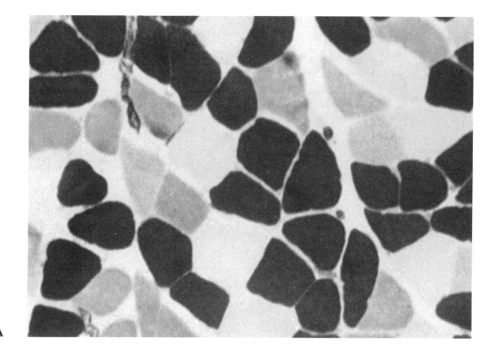

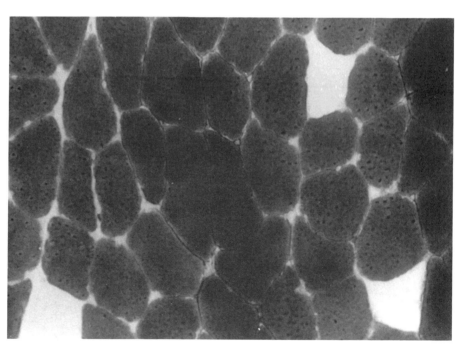

Fig. 5-5.   Fiber type distribution in scalene muscle control vs. TOS scalene muscle in myosin ATPase at pH 4.6 at 120× (original magnification, 160×). Type I fibers are dark stain; type IIA fibers are lightest, virtually clear stain; type IIB fibers are intermediate stain. **A:** Scalene control muscle. Note the presence of three fiber types. **B:** TOS scalene muscle. Note the lack of IIB fibers.

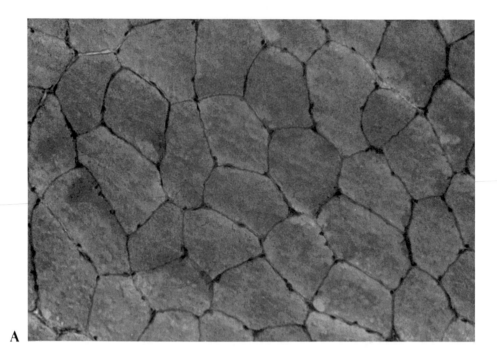

A

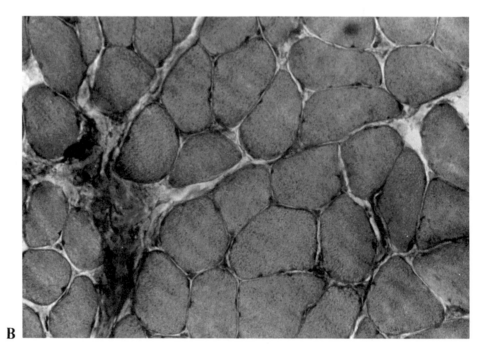

B

Fig. 5-6.   Connective tissue in scalene muscle control vs. TOS scalene muscle in VVG at 120× (original magnification, 160×). **A:** Normal scalene muscle. Note the minimal amount of connective tissue seen in the field. **B:** TOS scalene muscle. Note the increased infiltration of connective tissue.

Table 5–4.   **Connective Tissue**

Subjects	No. Muscles	Anterior Scalene		Middle Scalene	
		Range (%)[a]	Mean (%)	Range (%)[a]	Mean (%)
TOS patients	90	22–68	37.8	19–52 (± 10.4)[b]	34.1 (± 11.7)[b]
Controls	9	8–20 (± 4.9)[b]	14.5		

[a]Range of means/subject (Not range of individual fields).
[b]Values are means ± standard deviation.
$P < 0.001$ (TOS vs. control measurements).
(From Sanders RJ, Jackson CGR, Banchero N, Pearce WH. Scalene muscle abnormalities in traumatic thoracic outlet syndrome. Am J Surg 1990; 159:231–236. With Permission.)

Table 5–5.   **Summary of Findings**

Subjects	No. Patients	Type I (%)[a]	Type II Size	Connective Tissue (%)
Normal controls	5	53	Normal	14.5
Abnormal controls	4	78	Atrophy	<15
Traumatic TOS	45	78	Atrophy	36

[a]Values are means.
(From Sanders RJ, Jackson CGR, Banchero N, Pearce WH. Scalene muscle abnormalities in traumatic thoracic outlet syndrome. Am J Surg 1990; 159:231–236. With Permission.)

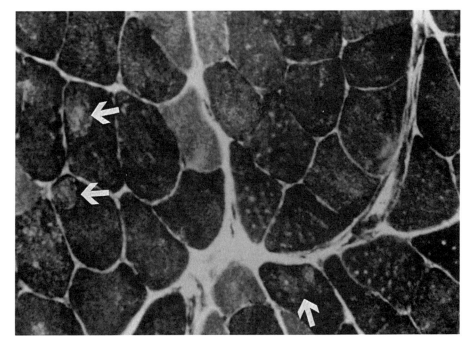

Fig. 5-7.   NADH-TR in TOS scalene muscle at 120× (original magnification, 160×). The arrows indicate cores and mottled appearance of selected fibers. Neither of these features is present in normal muscle.

Electron Microscopy

In TOS patients, the electron micrographs revealed Z-line streaming and disruption, increased amounts of lipid, and subsarcolemmal lipofuchsin granules. There was an increase in collagen bundles between myofibrils and there was active macrophage activity. Fibroblasts showed high levels of activity suggesting increased connective tissue formation. All of these observations indicate nonspecific deviations from normal.

Other Scalene Muscle Pathology

In four patients, three of whom had histories of neck trauma, the scalene muscles revealed unsuspected histological findings different from those of the traumatic TOS patients. In two patients, the findings were those of muscular dystrophy, and in one each, the diagnosis was sarcoidosis and mitochondrial abnormality. After the histological evaluation of the muscle, the patients were referred to other physicians for treatment of their generalized conditions. In these cases, the TOS symptoms improved because the brachial plexus had been decompressed, even though the systemic condition still existed. These conditions may have contributed to or caused the TOS symptoms; there is no way to know this with certainty.

Skeletal Muscle of TOS Patients

Random samples of sternocleidomastoid and omohyoid muscles were obtained from several TOS and control patients. That was done to determine if the histologic and histochemical changes observed in the scalene muscles of TOS patients were limited to those muscles and were not a part of a generalized muscle abnormality. The samples were processed in the same manner as the scalene muscles and all had the same fiber type properties, amount of connective tissue, and staining characteristics as normal limb skeletal muscle.

Comparison to Other Investigations

Machleder et al., in 1986, published the only other study on the histochemical properties of scalene muscles in TOS patients.[5] Using techniques similar to the ones described here, they performed histochemical and morphometric analyses of the scalene muscles from eleven female patients, seven with primary TOS and four with recurrent TOS.

The findings in TOS patients, type I fiber predominance and atrophy of type II fibers, were similar to our findings (Table 5–6). Although Machleder et al. did not report type II atrophy, the photomicrograph, the atrophy index, and the measured diameter as published in their manuscript are compatible with this conclusion.

Controls from the two studies were quite different and should be reviewed closely because the interpretations of abnormalities in TOS patients were based on

Table 5–6. Histological Features of Controls and TOS Patients: Comparison of Two Studies

	Machleder et al.			Sanders/Jackson et al.		
	Controls	TOS	Recurrent TOS	Undiseased Controls	Diseased Controls	TOS
No. Patients	4	7	4	5	4	37
Age	44–73	27–40	24–40	20–39	31–45	19–42 (76%)
	Avg. = 60	Avg. = 38	Avg. = 36	Avg. = 25	Avg. = 36	Avg. = 39
Sex	2M, 2F	F	F	4M, 1F	F	6M, 31F
Type I% (Avg.)	75%	85%	77%	50%	78%	78%
Type I Diam[a] (μm)	51	56	34	65M 51F	Normal	59M 45F
Type II Diam[a] (μm)	33	32	34	84M 80F	Atrophy	53M 34F

[a]Diam = diameter. Note that in Tables 5–1 and 5–3 the size of fibers in our data is recorded as fiber cross-sectional area in μm^2. For purposes of comparison to the data of Machleder et al., our data was converted to diameter in μm for *this table only*.

a comparison to respective control groups (Table 5–6). Machleder et al. included four patients, two male and two female, 44–73 years old, with an average age of 60 years, three of whom had vascular disease (data supplied by Dr. Machleder). The type I fibers of these controls averaged 75% with a mean diameter of 51 μm and type II fibers of 33 μm. The seven TOS patients averaged 85% type I fibers with a mean diameter of 56 μm and type II fibers of 32 μm. Based upon these four controls, the features of primary TOS were these: 1) type I fiber predominance (85% vs. 75%) and 2) type I fiber hypertrophy (56 μm vs. 51 μm).

In comparison, our controls differed significantly from those of Machleder et al.: ages 20–39, averaging 25 years old; type I fibers averaged 50% for males and 56% for the one female; the type I fibers were 65 μm for males and 51 μm for the female; and the type II fibers were larger than the type I fibers for both sexes (Table 5–6). Based on these controls, the features of primary TOS were as follows: 1) type I fiber predominance (78% TOS vs. 50% control); 2) no type I fiber hypertrophy (50 μm TOS vs. 51 μm control female, and 64 μm TOS vs. 65 μm control male); and 3) type II fiber atrophy (34 μm TOS female, 53 μm TOS male vs. 84 μm combined controls).

The finding of 75% type I fibers in the controls of Machleder et al. was explained by suggesting that those muscles have become specialized to assist in respiration and have converted to a higher type I fiber composition for that purpose. The observation that our normal controls had a lower type I fiber percentage of 50% suggests that scalene muscle is not specialized and is similar to other skeletal muscle. Supporting this contention is the observation that the type II fiber size in our normal controls was larger than the type I fiber size, similar to other skeletal muscle. Another point of difference was the type I fiber hypertrophy reported in the Machleder study, a finding that was not confirmed by our data.

Machleder et al. described four women with recurrent TOS following temporary success from transaxillary first rib resection, which included anterior scalene tenotomy (scalenotomy) as a part of the operation. The histochemical observations led to the conclusion that their muscles had 1) type I fiber atrophy (56 μm vs. 34 μm) and 2) transformation of type I fibers back to type II fibers (85% to 77%). The type I fiber atrophy following tenotomy is to be expected, since the muscle insertion is divided and the muscle no longer contracts the way it did before tenotomy. However, the apparent decrease in type I fibers, from 85% to 77%, is not necessarily a transformation to type II fibers but could represent a loss of type I fibers in the field.

To date our study is the only one in which the amount of connective tissue in a field was estimated in TOS patients. This finding offers a partial explanation of how the scalene muscles might compress the nerves of the brachial plexus when they contract, given that fibrosed muscle would be less flexible than normal. It is probably a result of injury, and, although there is no proof that this is the cause of TOS, the increased connective tissue was not present in any of the normal or diseased controls.

Clearly there is a need for more studies in this area, particularly to define the histochemical and morphometric features of normal scalene muscle as well as the features of trauma in other skeletal muscle.

References

1. Adson AW, Coffey JR. Cervical rib: a method of anterior approach for relief of symptoms by division of the scalenus anticus. Ann Surg 1927; 85:839–857.
2. Ochsner A, Gage M, Debakey M. Scalenus anticus (Naffziger) syndrome. Am J Surg 1935; 28:669–695.
3. Donald JM, Morton BF. The scalenus anticus syndrome with and without cervical rib. Ann Surg 1940; 111:709–723.
4. Sanders RJ, Monsour JW, Gerber FG, Adams WRA, Thompson N. Scalenectomy versus first rib resection for treatment of the thoracic outlet syndrome. Surgery 1979; 85:109–121.
5. Machleder HI, Moll F, Verity A. The anterior scalene muscle in thoracic outlet compression syndrome: histochemical and morphometric studies. Arch Surg 1986; 121:1141–1144.
6. Sanders RJ, Jackson CGR, Banchero N, Pearce WH. Scalene muscle abnormalities in traumatic thoracic outlet syndrome. Am J Surg 1990; 159:231–236.
7. Dubowitz V, Brooke M. Muscle biopsy: a modern approach, Philadelphia: W. B. Sanders, 1973.
8. Dubowitz V. Muscle biopsy: a practical approach. Philadelphia: Bailliere Tindall, 1985.
9. Jackson CGR, Dickinson AL. Adaptations of skeletal muscle to strength or endurance training. In: Granna WA, ed. Advances in sports medicine and fitness. Vol 1. Chicago: Year Book Medical Publishers, 1988; 45–60.
10. Saltin B, Gollnick PD. Skeletal muscle adaptability: significance for metabolism and performance. In: Peachey LD, ed. Handbook of physiology, Sect. 10: Skeletal muscle. Bethesda, MD: American Physiological Society, 1983;555–631.

11. Mahon M, Toman A, Willan P, Bagnall K. Variability of histochemical and morphometric data from needle biopsy specimens of human quadriceps femoris muscle. J Neurol Sci 1984; 63:85–100.

12. MacDougall J, Sale D, Alway S, Sutton J. Muscle fiber number in biceps brachii in bodybuilders and control subjects. J Appl Physiol 1984; 57:1399–1403.

13. Grimby G, Saltin B. Mini-review: The ageing muscle. Clin Physiol 1983; 3:209–218.

14. Maxwell L, Faulkner J, Lieberman D. Histochemical manifestations of age and endurance training in skeletal muscle fibers. Am J Physiol 1973; 224:356–361.

15. Tomonaga M. Histochemical and ultrastructural changes in senile human skeletal muscle. J Am Geriatric Soc 1977; 3:125–131.

16. Layzer RB. Complications of medical and surgical treatment. In: Neuromuscular manifestations of systemic disease. Philadelphia: FA Davis, 1985; 363–366.

17. Carpenter S, Karpati G. Pathology of skeletal muscle. New York: Churchill Livingston, 1984; 20–22.

6
Clinical Presentation

Richard J. Sanders

History
Traumatic TOS
Nontraumatic TOS

Symptoms
Neurological Symptoms
Musculoskeletal Symptoms
Vascular Symptoms
Upper and Lower Plexus Symptoms

Physical Examination
Supravascular Tenderness
Postural Maneuvers
Vascular Signs
Other Parts of Physical Examination

History

Traumatic TOS

The onset of TOS symptoms is often sudden but can be insidious. Over 80% of patients with TOS have a history of some type of trauma preceding the onset of their illness. That trauma can be an accident or a job-related activity that causes chronic strain in the muscles of the neck and arms.

The usual cause is an auto accident, most often a rear-end collision, but impacts from the front or side are fairly frequent causes. The common denominator is acute hyperextension of the neck (whiplash injury), even though most patients do not recall precisely what happened to their necks. Within 24 hours of the injury, headaches, neck pain, and neck stiffness develop. Dorsal spine pain and aching in the shoulders are other early symptoms. Numbness and tingling in the arms and fingers usually do not occur immediately but appear several days, weeks, or sometimes even a few months after the accident. Elevating the arms typically elicits or aggravates the symptoms.

Another type of injury is the result of a fall by slipping on a wet floor or patch of ice, or tripping over an obstacle. The exact cause is unimportant. It is the mechanism—an acute hyperextension of the neck—that precipitates the symptom complex begins.

People in certain occupations are predisposed to develop symptoms. Those occupations include keyboard jobs where typists or phone operators are constantly turning or flexing their necks several times a minute to gaze between their keyboards and monitor; sitting in a fixed position for long hours doing a repetitive job; working on an assembly line; performing tasks requiring lifting or holding the arms above the shoulders; or working with vibrating tools. A precise single incident that can be called an injury is lacking in many of these people, yet their symptoms often sound similar to those of patients who did have accidents.

Repeat questioning can help patients remember injuries that occurred a few years earlier but have been forgotten. An aggressive approach on the part of the examiner will sometimes elicit a history that otherwise would have been lost.

Nontraumatic TOS

A small number of patients have no history of injury or trauma. Their symptoms are insidious in onset and are often primarily in the arm and hand. Occasionally, the neck and head are also involved.

Symptoms

The specific symptoms vary considerably from one patient to another. No single symptom is pathognomonic for TOS, a fact that makes precise diagnosis difficult.

Reviewing the literature reveals significant differences in the reports of several authors and even in reports by the same authors at different times. Such differences are illustrated in Table 6–1 where the symptoms are listed over three

Table 6–1. Symptoms in TOS

	Author's Series			17 Reports (1964–1985)[1–17]		
				Number of		
	1964–1971	1972–1979	1980–1985	Reports	Range	Median
Number of Operations	76	261	223	17	22–433	120
History of Trauma	54%	89%	91%	7	21–72%	31%
Paresthesia	88%	88%	90%	17	46–100%	95%
Headaches	36%	74%	83%	6	13–66%	33%
Neck Pain	68%	92%	85%	13	58–100%	92%
Arm Pain	82%	83%	74%			
Chest Pain	14%	8%	9%	4	16–22%	19%
Weakness	39%	49%	29%	12	18–100%	40%
Raynaud's Phenome-non	4%	2%	2%	7	2–22%	5%
Swelling	4%	0%	1%	13	3–24%	10%
Shoulder Pain	74%	72%	68%	–	–	–
Facial Pain	7%	5%	4%	–	–	–
Vein Occlusion	4%	0%	1%			

% = Percent of patients with this symptom.

time periods from 1964 to 1985. When the symptoms between 1964 and 1971 were reviewed, neck pain in 68% and headache in 36% were unexpected findings, as was the 54% incidence of neck injuries. These complaints had been elicited from patients by simply asking what was bothering them. Postoperatively, several patients mentioned that their headaches were gone even though many had never mentioned their headaches preoperatively. The absence of history of headaches simply reflected an incomplete interview at the initial examination.

After 1971, our history taking improved. Patients were specifically asked if they had experienced injuries, neck pain, or headaches. A written questionnaire listing all possible symptoms was given to each patient prior to examination (Table 6–2). The result was more thorough interviews and significantly higher reported incidences of trauma (91%), headache (83%), and neck pain (85%) (Table 6–1).

Seventeen articles, published between 1964 and 1985, listed the incidence of various symptoms (Table 6–1). Although there are wide variations, it is possible to draw a rough consensus from them. A history of trauma was present in 21–72%, with a median of 31%. Paresthesia in the hand and pain in the arm or neck were present in over 90% of the patients in most series, although the incidence of even these common symptoms was as low as 50% in some reviews. The low figures could indicate incomplete history taking or they could reflect experiences in which there were a large number of patients with vascular TOS and fewer with neurologic TOS.

In comparing our experiences with those of other investigators, most categories are similar (Table 6–1).[1–17] Paresthesia and pain are the most common symptoms in both sets of reports, close to 90%, and the incidence of chest pain, arm weakness, Raynaud's phenomenon, and arm swelling are all in the same general range. The only points of difference are in the incidence of headache and

Table 6–2. **Questionnaire To Be Completed by TOS Patient Prior to Interview With Doctor**

Instructions: Circle YES or NO for each question
Circle RIGHT or LEFT or both RIGHT and LEFT if on both sides

1. Do you have pain in any of these areas:

Head (Headache)	Yes	No—If yes, back or front of head?		
Neck	Yes	No		
Between shoulders	Yes	No		
Shoulders	Yes	No	Right	Left
Arm	Yes	No	Right	Left
Elbow	Yes	No	Right	Left
Forearm	Yes	No	Right	Left
Hand	Yes	No	Right	Left

2. Do you have numbness or tingling in your:

A. fingers   Yes   No   If yes, circle which fingers
Right Hand—Thumb, Index, Middle, Ring, Baby
Left Hand—Thumb, Index, Middle, Ring, Baby

B. arm or forearm   Yes   No   Right   Left

3. Do you have weakness of your hand or arm?   Yes   No   Right   Left
4. Does elevating your hand over your head make symptoms worse?   Yes   No
5. Date of your accident? _____
6. Were any of your symptoms present prior to this accident?   Yes   No
7. Have you had any other accidents involving your head or neck before or after this one?   Yes   No   If yes, give date _____

history of trauma, and even for these, our statistics for the 1964 to 1971 period are very similar to the general consensus. It was only after changing methods of interviewing that the incidence of trauma and headache increased (1972 to 1985).

Patient referral patterns influence the incidence of various symptoms. When referrals are from people who deal with accidents and injuries, the number of patients with traumatic TOS, neck pain, and headache will be high. When patients are referred primarily because they have osseous abnormalities, vascular occlusion, and symptoms limited to the arm and hand, the incidence of traumatic TOS will obviously be lower.

Three groups of symptoms are seen: neurological, musculoskeletal, and vascular. Neurological symptoms are present in almost all patients while true vascular symptoms are infrequent.

Neurological Symptoms

There are only three symptoms of nerve involvement: paresthesia, weakness, and pain. The location of these symptoms in the upper extremity depends upon the portion of the brachial plexus that is being irritated or compressed. While the textbook description of TOS describes numbness and tingling in ring and baby fingers, more patients have involvement of all five fingers, with the fourth and fifth fingers often being worse (Table 6–3). In a smaller number of cases, only the first three fingers are involved.

Table 6–3.   Location of Paraesthesia and Headaches

Symptom	Author's Series—560 Operations		
	1964–1971	1972–1979	1980–1985
Paraesthesia			
1–3 Fingers	22%	11%	14%
4–5 Fingers	18%	25%	30%
All 5 Fingers	48%	52%	46%
No Paraesthesia	12%	12%	10%
Headaches			
Occipital	36%	63%	74%
Frontal	0%	3%	6%
Occipital & Frontal	0%	8%	3%
No Headaches	64%	26%	17%

Pain from brachial plexus irritation can be in the hand, forearm, elbow, arm, shoulder, over the scapula or on its medial edge, and occasionally in the axilla and anterior chest wall. Pain in other areas, such as the jaw and face, is sometimes seen with TOS, but is not the result of plexus compression. It is probably due to another problem such as temporomandibular joint abnormality.

Musculoskeletal Symptoms

Pain in the trapezius muscles, dorsal spine, parascapular area, neck, and occiput is commonly seen with traumatic TOS. The neck pain and headache can be due to tight scalene muscles or associated injuries in the cervical spine. Neck pain and headache are absent in patients with osseous abnormalities, unless trauma precipitated the onset of symptoms. Trapezius muscle, dorsal spine, and parascapular pain are sometimes caused by irritation of the suprascapular and dorsal scapular nerves (C-5 and C-6), but those symptoms are more often due to muscle injury and inflammation and are not a part of TOS.

Nontraumatic and nonosseous TOS patients may have neck and head symptoms if the underlying cause is scalene muscle inflammation or myopathy. If the cause is costoclavicular or pectoralis minor compression, then head and neck symptoms are usually absent.

Vascular Symptoms

The incidence of vascular symptoms in all TOS patients is small. Arterial symptoms include coldness, pallor, Raynaud's phenomenon (color changes), claudication, and gangrene of fingertips (from emboli). The etiology of such vascular symptoms is usually irritation of the sympathetic nerves accompanying the somatic nerves of the plexus;[18] therefore, they are indicative of neurologic compression. In only a few cases are those symptoms due to arterial compression or emboli. Venous symptoms are swelling, cyanosis, and aching.

Upper and Lower Plexus Symptoms

In 1944, Swank and Simeone divided their 15 patients with scalenus anticus syndrome into those who had upper and lower brachial plexus symptoms.[19] Upper plexus involvement, C-5, C-6, and C-7, features sensory changes in the first three fingers and muscle pain or weakness in the anterior chest, triceps, deltoid, parascapular areas and down the outer arm to the extensor muscles of the forearm. Lower plexus irritation, C-8 and T-1, involves numbness in the fourth and fifth fingers; muscle pain and weakness from the rhomboid and scapular regions to the back of the axilla, down the ulnar nerve distribution of the forearm, involving the elbow and flexors of the wrist and intrinsic muscles of the hand. In Swank and Simeone's small series, 60% had lower plexus involvement and 40% upper. Only a few patients had both types.

Roos, in 1982, elaborated on the separation of TOS symptoms into those of upper plexus, lower plexus, or both.[20] He added to the list of upper plexus symptoms pain in the neck, face, mandible, ear, and occipital headaches. Woods, in 1965, also noted dizziness, vertigo, and blurred vision in some patients with TOS.[1] However, it is quite possible that these additional symptoms in the head and neck are due to causes other than brachial plexus compression, since the branches of the brachial plexus do not innervate these areas.

Physical Examination

Physical examination is not as important in making a diagnosis of TOS as is history. In Table 6–4 are specific areas of the physical examination that we have found useful, and in Table 6–5 is a list of significant physical findings and their frequency. The only two physical findings that are present in over 90% of TOS patients are tenderness over the scalene muscles and reproduction of symptoms with the arms abducted to 90 degrees in external rotation (90-degree AER position), one of the postural maneuvers.

Table 6–4.   **Basic Physical Examination for TOS**

1. Hand strength measured with a dynamometer
2. Supraclavicular tenderness over scalene muscles
3. Brachial plexus pressure to elicit arm and hand symptoms
4. Tinel's sign over brachial plexus
5. Biceps/rotator cuff tenderness
6. Abducting arms to 180 degrees
7. Range of motion of neck in each direction
8. Head tilting
9. Trapezius and rhomboid muscle tenderness
10. Cervical spine and dorsal spine tenderness
11. Carpal tunnel evaluation—(Tinel's, Phelan's, and numbness)
12. Tinel's sign at elbows
13. Abducting arms to 90-degree AER noting pulses and symptoms
14. Bruits, supra- and infraclavicular
15. Neurological examination: gross sensation, strength, reflexes when appropriate

Table 6–5.   **Physical Findings**

	Author's Series			11 Reports (1964–1985)[2, 6–14, 17]		
	1964–1971	1972–1979	1980–1985	Number of Reports	Range	Median
Number of Operations	76	261	223	11	22–433	120
Physical Finding[a]						
Supraclav. tender.	64%	96%	95%	4	28–81%	31%
Symptoms @ 90-AER	94%	92%	94%	5	17–95%	76%
Pulse Decr. @ 90-AER	51%	31%	24%	7	20–91%	66%
Adson's Test	–	–	–	6	22–100%	31%
Reduced neck ROM	68%	92%	85%			
Bruit, supra/infra clavicular	24%	19%	–			

[a]Supraclav. tender. = supraclavicular tenderness; 90-AER = 90-degree abduction in external rotation. ROM = range of motion.

Supraclavicular Tenderness

The most important aspects of physical examination in establishing a diagnosis of TOS are palpation for supraclavicular tenderness and checking for symptoms with the arms in the 90-degree AER position. Even these areas of the examination have some variations. There are two spots in the supraclavicular area that can be checked. One is directly over the anterior scalene muscle, which lies about 3 cm lateral to the trachea and 2–3 cm above the clavicle (Fig. 6-1). Because normal people can be tender there, a comparison of the two sides is valuable. In bilateral disease, the diagnosis is more difficult because both sides are usually tender. On the other hand, non-tender scalenes are a strong point against a diagnosis of traumatic TOS, although in nontraumatic or osseous TOS the anterior scalene can be non-tender.

The second point to palpate in the supraclavicular space is directly over the brachial plexus, located only 1 cm posterior to the anterior scalene muscle. The thumb presses over the plexus of each side holding pressure for 20–30 seconds. A positive response is the onset of paresthesia or pain radiating to the arm and hand, similar to the patient's symptoms. Another way of observing the same response is by tapping over the brachial plexus with a finger or reflex hammer to elicit Tinel's sign. Either thumb pressure or tapping, when positive, indicate irritation of plexus.

In Table 6–5, supraclavicular tenderness in our cases refers to palpation over the scalene muscles, not the plexus. In the other reports the specific supraclavicular point is not stated. It has only been in the past few years that we have used Tinel's sign and direct pressure over the brachial plexus as part of our routine examination for TOS. Although statistics are not available, our impression is that both tests are positive in the majority of TOS patients, but not as frequently positive as muscle tenderness. Moreover, in patients with unilateral disease, Tinel's sign is sometimes positive bilaterally.

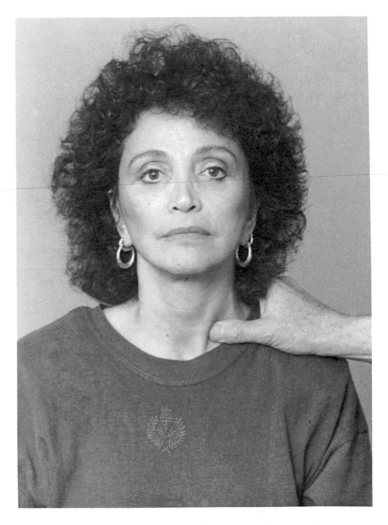

Fig. 6-1.   Examiner's thumb over the anterior scalene muscle presses to detect tenderness. Comparison of relative tenderness on each side is very helpful in unilateral disease.

Postural Maneuvers

Placing the arms in specific positions and noting pulse alterations and/or neurologic symptoms has been one of the important aspects of physical examination. Three specific positions, for diagnostic purposes, were described between 1927 and 1943: Adson's test,[21] shoulder bracing,[22] and the 90-degree AER position.[23] In 1963, Gilroy and Meyers compared the three positions in normal and TOS patients.[24] In all 11 TOS patients, there was obliteration of the radial pulse and production of symptoms in the various positions. In the control group of 40 patients, there were no symptoms in any position, although murmurs and pulse obliteration were observed in some positions in 69% of the control extremities.

The Adson Test

For decades, a positive Adson's test was regarded as THE single, most important finding in making a diagnosis of TOS. Some physicians still rely on it today. As described by Adson in 1927, and again in 1947, the test is performed with the patient's hands at the side: "The patient takes a long deep breath, elevates the chin, and turns it to the affected side. A decrease or obliteration of the radial pulse or blood pressure is a pathognomonic sign of scalenus anticus syndrome."[21, 25]

Adson's faith in this "infallible sign" has not been shared by most investigators. Disagreement began appearing in 1945 when Wright noted pulse obliteration in some patients turning their head to the same side, and in other patients turning their head to the opposite side.[26] Woods, in 1965, noted a positive Adson's test in 63% of TOS patients who turned their head to the contralateral side, and in only 22% who turned their head to the ipsilateral side.[1]

Other authors have noted normal Adson's tests in a large percentage of TOS patients.[27, 28] In Table 6–5, the incidence of positive Adson's tests ranged from 27%[11] to 100%,[12] with a median of only 31%. Further reducing the value of the Adson maneuver are the significant number of normal people who have positive tests. Gage, in 1947, noted an incidence of 50% positive tests in normals.[29]

Shoulder Bracing or Military Position

Retracting the shoulders backward and downward, also described as shoulder bracing or assuming a military position, was initially described in 1943 by Falconer and Weddell as a means of narrowing the costoclavicular space.[22] This maneuver is usually positive in the costoclavicular syndrome.[30] However, shoulder bracing reduces or obliterates the pulses in a significant proportion of the normal population. Falconer and Weddell found that to be so in 50% and 58% of normal men and women, respectively;[22] Telford and Mottershead noted it in 68% of normals.[31] Because of these findings, shoulder bracing, like Adson's test, cannot be relied upon.

Studies in Normals

Between 1980 and 1988, three studies were performed in normal subjects to determine the incidence of arterial compression in asymptomatic people. Two of the investigations employed sensitive fingertip devices connected to recorders to document reductions greater than 75% in pulse amplitudes[32] or flow;[33] in the third study,[34] both photoplethysmographic tracings and palpation of radial pulses were recorded (Table 6–6). The results of these studies further support the views of many earlier authors that positional maneuvers reduce arterial flow to the hand in many normal people. In addition, Warrens' study revealed poor correlation between clinical palpation and plethysmographic findings.[34]

90-Degree AER Position

In 1939, Eden noted in a case of costoclavicular compression that the radial pulse obliterated if the arm was raised to the level of the shoulder.[23] In 1963, Gilroy and Meyer found the "90 degree AER position" comparable to the other positional

Table 6–6.　　Arterial Compression Studies in Normal Subjects

Author	Yr.	No.	Adson's Test	Costocl. or Military[a]	Hyperabd.[b]	At Least One Pos. Test	Criteria
Gergoudis, Barnes[32]	'80	130	53%	14%	19%	60%	Decreased amplitude >75%
Colon, Westdrop[33]	'88	115	9%	8%	44%		Decreased flow >75%
Warrens, Heaton[34]	'87	64	15%	27%	19%	58%	Loss of palpable pulse

[a]Costocl. or Military = Costoclavicular compression or the military position with shoulders braced backward.
[b]Hyperabd. = Hyperabduction maneuver, abducting the arms 180 degrees above the head.

maneuvers.[24] In 1966, Roos claimed this to be one of the more reliable maneuvers for diagnosing TOS.[35]

The 90-degree AER position has reproduced symptoms in over 90% of the patients in all three of our series. Obliteration of the radial pulse is much less consistent, ranging from 24% to 51%. This is not surprising, as the large majority of TOS patients have neurological and not vascular symptoms. It is a more reliable maneuver than shoulder bracing or Adson's test because positive responses in normal patients are only 5% to 10%.[24, 36, 37]

The 90-degree AER position has some variations. The degree of shoulder flexion (forward) or extension (backward) is critical (Fig. 6-2, A–C). The arm position should be straight with the elbows in line with the shoulder, in such a way that if the patient were standing with his/her back against a wall, the abducted, externally rotated arms would lie flat against the wall too. If the arms are held forward, away from the wall, standardization is lost and a false negative response can occur. The neck should be extended when performing this maneuver. Roos describes exercising the fingers in this position, but our experience suggests that a positive response will occur as easily without exercise.[35]

Conclusions

Favorable clinical experiences and the low incidence of positive tests (defined as production of symptoms *or* pulse obliteration) among normals have led us to rely on the 90-degree AER test and to abandon shoulder bracing and the Adson maneuver. A positive 90-degree AER test is very helpful in unilateral and bilateral disease, but is not pathognomonic. A negative test makes a diagnosis of TOS less likely.

Vascular Signs

In patients with symptoms of arterial insufficiency such as Raynaud's phenomenon, ischemic fingers, or claudication, more attention is paid to documenting arterial obstruction. The measurement of blood pressure in each arm at rest and

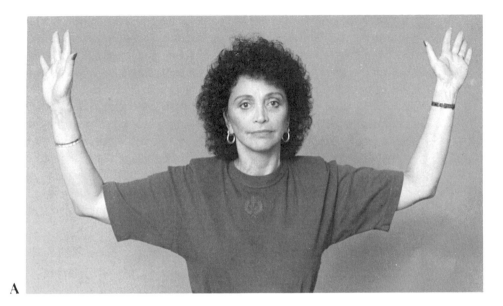

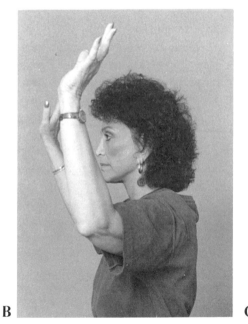

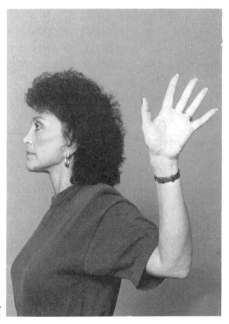

Fig. 6-2.   90-degree abduction external rotation position (90-degree AER): The patient is asked to hold arms in this position for three minutes. Reduction or obliteration of each radial pulse is noted. The development of paresthesia, pain, weakness, and fatigue is recorded. **A:** Correct position with elbows in plane of shoulders. **B:** Arms are too far forward, too much shoulder adduction. **C:** Arms are too far back, too much shoulder hyperextension.

in the 90-degree AER position can document arterial cutoff, but the same objective sign can be detected by feeling the radial pulse in each position and listening for a bruit above or below the clavicle as the arm is raised from resting to 90 degrees. When listening for such a bruit, the listener should begin with the arm at rest and continue listening as the arm is slowly raised. The bruit may be heard in some positions, then disappear. That is due to arterial compression going from partial to complete occlusion or to the lumen being narrowed as the arm goes up and then enlarging as the arm is raised further. What actually happens to the subclavian artery is determined by the relationship of the clavicle to the first rib or to cervical ribs, when present. The clavicle is as apt to be the compressing structure as is the first rib, as has been demonstrated in many patients whose pulses continue to be obliterated following first rib resection in spite of symptomatic relief.

Other Parts of Physical Examination

Hand strength is determined to provide an objective measurement for follow-up. It does not influence the diagnosis. About half of TOS patients demonstrate weakness in the affected hand.

Range of motion of the neck is measured with the patient sitting on a table and turning the head as far as possible to each side. The examiner holds the patient's shoulders to prevent rotation. A normal range of motion is 90–110 degrees to each side. Reduction in range is estimated as a percentage of normal. The majority of traumatic TOS patients demonstrate reduced neck motion, which is usually due to tight scalene muscles, but can be due to associated cervical spine strain, arthritis, or previous cervical spine surgery.

Head tilting, performed by having the patient sit erect and tilt the head to one side by trying to touch the shoulder with the ear, stretches neck muscles on the contralateral side. In patients with TOS, this maneuver often elicits pain referred to the opposite side.

Checking for tenderness over the cervical and dorsal spine, trapezius and rhomboid muscles, and the ligaments and tendons around the shoulder joint is done to detect associated conditions that frequently accompany TOS. Asking the patient to abduct the arms to 180 degrees is another helpful maneuver to check the integrity of the shoulder joint. Inability to reach 180 degrees is an indication for orthopedic evaluation of the shoulder joint (Table 6–4).

References

1. Woods WW. Personal experiences with surgical treatment of 250 cases of cervicobrachial neurovascular compression syndrome. J Int Coll Surg 1965; 44: 273–283.
2. Urschel HC, Paulson DL, McNamara JJ. Thoracic outlet syndrome. Ann Thorac Surg 1968; 6:1–10.
3. Urschel HC, Razzuk MA, Wood RE, Parekh M, Paulson DL. Objective diagnosis (ulnar nerve conduction velocity) and current therapy of the thoracic outlet syndrome. Ann Thorac Surg 1971; 12:608–620.

4. Hoofer WD, Burnett AD. Thoracic outlet relief. J Kansas Med Soc 1973; 74: 329–331, 352.

5. Johnson CR. Treatment of TOS by removal of first rib and related entrapments through posterolateral approach: a 22 year approach. J Thorac Cardiovasc Surg 1974; 68:536–545.

6. Dale WA. Management of thoracic outlet syndrome. Ann Surg 1975; 181:575–585.

7. Stanton PE Jr, McClusky DA Jr, Richardson HD, Lamis PA. Thoracic outlet syndrome: a comprehensive evaluation. South Med J 1978; 71:1070–1073.

8. Thomas GI, Jones TW, Stavney LS, Manhas DR. Thoracic outlet syndrome. Am Surg 1978; 44:483–495.

9. Woods WW. Thoracic outlet syndrome. West J Med 1978; 128:9–12.

10. Kelly TR. Thoracic outlet syndrome: current concepts of treatment. Ann Surg 1979; 190:657–662.

11. McGough EC, Pearce MB, Byrne JP. Management of thoracic outlet syndrome. J Ther Card Med 1979; 77:169–174.

12. Murphy TO, Clinton AP, Kanar EA, McAlexander RA. Subclavicular approach to first rib resection. Am J Surg 1980; 139:634–636.

13. Hempel GK, Rucher AH Jr, Wheeler CG, Hunt DG, Bukhari HI. Supraclavicular resection of the first rib for thoracic outlet syndrome. Am J Surg 1981; 141:213–215.

14. Daskalakis MK. Thoracic outlet compression syndrome: current concepts and surgical experience. Int Surg 1983; 68:337–344.

15. Sallstrom J, Gjores JE. Surgical treatment of the thoracic outlet syndrome. Acta Chir Scand 1983; 149:555–560.

16. Heughan C. Thoracic outlet syndrome. Can J Surg 1984; 27:35–36.

17. Qvarfordt PG, Ehrenfeld WK, Stoney RJ. Supraclavicular radical scalenectomy and transaxillary first rib resection for the thoracic outlet syndrome, a combined approach. Am J Surg 1984; 148:111–116.

18. Telford ED, Stopford JSB. The vascular complications of cervical rib. Br J Surg 1930; 18:557–564.

19. Swank RL, Simeone FA. Scalenus anticus syndrome. Types; their characterization, diagnosis and treatment. Arch Neurol Psych 1944; 51:432–445.

20. Roos DB. The place for scalenectomy and first rib resection in thoracic outlet syndrome. Surgery 1982; 92:1077–1085.

21. Adson AW, Coffey JR. Cervical rib: a method of anterior approach for relief of symptoms by division of the scalenus anticus. Ann Surg 1927; 85:839–857.

22. Falconer MA, Weddell G. Costoclavicular compression of the subclavian artery and vein. Lancet 1943; 2:539–543.

23. Eden KC. Complications of cervical rib. Vascular complications of cervical ribs and first thoracic rib abnormalities. Br J Surg 1939–40; 27:111–139.

24. Gilroy J, Meyer JS. Compression of the subclavian artery as a cause of ischemic brachial neuropathy. Brain 1963; 86:733–745.

25. Adson AW. Surgical treatment for symptoms produced by cervical ribs and the scalenus anticus muscle. Surg Gynecol Obstet 1947; 85:687–700.

26. Wright IS. The neurovascular syndrome produced by hyperabduction of the arms. Am Heart J 1945; 29:1–19.

27. McGowan JM, Velinsky M. Costoclavicular compression: relation to the scalenus anticus and cervical rib syndrome. Arch Surg 1949; 59:62–73.

28. Holden WD, Murphy JA, Portmann AF. Scalene anticus syndrome: unusual diagnostic and therapeutic aspects. Am J Surg 1951; 81:411–416.

29. Gage M, Parnell H. Scalenus anticus syndrome. Am J Surg 1947; 73:252–268.

30. Rosati LM, Lord JW. Neurovascular compression of the shoulder. Modern Surgery Monographs. New York: Grune and Stratton, 1961.

31. Telford ED, Mottershead S. Pressure at the cervico-brachial junction: an operative and anatomical study. J Bone Joint Surg 1948; 30:249–265.

32. Gergoudis R, Barnes RW. Thoracic outlet arterial compression: prevalence in normal persons. Angiology 1980; 31:538–541.
33. Colon E, Westdrop R: Vascular compression in the thoracic outlet: age dependent normative value in noninvasive testing. J Cardiovasc Surg 1988; 29:166–171.
34. Warrens A, Heaton JM. Thoracic outlet compression syndrome: the lack of reliability of its clinical assessment. Ann R Coll Surg Engl 1987; 69:203–204.
35. Roos DB, Owens JC. Thoracic outlet syndrome. Arch Surg 1966; 93:71–74.
36. Winsor T, Brow R. Costoclavicular syndrome, its diagnosis and treatment. J Am Med Assoc 1966; 196:109–111.
37. Telford ED, Mottershead S. The costoclavicular syndrome. Br Med J 1947; 1:325–328.

7
Diagnostic Studies

Richard J. Sanders
Richard Smith

Imaging
       X-rays
       CAT Scans and MRI

Noninvasive Vascular Studies

Angiography
       Arteriography
       Technique of Arteriography
       Venography

Duplex Scanning

Neurophysiologic Studies
       Electromyography (EMG)
       Nerve Conduction Velocity (NCV)
       Cervical Root Stimulation
       F-waves
       Somatosensory Evoked Potentials (SSEP)

Scalene Muscle Block

Advances in technology in the last half of the twentieth century have provided the clinician with a variety of tests employing sophisicated, expensive equipment that can be used to evaluate compression in the thoracic outlet area. Unfortunately, most of the available tests are of limited value in diagnosing TOS. Special tests should be ordered only for specific indications.

Imaging

X-rays

Roentgenograms of the chest and cervical spine should be obtained on all patients with symptoms of TOS. Those x-rays will precisely diagnose the presence or absence of cervical ribs, abnormal first ribs, or healed fractures of ribs or clavicle. The existence of osseous abnormalities will assist in determining the need for other diagnostic tests.

Small cervical ribs, 1 to 2 cm long, are often thin and can be missed on anterior-posterior projections of the cervical spine. This is particularly true if the films are over-exposed. Oblique views of that region can more clearly demonstrate the existence of such anomalies (Fig. 7-1, A and B). X-rays are also of value in detecting significant cervical spine abnormalities such as arthritis or degenerative disc disease.

CAT Scans and MRI

Computerized axial tomography (CAT scan) and magnetic resonance imaging (MRI) are currently the most sensitive noninvasive diagnostic tools for evaluating the cervical spine for disc displacement, disc degeneration, and cervical spine stenosis. These tests do not reveal any characteristic findings in patients with TOS; they are used as aides in differential diagnosis.

Noninvasive Vascular Studies

The place for noninvasive vascular lab studies in TOS is limited. They have no role in diagnosing neurogenic TOS. In the 1960s, when many cases of TOS were thought to be of vascular origin, plethysmography, pulse volume recordings, and arm pressure measurements were used to document reduction in arterial blood flow when the arms were raised from a resting position to an elevated one.[1] In the ensuing years, it became apparent that signs of arterial compression were unreliable for diagnosing neurogenic TOS. Too many normal asymptomatic people compress their subclavian arteries during arm elevation (Chapter 6, Table 6–6). Furthermore, noting diminished radial pulses by palpation during positional maneuvers of the arm can provide the same information as noninvasive lab studies.

In cases where arterial stenosis or occlusion is suspected, noninvasive vascular lab studies are helpful to quantify the hemodynamic disturbance and to establish a baseline for future comparisons. There are several instruments available today that can perform this assessment equally well.

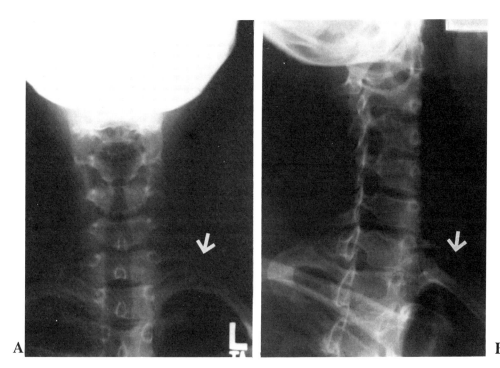

Fig. 7-1.   X-rays of neck in TOS patients with a 1-cm cervical rib on the left side. **A:** PA view in which cervical rib is barely seen. **B:** Oblique view of same patient that projects the cervical rib away from the first rib making it more distinguishable.

Subclavian vein occlusion can sometimes be detected by noninvasive venous plethysmography. However, this test is unreliable and can too often give false-negative results. When venous obstruction is suspected, venography is the preferred diagnostic test.

Angiography

Arteriography

This procedure is indicated for the diagnosis of subclavian artery aneurysms, stenosis, or occlusion. Clinical findings that suggest those arterial abnormalities include the absence or decrease of peripheral pulses, lower blood pressure on the involved side with the arms *at rest*; a bruit above or below the clavicle *at rest*; a pulsatile lump in the supraclavicular area; ischemia of the hand; or a history of emboli to the hand. Obliteration of the pulse by positional maneuvers on physical examination is not, by itself, an indication for arteriography. Since arterial damage in patients with TOS is rarely seen without a bony abnormality, arteriography is seldom indicated in the absence of an osseous defect. In the case of cervical ribs, it is more often a complete cervical rib that is associated with arterial injury. Incomplete ribs, 1 to 2 cm long, rarely cause permanent arterial wall damage. They are not near the artery.

Technique of Arteriography

Digital subtraction angiography (DSA) by the intravenous route often provides adequate visualization to make a diagnosis. If the films are of poor quality, transfemoral arterial catheterization with a direct injection into the subclavian artery is the next route of choice. If the artery is normal with the arms at rest, additional injections with the arms raised and shoulders abducted will not be of clinical value. This is true for two reasons: First, positional arteriography can demonstrate subclavian artery stenosis or occlusion in many asymptomatic people, so that demonstrating compression with positional maneuvers is not diagnostic of TOS. Second, it is not possible to determine whether the compressing structure is clavicle, first rib, scalene muscle, or a ligament. Anatomicaly, all of those structures lie too close to each other to distinguish, with certainty, the offending element. In early experiences with TOS, many arteriograms were performed to determine the point of compression,[2] a procedure that is now regarded as unnecessary in neurogenic TOS. The cause of arterial compression may not be the cause of the patient's symptoms. The only value of arteriography is to determine the state of the subclavian artery with the arms at rest.

Venography

Upper extremity venography is the best test to diagnose subclavian vein obstruction. Venography is easily performed by injecting dye into a peripheral vein in the hand or forearm. A regular x-ray table, using single 14×17 inch films changed once by hand, will often do as complete a job for venous disease as a multiple film changer. If the film taken at rest is normal, repeat injection should be done with the arm elevated and the shoulder abducted. Delayed emptying of dye from the arm and the presence of dilated collaterals are indicative of obstruction, which may be partial or complete. It is important to continue filming to make sure that the normal-appearing veins empty after a few seconds.

Duplex Scanning

The use of ultrasound combined with Doppler velocity waveforms can be of help in evaluating subclavian arterial or venous disease. Subclavian aneurysms can be checked for mural thrombus; the hemodynamics of subclavian artery stenosis can be measured; and partial axillosubclavian vein obstruction can be calibrated.

Neurophysiologic Studies

Neurophysiologic studies include both indirect assessment of nerves by observing electrical activity of muscles (electromyography—EMG) and direct assessment by measuring the responses to various forms of nerve stimulation—late F-wave responses, nerve conduction velocities (NCV), and somatosensory evoked potentials (SSEP). Positive results are nonspecific: They indicate an abnormality in nerve function, but do not give the specific cause. A diagnosis is established by combining a positive test with clinical information from an individual's history and physical examination.

Electromyography (EMG)

EMG examines the electrical characteristics of muscle in three states: at rest, with weak voluntary contraction, and with maximum voluntary contraction. Abnormal patterns are separated into those of muscle disease (myogenic) or nerve disease (neurogenic).

The technique involves placing a needle electrode into a muscle and observing the muscle activity at the moment of insertion and at rest. The changes in electric potential (voltage) can be visualized on an oscilloscope or transformed into auditory signals and heard through a speaker. The visual responses can be copied and preserved, but in many clinical laboratories, the electromyographer interprets the data qualitatively without producing a permanent record. (Permanent records are usually only made for NCVs.) The patient is asked to gently move the test muscle by voluntarily contracting it while the electrical activity of the muscle is displayed. Maximal muscle activity (recruitment) is determined by asking the patient to push or pull as hard as possible against a fixed object such as a table or the examiners hand.

The patterns recorded from these three states are compared to the patterns of normal people and patients with various muscle and nerve disorders. A general impression can be made from EMG but the findings often require correlation with other direct nerve tests and clinical features to obtain a specific diagnosis and to localize the abnormality.

EMG is a measure of motor, not sensory, function. It detects abnormalities of the lower motor neuron, the neuromuscular junction, and the muscle fibers. In the few TOS patients with muscle wasting, EMGs of the small hand muscles are abnormal.[3] However, since the majority of TOS patients do not have muscle atrophy, symptoms are sensory, not motor, and EMG results are usually normal. Perhaps the main value of EMG in thoracic outlet syndrome is to help exclude other diagnoses.[4]

Nerve Conduction Velocity (NCV)

The time required for an impulse to travel the length of a nerve segment is the *latency* of that segment; the distance traveled in a unit of time is the *nerve conduction velocity*. Latency is determined by measuring the time it takes an impulse to travel between two electrodes, one stimulating and one recording. Nerve conduction velocity is determined by dividing the measured distance an impulse travels by the latency. NCVs are measured for both sensory and motor nerves using the same principles.

In measuring NCVs through the thoracic outlet area, one electrode must be placed on or near a nerve proximal to the brachial plexus. This can be done at Erb's point, located at the base of the neck, or at the foramina of the cervical spine. The distal electrode is placed on a finger or hand muscle.

Injury or simple extrinsic pressure against a nerve can slow conduction time (or prolong the latency). If a nerve is only mildly irritated, it may not be compressed enough to slow conduction, yet pain and paresthesia may be present. This could be the reason that many TOS patients have normal nerve conduction times.

Following the introduction of nerve conduction velocity measurements by Jebson in 1967,[5] Urschel et al.,[6] and Caldwell, et al.[7] popularized nerve conduction studies in TOS, reporting that the normal ulnar nerve conduction velocity (UNCV) had a mean of 72 meters per second (m/s) while TOS patients averaged 57.8 meters per second (m/s). However, several clinicians who have used UNCVs have found the results no different from those in control patients[8–10] and other investigators disagree as to the range of normal. For example, Cherington studied 213 normal subjects and found an average proximal UNCV of 59 m/s,[11] which is similar to the value of Urschel's TOS patients. Subsequently, discrepancies have been pointed out in some of this work.[12, 13] Since many TOS patients have responded well to surgical treatment in spite of normal nerve conduction studies, a normal study does not rule out the diagnosis of TOS.

Cervical Root Stimulation

This is another method of studying nerve conduction velocity across the thoracic outlet. The stimulus is more specific than at Erb's point where the entire brachial plexus is often stimulated. However, this method is neither more sensitive nor more specific in the diagnosis of TOS than other techniques.[14, 15]

F-waves

An F-wave is a small-motor response that is obtained by stimulating a nerve antidromically (for motor nerves, antidromic is from the periphery toward the spinal cord). The stimulus travels from wrist or elbow to anterior horn cells in the spinal cord and then returns down the arm to the recording electrode on the hand. The time from stimulation until the F-wave appears, the F-wave latency, is measured.[16]

In normal subjects, F-waves are often absent, and when present, have a wide range of normal values. In TOS patients, F-wave latency may be prolonged, although this is nonlocalizing. Other limitations of F-wave measurements are that they assess motor nerve functions only and are abnormal in a variety of brachial plexus and peripheral nerve injuries.[10]

Somatosensory Evoked Potentials (SSEP)

Somatosensory evoked potentials are responses of the brain produced by stimulating a peripheral nerve. The time for the response to reach the brain is determined. The size of the response is quite small and requires the use of a computerized system to average the signal.

Median or ulnar nerves can be studied and responses recorded from Erb's point, the cervical spine, and the scalp. Prolongation of the latency from wrist to Erb's point can indicate compression of the lower trunk of the brachial plexus, as would be present in neurogenic TOS. However, such an abnormality is nonlocalizing since it could be due to pathology at any point between the wrist and brachial plexus.

Glover et al. were first to report the use of SSEP for the diagnosis of TOS.[17] Machleder et al. observed that 86% of TOS patients with abnormal SSEP test results had good responses to surgical treatment.[18] However, another group of TOS patients with normal SSEP tests also had good responses to surgical treatment (76% good to excellent). Thus, like nerve conduction velocity studies, SSEP has a low sensitivity. Other studies of SSEPs in TOS have not provided evidence of a characteristic abnormality that is clinically useful.[4]

Scalene Muscle Block

The injection of procaine hydrochloride and subsequently lidocaine into the anterior scalene muscle of patients with a diagnosis of TOS was reported by Gage in 1939.[19] The test is performed by infiltrating 4–5 cL of 1% lidocaine into the muscle belly with the patient recumbent or sitting and the neck hyperextended (Fig. 7-2). A good response to the injection is improvement in range of motion of the neck and fewer symptoms of pain and paresthesia when the arm is abducted to 90 degrees in external rotation. Sometimes, patients with paresthesia or headache at rest notice improvement in these symptoms too.

The sign of a successful block is loss of tenderness over the anterior scalene muscle. If the patient had no tenderness here preoperatively, it is impossible to be sure that the block was successful. However, if the signs on physical examination improve after the block, this can be regarded as a positive or good response. In patients with tenderness over their scalene muscles, if the tenderness persists after the injection, the injection should be repeated. If the tenderness is not relieved, it is probable that the anterior scalene muscle was missed or the scalene muscle is not the source of pathology.

The scalene block is not always successful. In about 5–10% of blocks, a portion of the anesthetic reaches the brachial plexus and causes a weak, numb arm. This usually disappears within 10 minutes, but it renders the block unsuccessful and of no diagnostic value. In these patients, the diagnosis is made on the basis of other clinical criteria.

Improvement following the block correlated with a good response to surgery in 80% of 132 patients receiving scalenectomy and in 92% of 19 patients who underwent first rib resection. In contrast, when there was a poor response to the block, only 33% of 22 patients had good results following scalenectomy or rib resection.[20]

On the basis of these data, we have used the scalene block in most TOS patients in the past several years. A good response to the block is used to support a

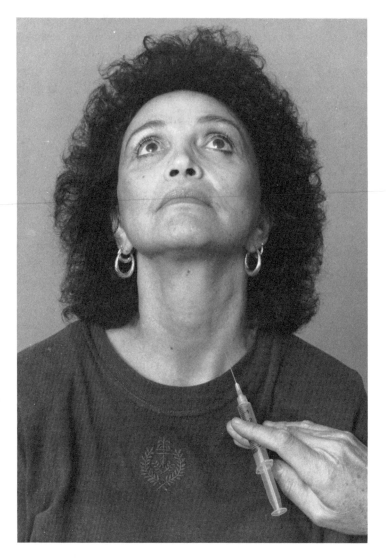

Fig. 7-2.   Scalene muscle block. The needle is inserted where shown, about 3 cm lateral to the midline and 2 cm above the clavicle. The anterior scalene muscle can usually be palpated through the skin if the patient hyperextends the neck. About 4 cc of 1% lidocaine is infiltrated into the anterior scalene muscle, constantly moving the needle throughout the injection. Aspiration prior to injection is usually not performed. To date, we have seen no sequelae from directly injecting a small amount of lidocaine directly into a major vessel, which presumably has been done in view of the several hundreds of patients we have injected.

diagnosis of TOS, which can be helpful in patients with borderline clinical criteria. A negative response to the block, assuming a good block was achieved, makes a diagnosis of TOS less likely; surgery is not considered in negative-response patients unless there are several other positive clinical criteria upon which to base a diagnosis.

The correlation between the results of the scalene block and TOS surgery are summarized in Table 7–1. They indicate a 94% improvement rate following

Table 7–1. **Correlation Between Results of Scalene Block and TOS Surgery**

Response to Block[a]	No. Cases	Good Response to Surgery	Poor Response to Surgery
Positive (improved)	442	415 (94%)	27 (6%)
Negative (no improvement)	21	18 (86%)	3 (14%)

[a] Response to the scalene block is the early success rate, in the first 3 months. Later failures did occur in some of these patients, but these were probably the result of scar tissue formation in the healing process. The diagnosis was regarded as correct if there was early improvement.

surgery for 442 patients with good responses to the block. Only 21 patients with poor responses to the block were operated upon. Although many times this number of patients have had negative responses, most did not undergo surgery and do not appear in the statistics. In the patients operated upon, other clinical criteria were used to establish a diagnosis and 86% improved postoperatively. Therefore, a good response to the block continues to have a high correlation with improvement following surgery while a poor response to the block does not rule out the diagnosis.[21]

References

1. Sanders RJ, Monsour JW, Baer SB. Transaxillary first rib resection for the thoracic outlet syndrome. Arch Surg 1968; 97:1014–1023.
2. Lang EK. Arteriographic diagnosis of the thoracic outlet syndrome. Radiology 1965; 84:296–303.
3. Smith T, Trojaborg W. Diagnosis of thoracic outlet syndrome: value of sensory and motor conduction studies and quantitative electromyography. Arch Neurol 1987; 44:1161–1163.
4. Veilleux M, Stevens JC, Campbell JK. Somatosensory evoked potentials: lack of value for diagnosis of thoracic outlet syndrome. Muscle Nerve 1988; 11:571–575.
5. Jebsen RH. Motor conduction velocities in the median and ulnar nerves. Arch Phys Med 1967; 48:185–194.
6. Urschel HC, Paulson DL, McNamara JJ. Thoracic outlet syndrome. Ann Thorac Surg 1968; 6:1–10.
7. Caldwell JW, Crane CR, Krusen EM. Nerve conduction studies, an aid in the diagnosis of the thoracic outlet syndrome. South Med J 1971; 64:210–212.
8. Daube JR. Nerve conduction studies in thoracic outlet syndrome. Neurology (Minneap) 1975; 25:347.
9. Ryding E, Ribbe E, Rosen I, Norgren L. A neurophysiologic investigation of thoracic outlet syndrome. Acta Chir Scand 1985; 151:327–331.
10. Aminoff MJ, Olney RK, Parry GJ, Raskin NH. Relative utility of different electrophysiologic techniques in the evaluation of brachial plexopathies. Neurology 1988; 38:546–549.
11. Cherington M. Ulnar conduction velocity in thoracic outlet syndrome. N Engl J Med 1976; 294:1185.
12. Wilbourn AJ. Evidence for conduction delay in thoracic outlet syndrome is challenged. N Engl J Med 1984; 310:1052–1053.
13. Urschel HC. Evidence for conduction delay in thoracic outlet syndrome is challenged. N Engl J Med 1984; 310:1052–1053.

14. Livingstone EF, DeLisa JA, Halar EM. Electrodiagnostic values through the thoracic outlet using C8 root needle studies, F-waves, and cervical somatosensory evoked potentials. Arch Phys Med Rehabil 1984; 65:726–730.
15. Berger AR, Busis NA, Logigian EL, Wierzbicka M, Shahani BT. Cervical root stimulation in the diagnosis of radiculopathy. Neurology 1987; 37:329–332.
16. Hongladhrom T. "F"-wave conduction velocity in thoracic outlet syndrome. N Engl J Med 1976; 295:1382–1383.
17. Glover JL, Worth RM, Bendick PJ, Hall PV, Markand OM. Evoked responses in the diagnosis of thoracic outlet syndrome. Surgery 1981; 89:86–93.
18. Machleder HJ, Moll F, Nuwer M, Jordan S. Somatosensory evoked potentials in the assessment of thoracic outlet compression syndrome. J Vasc Surg 1987; 6:177–184.
19. Gage M. Scalenus anticus syndrome. A diagnostic and confirmatory test. Surgery 1939; 5:599–601.
20. Sanders RJ, Monsour JW, Gerber FG, Adams WRA, Thompson N. Scalenectomy versus first rib resection for treatment of the thoracic outlet syndrome. Surgery 1979; 85:109–121.
21. Sanders RJ, Pearce WH. The treatment of thoracic outlet syndrome: a comparison of different operations. J Vasc Surg 1989; 10:626–634.

8
Differential and Associated Diagnoses

Richard J. Sanders
Angelika Voelkel

Compression Syndromes
Double Crush Nerve Compression

Biceps/Rotator Cuff Tendinitis or Impingement Syndrome

Cervical Spine Strain/Sprain

Fibromyositis

Cervical Disk Disease and Spinal Stenosis

Cervical Arthritis

Brachial Plexus Injury

Pectoralis Minor Syndrome

Temporomandibular Joint Abnormalities

Other Conditions

In discussing TOS, the term "associated diagnosis" is more appropriate than differential diagnosis because TOS is usually associated with at least one other condition. Since a large majority of TOS patients develop their symptoms following neck trauma, other structures in the neck, dorsal spine, shoulder girdle, or upper extremity are often damaged during the same accident.

Compression Syndromes

Carpal tunnel, ulnar tunnel, pronator tunnel syndromes, and ulnar nerve entrapment at the elbow are all disorders that arise from repetitive trauma, arthritis of the upper extremity, or rarely from endocrinopathies.[1] These conditions produce pain and paraesthesia in the fingers, hand, and forearm, but only occasionally cause symptoms in the shoulders or neck. Neurophysiologic diagnostic studies are of greater value and are more reliable in diagnosing these conditions than in diagnosing TOS.

Carpal tunnel syndrome is the most common differential condition. It usually involves the median nerve and produces paraesthesia in the first three and one half fingers. TOS, in contrast, usually involves the ulnar nerve as well as the median nerve, and commonly includes pain the shoulder, neck, and occiput. Carpal tunnel syndrome is associated with TOS in 21–30% of TOS cases and with ulnar nerve compression at the elbow in 6–10%.[2,3] Treatment in such cases has been arbitrary. If hand symptoms are predominant, the carpal tunnel is treated first, while if shoulder and neck pain are the major problem the TOS is treated first. On occasion, both areas have been operated upon simultaneously, but this is not encouraged.

Double Crush Nerve Compression

The term double crush syndrome was first suggested by Upton and McComas in 1973 to indicate the existence of more than one area of nerve compression in an extremity.[4] In 1990, Wood reported 165 cases of TOS in whom there was a 44% incidence of another compression distally as shown by neurophysiologic studies.[5]

Biceps/Rotator Cuff Tendinitis or Impingement Syndrome

Inflammation of the biceps/rotator cuff area frequently accompanies TOS. The diagnosis is made by the presence of localized tenderness over the short head of the biceps or rotator cuff and by a painful arc on abduction of the arm above shoulder level. This condition is treated with anti-inflammatory drugs, local heat, ultrasound, range of motion exercises, and cortisone injections. If symptoms are severe enough and do not respond to conservative treatment, magnetic resonance imaging (MRI), arthrography, arthroscopy, and sometimes surgical exploration to repair the tendons is indicated. Relief from symptoms of tendinitis may result in enough symptomatic improvement that surgical treatment of coexistent TOS can be avoided.

Cervical Spine Strain/Sprain

Cervical spine strain results from stretching the muscles and ligaments along the cervical spine. It occurs from the same type of hyperextension neck injuries that produce TOS, with which it coexists in many TOS patients. Its main symptom is limited to neck pain and stiffness. Physical examination reveals tenderness over and adjacent to the cervical spine. The only supportive diagnostic test for cervical spine strain is straightening of the normal curvature in the cervical spine on a lateral neck x-ray, but this is nonspecific (Fig. 8-1, A and B).

Cervical sprain is a more extended neck injury: In addition to neck pain and stiffness, symptoms include numbness and tingling in the arm and hand, occipital headaches, and radicular pain. Physical examination reveals not only tenderness over the cervical spine but also objective findings of limitation of range of motion of the neck and spasticity.

Treatment of cervical spine strain/sprain is conservative: muscle relaxers, anti-inflammatory drugs, heat, ice, massage, ultrasound, and time (weeks to months). Neck collars are recommended by some physicians but should only be used in the acute phase. Neck traction and manipulations of the spine may or may not be helpful. Cervical strains clear up in a few days to weeks. If symptoms persist beyond two months, the diagnosis should be changed to sprain. In patients undergoing surgery for TOS, the failure of neck pain to be relieved postoperatively may be due to the coexistence of cervical neck sprain that did not respond to conservative treatment. Unfortunately, there is no adequate way to completely differentiate the symptoms of TOS from those of cervical neck sprain; in general, neck pain in TOS is more anterior and in cervical sprain more posterior in the neck.

Fibromyositis

Inflammation of the trapezius, rhomboid, supraspinatus, or infraspinatus muscles is another common disorder that frequently accompanies TOS as a result of trauma to the dorsal spine, neck, and shoulder girdle areas. The main symptom is pain over and around the scapula and neck, with diffuse pain and paresthesia radiating into the arm. The diagnosis is made by demonstrating tenderness and fibrocystic nodules over these muscle groups.

It is usually impossible to differentiate pain due to fibromyositis from the pain of anterior scalene muscle entrapment of brachial plexus branches going to the scapula. Regardless of the cause, initial treatment is conservative.[6] When parascapular pain persists after TOS surgery, it usually means the pain in this area was caused by muscle inflammation rather than TOS.

Cervical Disc Disease and Spinal Stenosis

Herniation of a cervical disc or spinal stenosis are two conditions that must be differentiated from TOS. The most common location of a displaced cervical disc is

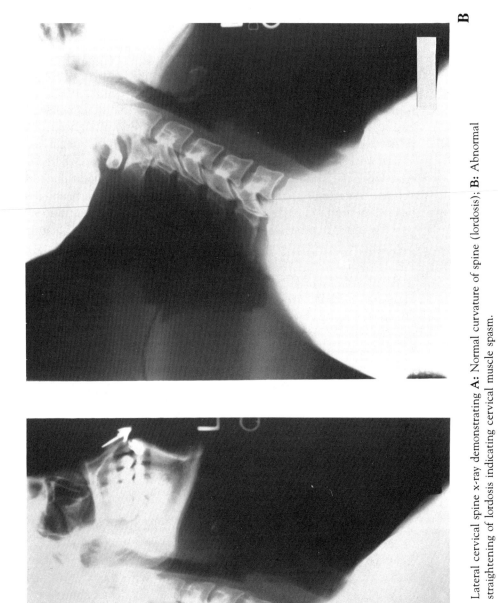

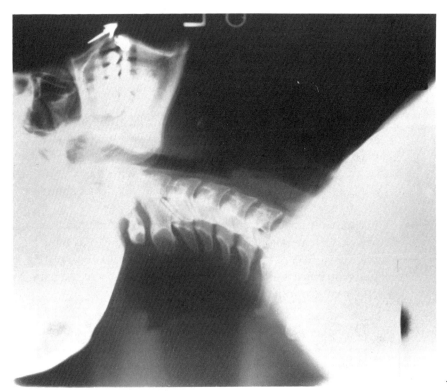

Fig. 8-1.   Lateral cervical spine x-ray demonstrating **A:** Normal curvature of spine (lordosis); **B:** Abnormal straightening of lordosis indicating cervical muscle spasm.

at C5–6. Symptoms are similar to TOS and include neck pain and stiffness, arm weakness, and paresthesia that involves the thumb and index finger rather than the ring and little finger, as in TOS. These symptoms are often improved by elevating the arm, an important differential from TOS in which symptoms are aggravated by arm elevation. Magnetic resonant imaging (MRI), computerized axial tomography (CAT scan), and myelography are often necessary to diagnose at displaced cervical disc or spinal stenosis (Figs. 8-2, 8-3, 8-4). When TOS and cervical disc disease or spinal stenosis coexist and symptoms have not responded to conservative therapy, surgery on the spine is usually recommended first because its diagnosis is more objective and reliable.

Cervical Arthritis

Some degree of cervical arthritis is present in most people over age 50 and minor arthritic changes are frequent in the 30- to 50-year age group. Most people with radiologic changes of arthritis have few or no symptoms. When symptoms occur, they usually are limited to neck pain and stiffness. Arm pain and hand paraesthesia can occur but are infrequent. The nature of the onset of symptoms is an important differential in separating TOS symptoms from those of arthritis. When symptoms develop in close proximity to a neck injury, are aggravated by elevating the arms, and there is scalene muscle tenderness on physical examination, TOS is probably present. If neck x-rays in such a case reveal arthritic changes, the two conditions probably coexist. If conservative therapy is unsuccessful, surgical treatment of the TOS can be considered in patients with preexisting cervical arthritis whose symptoms were aggravated by a neck injury.

Brachial Plexus Injury

Injury to the nerves of the brachial plexus occurs from direct blows to the shoulder or stretch injuries to the arm. The symptoms are similar to those of TOS: pain and weakness in the arm and paraesthesia in the hand. Unlike TOS, the symptoms from plexus injuries are usually constant, rather than intermittent. Neurophysiologic diagnostic studies are abnormal in plexus injuries.

Only conservative treatment is available for direct nerve injuries (see Chapter 11). The importance in recognizing nerve injuries is to avoid unnecessary operations for TOS that obviously will be unsuccessful.

Pectoralis Minor Syndrome

Hyperabduction, or pectoralis minor, syndrome is uncommon. It is manifest by paresthesia in the hands brought on by elevating the arms to 180 degrees. It is not associated with neck pain, occipital headaches, and only rarely with shoulder pain. The symptoms occur primarily at night and are related to sleeping with the arms above the head. There is no history of trauma.

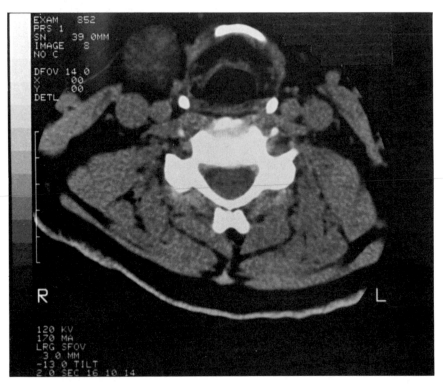

A

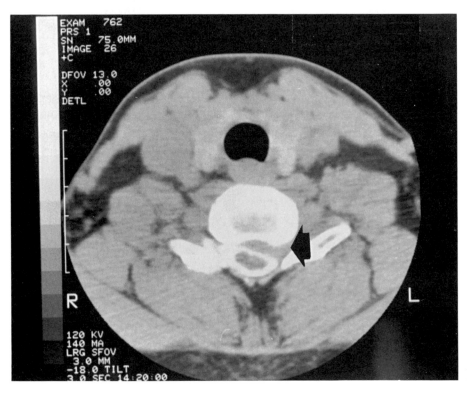

B

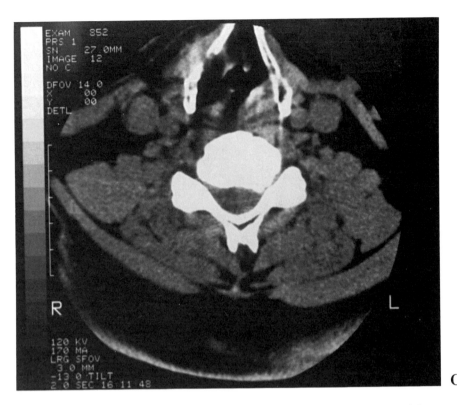

C

Fig. 8-2.   Computerized axial tomography (CAT scan) of cervical spine. **A:** Normal. **B:** Cervical disc compressing left side of spinal cord (arrow). **C:** Cervical spinal stenosis demonstrating diffuse osseous compression of spinal cord.

This condition is included as one of the disorders that can produce TOS. However, its anatomy is lateral to the scalene triangle and it should be separated from the other conditions. It is usually treatable by conservative measures, particularly by instructing patients to sleep with their arms at the side and even tying their hands to the foot of the bed if necessary. Rarely are symptoms severe enough to require surgery. In such cases, division of the pectoralis minor tendon, a simple procedure, is all that is needed.

Temporomandibular Joint Abnormalities

Injury and inflammation in the temporomandibular joint (TMJ) is frequently seen following head and neck injuries. The symptoms are pain in the jaw, headaches, dizziness, tinnitus, and parasthesia in the neck, face, and ear. While headaches are common in TOS, vertigo, jaw pain, and paresthesia in the neck and face are not. This condition can accompany TOS and must be differentiated from it as it requires separate treatment by a dentist. TMJ abnormalities are usually treated before surgery is considered for TOS.

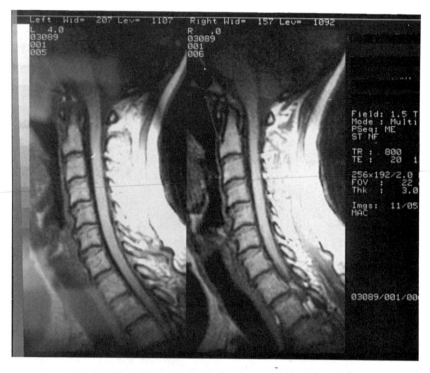

A

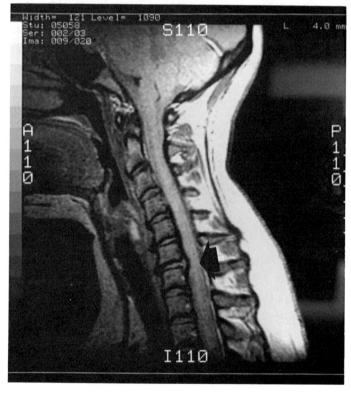

B

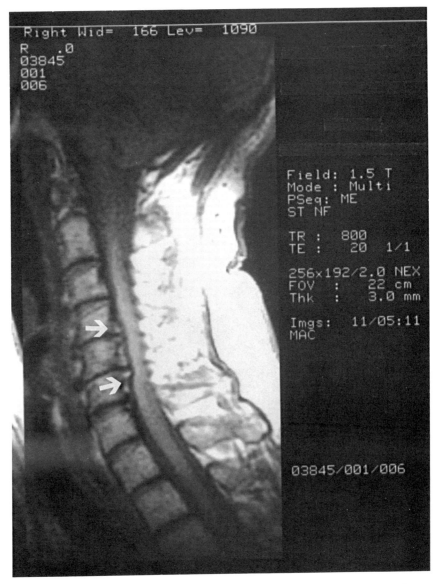

C

Fig. 8-3.   Magnetic resonance imaging (MRI) of cervical spine. **A:** Normal. These adjacent sagittal sections of cervical spine demonstrate mild arthritic changes anteriorly but no posterior encroachment against the spinal cord. **B:** Cervical disc at C5–6 compressing spinal cord (arrow). **C:** Spinal stenosis demonstrating osseous encroachment against the spinal cord between C-4 and C-6 (arrow).

Other Conditions

A variety of other neurological conditions should be considered. These include spinal tumors, multiple sclerosis, and reflex sympathetic dystrophy. Chest pain is occasionally the primary symptom in TOS, but this must be differentiated from angina, pleuritis, or costochondritis.

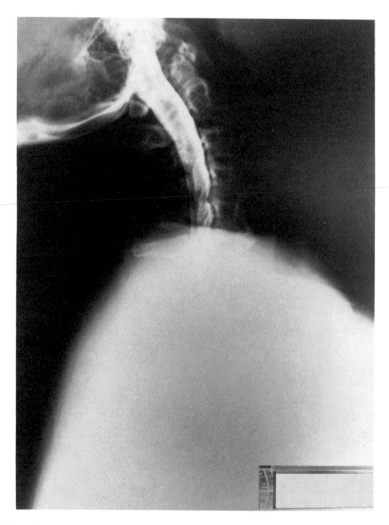

Fig. 8-4.   Cervical myelogram. Cervical disc compressing spinal cord at C4–5.

References

1. Johnson EW. Practical electromyography. Second edition. Baltimore: Williams & Wilkins, 1988.
2. Narakas A, Bonnard C, Egloff DV. The cervico-thoracic outlet syndrome. Ann Chir Main 1986; 5:185–207.
3. Wood VE, Twito R, Verska JM. Thoracic outlet syndrome: the results of first rib resection in 100 patients. Orthop Clin North Am 1988; 19:131–146.
4. Upton ARM, McComas AJ. The double crush in nerve-entrapment syndromes. Lancet 1973; 2:359–362.
5. Wood VE, Biondi J. Double-crush nerve compression in thoracic outlet syndrome. J Bone Joint Surg 1990; 72A: 85–87.
6. Travell JG, Simons DG. Myofascial pain and dysfunction: the trigger point manual. Balitmore: Williams & Wilkins, 1983: 331–476.

9
Conservative Treatment

Angelika Voelkel

Diagnosis
Stages

Treatment
Goals
Plan of Therapy
Control of Symptoms
Long-Term Maintenance

Prognosis

Work Capacity Evaluation
Sports and Hobbies

Rating Maximal Medical Improvement
Impairment Rating
Disability Rating

Conservative therapy for thoracic outlet syndrome (TOS) includes a variety of treatment forms. The initial interview with a patient being treated for TOS should include an explanation of the nature of the condition, how it develops, and how compression symptoms are produced. An outline should be given to the patient that includes the goals of therapy and how the treatment plan will progress from working with the therapist to eventual home care. A contract for a set time frame is defined for each patient. Establishing such a contract with time limits creates a better chance for obtaining patient compliance.

In obtaining an initial history, it often occurs that some patients have already received extensive, complete, and thorough therapy over several months. In such patients, additional conservative therapy will probably not be successful and the patient should be so advised.

Diagnosis

As with any illness, a working diagnosis should be established. The diagnosis is continually reviewed for additional diagnoses or secondary conditions. Conditions that can influence complaints—psychological factors (e.g., anxiety or depression), secondary gain, malingering, litigation—should be sought out.

Stages

The choice of treatment will depend upon whether the TOS symptoms are in the acute, subacute, or chronic stage.

Acute Stage: constant pain, reduced ROM, inability to perform activities of daily living

Subacute Stage: constant pain, normal ROM, limited performance of activities of daily living

Chronic Stage: intermittent pain, full ROM, minimal to no interference of performance of activities of daily living

Treatment

Goals

The goals of therapy include these:

1. Relief or control of symptoms
   a. modalities/physical therapy
   b. delayed recovery/additional diagnoses
   c. medication
   d. termination of therapy (weaning)

   2. Long-term maintenance

      a. independent home program

      b. return to activities of daily living, restrictions, and limitations

      c. managing recurrent symptoms

   3. Work capacity evaluation

   4. Participation in activities, sports, and hobbies

Plan of Therapy

Acute and Subacute Stage

The patient should be seen by a physician on a weekly basis for the first six weeks to monitor medication and response to therapy. A program frequency often used is daily therapy for the first week, then therapy three times weekly for three to six weeks. After six weeks, therapy usually changes from passive therapeutic modalities and stretching to active exercises.

After the first few months, patients will fall into three groups: recovered, improved, or unimproved. Recovered patients can be discharged; improved patients are weaned and followed on a home exercise program for a few more months with monthly visits; unimproved patients, depending upon the severity of their symptoms and dysfunction, have the options of learning to live with their symptoms or seeking relief through surgical intervention.

When First Seen Months After Injury

Patients who have received no therapy in the first few months post-injury are managed in the same way as outlined for the acute stage. Therapy is continued until the symptoms show no further improvement and have reached a plateau, as determined subjectively and objectively, for a few weeks.

Chronic Stage

Patients in the chronic stage, who are not candidates for surgery, are managed by a home exercise program and nonaddicting medication.

Control of Symptoms

Modalities

The primary purpose of therapy is to increase the space in the thoracic outlet and reduce neurovascular compression. The first, and possibly the most important, aspect of treatment is correction of postural faults and poor body mechanics. The second aspect involves manual therapy: manipulation and mobilization of sterno- and acromioclavicular joints, scapula, and scalene, trapezius, and pectoral muscles. The third aspect emphasizes stretching of the neck and strengthening of the shoulder girdle.

There are many approaches to therapy, and all usually lead to improvement or resolution of complaints. Progress is monitored by both subjective complaints and objective findings. The therapist may direct the patient to keep a daily diary and record subjective symptoms on a pain scale of 1–10. Objective criteria of improvement can be monitored by increased range of motion (ROM) of neck and shoulders; increased strength, endurance, and workload measured by grip dynamometers and computer programmed instruments (e.g., Cybex, Biodex, BTE); and increased daily activity level at home and work.

Physical therapy, often with the addition of medication, is used to relieve symptoms. At the initial visit with the physical therapist, the frequency of visits and the duration of therapy is discussed with the patient by the therapist, and the time limits established with the physician are reviewed. The modalities available for symptom relief are as follows:

1. Therapeutic modalities of heat, cold, and contrast therapy. Heat usually includes hot packs and ultrasound; cold includes ice packs, ice massage, and fluorimethane sprays (Fig. 9-1).

2. Stretching exercises to improve and maintain ROM parameters.

3. Strengthening exercises for arms, shoulders, and neck. This includes in progression: passive strengthening using electrical stimulation; active strengthen-

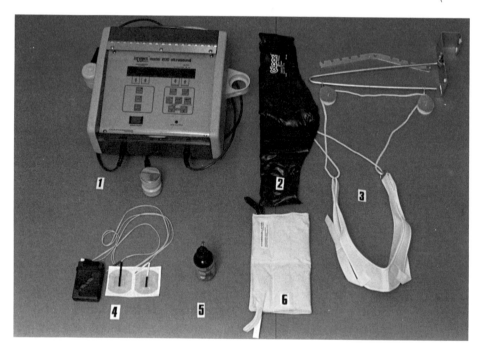

Fig. 9-1.   Common therapeutic modalities. 1: Ultrasound—deep heat to relieve pain and increase circulation to muscles. 2: Cold packs—to relieve pain and increase circulation after pack removal. 3: Cervical traction—to stretch spastic muscles and facet capsules. 4: Transcutaneous nerve stimulation (TNS) unit—to relieve pain and extinguish hypersensitive nerve fibers. 5: Spray and stretch—spray gives temporary pain relief to allow subcutaneous stretching of connective tissue. 6: Hot packs—superficial heat to relieve pain and increase circulation.

ing using multiangle progressive resistive exercises (PRE) with a therapist; and free weights and exercise equipment used independently, with supervision by a therapist. In TOS patients, strengthening is done to shoulder level only, avoiding overhead exercises, to prevent muscle hypertrophy in the shoulder and neck quadrants (see Appendix to this chapter).

4. Medication administered by phonophoresis, iontophoresis, and local injections.

5. Massage, both deep and superficial.

6. Transcutaneous nerve stimulator (TNS unit) (Fig. 9-1).

7. Manipulation and mobilization.

The modalities, as well as stretching and strengthening, are the mainstays of therapy. Cold therapy is used in the acute phase while heat therapy is more effective in the chronic phase. In the acute and subacute stage, alternating heat and cold (contrast therapy) is usually the appropriate choice. Range of motion and progressive resistive exercises are used in all phases. In the acute phase, these are applied gently and cautiously, while in the chronic phase, more vigorous and extensive forms are used. For resistant cases, the other modalities listed above are added.

Delayed Recovery

Ongoing evaluation. When symptoms do not improve, other diagnoses are sought. Evaluation for secondary involvement of additional structures is performed regularly. Additional structures include biceps and rotator cuff tendons and several joints—cervical and dorsal spine, acromioclavicular, shoulder, and temporomandibular joints. Muscles in those areas can develop inflammation or fibrocystic nodules. Spasm of muscles and tension headaches also can occur. Secondary involvement is thought to be the result of compensation by uninvolved muscles and tendons in the same quadrant as the initially injured muscles. Secondary involvement symptoms usually develop one to six weeks after an injury.

Increase in intensity of symptoms. It is common in the first two weeks of therapy for symptoms to increase in intensity due to exacerbation of secondary musculoskeletal problems. When this occurs, additional diagnostic tests and/or review of already performed tests are done to detect other diagnoses. Medications are adjusted to deal with the increased symptoms. Continuous contact between physician, patient, and therapist takes place on a weekly basis to prevent the patient from being discouraged with slow progress in the early weeks. It is emphasized to the patient that slow progress is a normal pattern that will lead to stabilization and, hopefully, to recovery.

Secondary inflammatory conditions. The neck and arm pain caused by TOS can lead to disuse of the upper extremity. This, in turn, is often accompanied by tendinitis, bursitis, and capsulitis in the joints and tendons of the limb. The most frequent triad of involvement is lateral elbow epicondylitis, biceps/rotator cuff tendinitis, and scapular fibromyositis. These associated conditions are treated by the same conservative modalities as are used to control symptoms.

Medication

Drugs, individually or in combination, are chosen to treat specific symptoms. There are four areas in which drugs are beneficial: 1) acute pain, 2) chronic pain with related depression, 3) muscle spasm, and 4) sleep disturbances.

Acute pain. For acute pain, nonaddicting, anti-inflammatory drugs are selected. Narcotics should be avoided because therapy may extend for weeks or months and addiction can occur. Drugs used for acute pain include nonprescription and prescription medications (nonsteroidal anti-inflammatory drugs). In occasional instances, steroids are tried on a short-term basis (two weeks).

Chronic pain and related depression (Somataform Disorder). It is postulated that chronic pain can lead to neurotransmitter imbalance in the central nervous system resulting in a reduction in endorphins. Secondary contributing factors, such as reduction of activities at home or at work, leads to situational depression. These psychological factors, which affect the physical condition of the body, result in weight gain, weight loss, sleep disturbances, and pain throughout the body. The goal of drug therapy is to control pain and reverse depression. The drugs used are the first-to-third generation antidepressants. For chronic pain, anti-inflammatory drugs, including short term steroids, are used.

Muscle spasm. Muscle spasm is treated with muscle relaxers that act at one of three levels: muscle, spinal, or central nervous system. The drugs used are a matter of trial and error.

1. Muscle level: cyclobenzaprine, chloroxazone, dantrolene

2. Spinal level: baclofen

3. Central level: These drugs should be monitored for response and/or side effects on an ongoing basis. If there is no response, drugs should be discontinued in four to six weeks.

      a. phenytoin, carbamazin

      b. benzodiazapen (long-acting)

      c. aprazolam (short-acting)

      d. amantadine (for rigidity)

Sleep disturbance. It is postulated that sleep disturbances are common with chronic pain. They are best managed with mild sedatives that are nonaddicting, have a limited period of action, and have no residual effects. These drugs—e.g., Dalmane, Restoril, and the benzodiazapan group—are used on a short-term basis and are fairly safe. Strong sedatives, such as barbiturates and chloral hydrate, should not be used.

Weaning From Modalities

The maximal therapeutic response is usually reached in six to twelve weeks, which equates to 20–60 patient/therapy contacts. In general, therapy beyond this time has been shown to have little or no effect. Weaning is a transition from clinic and therapist management to home or independent programs. The time required for weaning depends upon the intensity of the TOS symptoms, associated diagnoses, and secondary factors. Extended therapy is frequently required for complicated and multiple areas of involvement, particularly in secondary areas. During the weaning period, the effectiveness of therapy should be evaluated weekly.

Long-Term Maintenance

Independent Home Program and Management of Recurrent Symptoms

Following a supervised course of physical therapy or surgery for TOS, an independent home program is established to manage persistent or recurring symptoms. Home programs address the three fundamental principles of exercise: stretching, strengthening, and range-of-motion. Specific programs are individualized and directed to muscles of the neck, shoulders, arms, and upper back as is appropriate to fit the symptoms. Ideally, home exercise programs are performed twice a day, five days a week, and continue indefinitely to control symptoms and prevent recurrence.

Returning to Activities of Daily Living—Restrictions and Limitations

The goal of therapy is not only to relieve symptoms, but also to return the patient to the functional activities of daily living. Ideally, this means a return to preinjury level of activity, but that is not always possible.

During the last phases of physical therapy, the patient is encouraged to resume normal activities on a graduated basis (with guidance from physician or therapist). When progression is slower than expected, objective muscle testing is employed using instruments capable of measuring specific muscle groups for strength, endurance, efficiency, and workload.

In general, certain events and activities are recognized to cause recurrent symptoms. These include repetitive activities with the hands, working with the arms above the head, and repeated trauma to the neck. From a practical point of view, some patients will return to previous occupations that involve such activities. They should be informed that this increases the likelihood of recurrent symptoms. However, the only way to know with certainty is by trial and error when returning to work, sports, and hobbies.

Modifications based upon occupational, recreational, and sleeping habits should be considered. If possible, patients should avoid carrying heavy objects in the involved hand or over the shoulder. Patients with increased pain at night should avoid sleeping on their stomach or rotating and extending their neck. When sitting, arms should be supported and overhead activity kept to a minimum.

Appropriate Medical Follow-up and Managing Recurrent Symptoms

Recurrent symptoms may be chronic, subacute, or acute. Chronic and subacute symptoms can be managed by home programs and medication. Acute flare-ups are a signal for the patient to seek medical assistance for medication adjustments and/or return to physical therapy.

Recurrent symptoms are defined as follows:

Chronic: intermittent pain associated with an activity, relieved by stopping that activity, and not interfering with daily activities

Subacute: pain elicited by specific activity but not relieved by stopping that activity

Acute: pain elicited by specific activity, not relieved by stopping that activity, and accompanied by a decrease in range-of-motion beyond prior limitation, with little or no response to home program or medication

Prognosis

The prognosis for conservative treatment of TOS depends upon how long symptoms have been present at the time the patient is first seen. Most TOS patients improve on a conservative program. For example, McGough, Pearce, and Byrne treated 1,200 patients for TOS during a five-year period. All patients initially were treated with a conservative program. Only 113 patients, 9%, required surgery.[1]

The results of conservative treatment are better when therapy is started early, when symptoms first begin, rather than several months later. In cases of traumatic TOS, when symptoms have been present for over a year, it is likely that conservative therapy will do little more than provide temporary relief.

It is difficult to fully evaluate the role of conservative therapy on TOS itself because many of the symptoms of pain in the head, neck, and shoulder areas are due to injury of muscles other than the scalenes. Because therapy includes these areas too, improvement in symptoms can be interpreted in many ways.

Work Capacity Evaluation

In the 1940s, the Federal Government published job titles in a dictionary of occupational titles (DOT) and established five work levels (Table 9–1).[2] This dictionary has been revised every several years. Unfortunately, the categories in the DOT did not address functional issues of frequency and cardiovascular endurance; a work capacity classification was still needed. Physicians were receiving requests for such information from patients, employers, vocational counselors, and the legal system. They required impairment evaluation and assignment of restrictions and limitations in the work place, home, athletics, and other activities, but providing these was difficult because there were no objective standards.

In the late 1970s and early 1980s the Federal Government of the United States committed research funds to study bioengineering of the human body (ergonomics). The results of this study by Chaffin established a foundation upon which muscle capacity could be evaluated and applied to the work force.[3] On the basis of the information in the Chaffin study, Matheson expanded the five job

Table 9–1.   Dictionary of Occupational Titles—Work Levels

Work Level	Maximum Lift	Type of Work Load
Sedentary	10 lbs	Occasionally carry small objects
Light	20 lbs	Frequently lift/carry up to 10 lbs
Medium	50 lbs	Frequently lift/carry up to 10 lbs
Heavy	100 lbs	Frequently lift/carry up to 10 lbs
Very Heavy	over 100 lbs	Frequently lift/carry up to 10 lbs

(*From Dictionary of occupational titles, 4th edition; Washington, DC: US Dept. of Labor Employment Training Administration, 1977*)

classification into eight categories that consider the needs for static and dynamic strength and cardiovascular endurance (Table 9–2).[4]

Two types of methods have been developed to evaluate work capacity: direct and indirect. The direct method is a practical approach that includes work simulation and work stations in a free open setting. Examples of direct measurements are the Key[5] and the West[4] systems for work evaluation.

The indirect methods utilize computerized machines to supply the data to permit placing patients in the eight work categories. These machines can measure static and dynamic strength and endurance, provide a validity scale (which tells if the patient is giving his/her best effort consistently), provide an injury pattern, and compare the result to the general population norm for age, gender, height, and weight. Examples of the machines are B200 (200 Technologies Inc, Hillsborough, NC), Cybex (Ronkonkoma, NY), BTE (Baltimore Therapeutic Equipment, Baltimore, MD), ISTU (Isometric Strength Testing Unit, Ann Arbor, MI), KinKom (Kinesiology Komputer, Chattanooga, TN), Biodex (Shirley, NY), and the treadmill.

In returning the patient to work, many jobs do not strictly conform to the *job title* of the DOT. Therefore, a *job description* can be obtained from employer or employee to determine into which of the eight categories the job falls. If there is uncertainty or discrepancy regarding job category, a *job analysis* can be acquired from an independent evaluator, industrial hygienist, or vocational rehabilitation counselor.

Sports and Hobbies

Returning to sports and hobbies is accomplished by gradual introduction of the activity. Those activities that require functioning at or above shoulder level and sports with body contact can aggravate or reinjure the neck by hyperextension. Actions that can lead to inadvertent hyperextension of the neck should be avoided.

Sports can be divided into three categories: low-, medium-, and high-impact. The assignment of sports and activities to impact groups is arbitrary, depending

Table 9–2.   **Physical Demand Characteristics of Work**

Level	Weight Lifted	Frequency of Lift	Walking/Carrying	Typical Energy Required
Sedentary	10 lbs or less	Infrequently	None	1.5 mets
Sedentary-Light	15 lbs	Infrequently	Intermittent self-paced	2.0 mets
	10 lbs or less	Frequently	No load	
Light[a]	20 lbs	Infrequently	2.5 mph. No grade or	
	10 lbs or less	Frequently	slower speed with 10 lbs or less	2.5 mets
Light-Medium	35 lbs	Infrequently	3.0 mph. No grade or	
	20 lbs or less	Frequently	slower speed with 20 lbs or less	3.0 mets
Medium	50 lbs	Infrequently	3.5 mph. No grade or	
	25 lbs or less	Frequently	slower speed with 25 lbs or less	3.5 mets
Medium-Heavy	75 lbs	Infrequently	3.5 mph. No grade with 35 lbs load or	
	35 lbs or less	Frequently	115 lbs wheelbarrow 2.5 mph. No grade	4.5 mets
Heavy	100 lbs	Infrequently	3.5 mph with	6.0 mets
	50 lbs or less	Frequently	50 lbs or less load	
Very Heavy	Over 100 lbs	Infrequently	3.5 mph with	7.5–12.0 mets
	50 to 100 lbs	Frequently	50 lbs or more load	

[a]Even though the weight lifted may be negligible, a job is considered "light" if it requires a significant amount of walking or standing or frequent use of arm and/or leg controls.
(*From Matheson, LN. Work capacity evaluation. Anaheim, CA: Employment Rehabilitation Institute of California; 1160 Gilbert St, 1984*)

upon the level of participation, intensity, and length of action. Examples of assignments are these:

Low-impact sports/hobbies: golf, sedentary fishing, board and card games, painting

Medium-impact sports/hobbies: softball, badminton, bowling, swimming, fly fishing, ceramics, knitting, needle point, crocheting, and other activities of repetitive motion

High-impact sports/hobbies: boxing, football, lacrosse, baseball, tennis, canoeing, wind surfing, skiing, rock climbing, bicycling

To aid in pacing a patient's return to an activity, the activity is simulated on exercise equipment. Grips are enlarged one size, weights are reduced where possible, and the time of performance is gradually increased as tolerated.

Rating Maximal Medical Improvement

Impairment Rating

"Impairment rating" is a medico-legal term that assigns a percentage of medical impairment using a standard guide such as the American Medical Association (AMA) guidelines. The rating can be in terms of either loss of extremity or loss of whole body and is used when there are legal issues to be resolved. Considerations for impairment ratings include the following:

1. pain
2. loss of ROM, active versus passive
3. disfiguration
4. sensory change—neuritis, dysesthesia, hypesthesia
5. dominance

Pain and dominance are not listed as factors in impairment rating in the AMA guidelines but are listed in other guidelines. In TOS patients, they can be significant factors.

Disability Rating

"Disability rating" is a more inclusive medico-legal term than impairment rating. It considers both the medical impairment and vocational issues of functional loss, which include

1. reentry into the work force
2. wage loss
3. access to activities outside the work areas (sports, hobbies, loss of joy of life
4. cost of long term medical care

The final determination of disability rating is a legal act performed through the judicial system. The precise rating will vary, depending upon the legal jurisdiction (state or local) and the standards and customs within that jurisdiction. There may be large differences between the impairment and disability determinations, depending on a variety of factors.

References

1. McGough EC, Pearce MB, Byrne JP. Management of thoracic outlet syndrome. J Ther Card Med 1979; 77:169–174.
2. Dictionary of occupational titles, 4th edition; Washington, DC: US Dept. of Labor Employment Training Administration, 1977.
3. Chaffin DB, Andersson G. Occupational biomechanics. New York: Wiley Inter-science, 1984.
4. Matheson LN. Work capacity evaluation. Anaheim, CA: Employment Rehabilitation Institute of California, 1984.
5. Key G. Key functional assessment policy procedure manual. Minneapolis: Key Functional Associates, 1984.

Appendix

*Stretching and Strengthening Exercises**

General Comments

Progression of exercises depends upon the patient's complaints. In TOS patients, exercises begin with low resistance range of motion and stretching, and all exercises are done to insure the patients ability to perform these in all anatomical planes.

Progressive resistive exercises are added against gravity with progression to weights and/or exercise equipment. Overhead strengthening is avoided to prevent hypertrophy of muscles comprising the thoracic outlet triangle.

Occupational Work-Site Adjustments

Patients are encouraged to maintain their jobs and modify their work environment to minimize symptoms. They can do so by pacing their daily tasks, adjusting body position at their worksite, and adaptive equipment (Fig. 9-2).

TOS patients should be started on all three groups of exercises, for the neck, scapula, and shoulders. Programs are modified on the basis of periodic evaluations. The exercises are described in Figures 9-3 through 9-6.

---

* The exercises were assembled with the assistance of the physical therapists at Rose Medical Center, Presbyterian Hospital, Aurora Presbyterian Hospital, and Veterans Administration Hospital, Denver, Colorado.

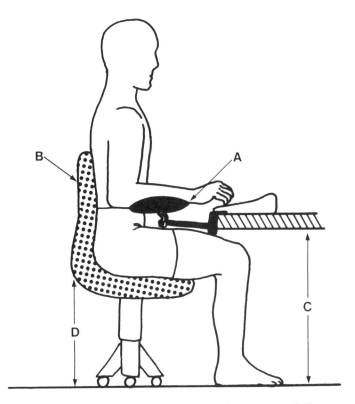

Fig. 9-2.   **A**: Forearm platform, or keyboard wrist rest, is alternative to chair armrests. **B**: Ergonomic chair with back support maintains good posture. **C**: Desk height adjusted to distance of floor to elbow. **D**: Chair height adjusted to permit feet to be flat on floor or slightly elevated and knees at 90 degree flexion to maintain proper sitting posture. Other helpful desk aides include an angulated desk top, adjustable foot rest, and swivel or tilt terminals.

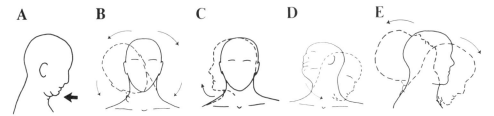

Fig. 9-3.   Neck exercises. **A**: Chin tucks—to stretch and strengthen cervical extensors. **B**: Cervical side-bends—to stretch lateral neck muscles. **C**: Cervical rotation—to stretch neck rotators. **D**: Oblique stretching: combined muscle stretching of the three scalene muscles. **E**: Flexion/extension—to stretch neck supporting muscles.

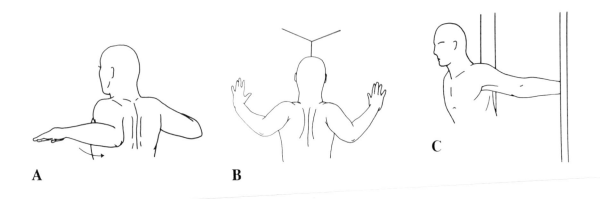

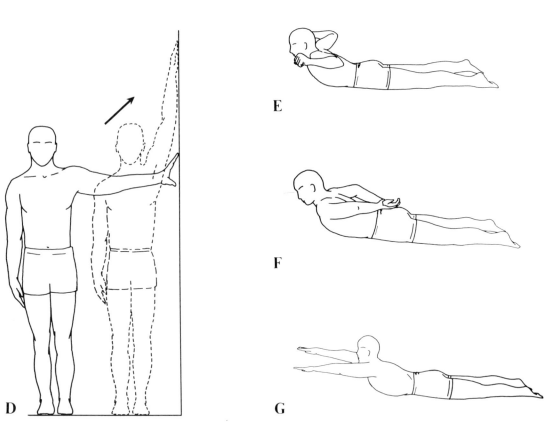

Fig. 9-4.   Scapula exercises. **A**: Scapula adduction—to stretch and strengthen rhomboid and trapezius muscles.
B: Corner stretch—to stretch pectorals and strengthen scapula adductors. **C**: Door jamb stretch—
another way to stretch pectorals and strengthen scapula adductors. **D**: Wall climbing—stretches
latissimus dorsi. **E**: Chicken wing exercises—to stretch and strengthen scapula adductors, back
extensors, and strengthen shoulder muscles with the addition of gravity. **F**: Prone extension—another
way to stretch and strengthen the scapula adductors, back extensors, and shoulder muscles with the
addition of gravity. **G**: Superman extension—a third way to stretch and strengthen the scapula adductors, back extensors, and shoulder muscles with addition of gravity

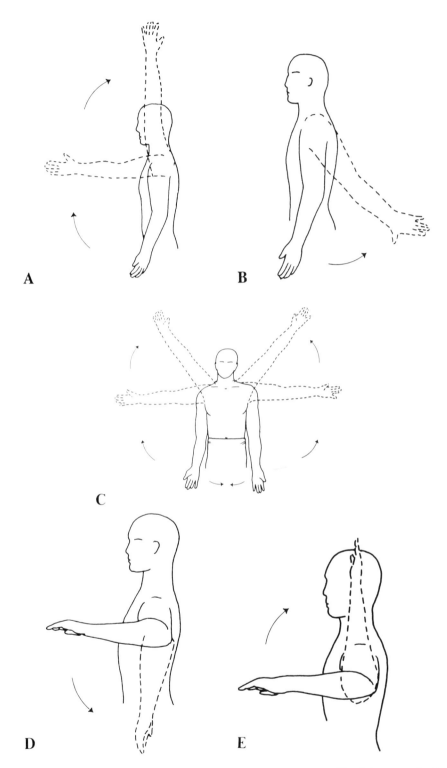

Fig. 9-5.   Shoulder exercises. Range of motion (ROM) in flexion (**A**), extension (**B**), abduction and adduction (**C**), internal rotation (**D**), external rotation (**E**)—to stretch shoulder girdle muscles.

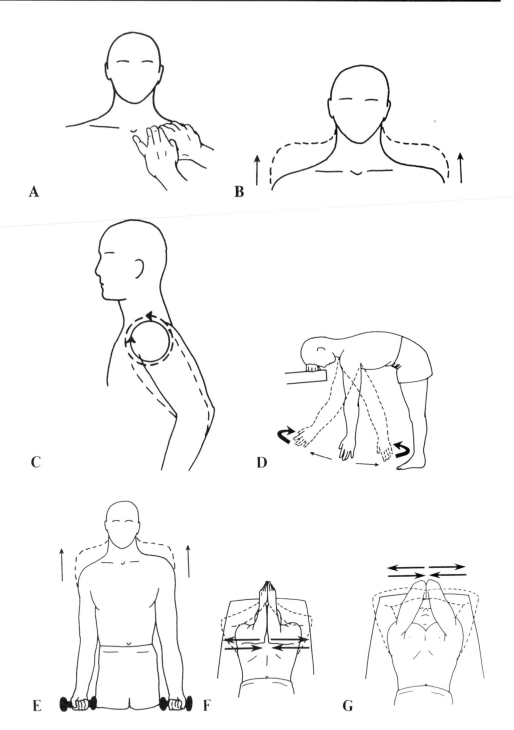

Fig. 9-6.   More shoulder exercises. **A:** Clavicle mobilization—to achieve full mobility of tight joint capsules. **B:** Shoulder shrugs—to loosen upper trapezius muscles. **C:** Shoulder circles (rotation)—to loosen deltoid muscles and shoulder capsule. **D:** Pendulum exercises—to loosen shoulder capsule. **E:** Shoulder elevation—to strengthen shoulder elevators. **F:** Shoulder stretch middle trapezius—to stretch middle trapezius.

10
Surgical Treatment

Richard J. Sanders

Anterior and Middle Scalenectomy

Brachial Plexus Neurolysis for Recurrence After Scalenectomy

First Rib Resection

Dorsal Sympathectomy

Several operations have been used to treat TOS: first rib resection, anterior scalenotomy, anterior and middle scalenectomy, and combinations of scalenectomy and rib resection. To some extent, the choice of procedure depends upon the etiology of TOS. If there are symptoms of venous or arterial compression or if the etiology is an osseous abnormality, operation should include resection of the first rib and/or cervical rib. When there is no evidence of bony involvement and there is a history of neck trauma, scalenectomy will probably be enough.

Vascular involvement requires that the vascular complication, in addition to the osseous abnormality, be corrected. Evidence of a subclavian artery aneurysm or distal emboli to the arm should be treated by subclavian artery repair or replacement, in addition to removal of the cervical and/or first rib.

Symptoms of venous obstruction—arm swelling, aching, and/or cyanosis— are indications to remove the first rib up to the costochondral junction. In addition, the subclavian vein should be examined to detect evidence of extrinsic pressure that can be relieved by dividing the costoclavicular ligament. In cases of axillosubclavian venous occlusion, either a venous bypass or venous endovenectomy may be necessary.

The techniques of those procedures are described in the paragraphs that follow. The operations for vascular repair are described in the chapters on arterial and venous TOS, Chapters 14 and 15.

Anterior and Middle Scalenectomy (Fig. 10-1, A through L)*

Positioning the Patient; Making the Incision (Fig. 10-1A)

Following general anesthesia and endotracheal intubation, a rolled towel is placed under the dorsal spine with the towel running vertically, parallel to the spine. This placement extends the neck and lowers the shoulders. The patient should be draped in such a way that the shoulder of the operated side can be elevated and brought forward during the operation, a maneuver that can help lift the clavicle out of the way to improve subclavicular exposure. The skin incision is made 2–3 cm above and parallel to the clavicle, in a skin fold if possible. The incision begins 1 cm lateral to the midline and extends 8–10 cm.

Elevating the Skin Flap (Fig. 10-1B)

Upper and lower skin flaps are elevated in the plane immediately above the sternocleidomastoid (SCM) muscle. Small nerves may be identified in this plane and should be preserved if possible. Injury to them results in numbness and paresthesia above and below the incision.

* (*Figures 10-1A to 10-1I and 10-2A to 10-2G are modified from Sanders RJ, Raymer S: The supraclavicular approach to scalenectomy and first rib resection: description of technique. J Vasc Surg 1985; 5:751–6. With permission.*)

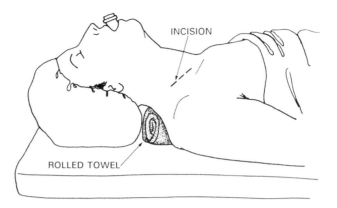

Fig. 10-1A.   Position with rolled towel or sandbag running vertically under the dorsal spine. Incision is 8–10 cm long and 2–3 cm above clavicle.

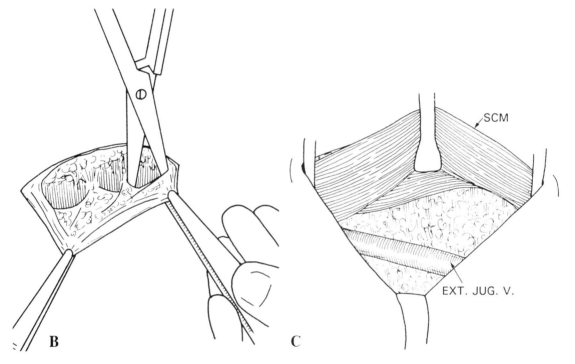

Fig. 10-1B.   Upper and lower skin flaps are elevated as far as possible. The plane of dissection is immediately superficial to the sternocleidomastoid muscle (SCM).

Fig. 10-1C.   Lateral edge of SCM is mobilized the length of the incision, at least 5 cm, and is retracted with a small Richardson retractor.

Mobilizing SCM (Fig. 10-1C)

The lateral edge of SCM is mobilized over as long a length as possible, at least 5 cm, and retracted medially with a small Richardson retractor. Although some surgeons advocate division of the clavicular head of SCM, mobilizing and retracting it medially is more physiologic and preserves the muscle to cover the area postoperatively. Only on rare occasions has it been necessary to divide a portion of this muscle.

The external jugular vein lies near the lateral edge of SCM. If the vein's position prevents good exposure of the lateral edge of SCM, enough of the vein is dissected free to allow safe dissection of the muscle. The vein is then gently retracted laterally. Division of the external jugular vein should be avoided, particularly in thin women, because the ligated end may produce an undesirable prominent bulge in the neck.

Dividing the Omohyoid Muscle (Fig. 10-1D)

The omohyoid muscle usually lies in the scalene fat pad below SCM. The omohyoid is divided and no attempt is made to resuture it on closing.

Dissecting the Scalene Fat Pad (Fig. 10-1E)

The anterior scalene muscle is located by palpating a round bulge below the scalene fat pad. A hole is made in the fat pad by blunt dissection over the lateral edge of the anterior scalene muscle. If the internal jugular vein comes into view, the dissection has proceeded too far medially.

Freeing the Phrenic Nerve (Fig. 10-1F)

The anterior scalene muscle lies exposed beneath the fat pad with the phrenic nerve on its surface, usually on the medial edge. The nerve passes obliquely across the anterior scalene muscle, usually running from the lateral side of the muscle cephalad, crossing the muscle, to the medial side caudad. The nerve is freed on its

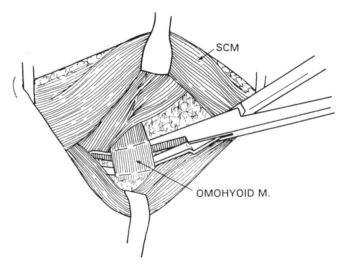

Fig. 10-1D.   Omohyoid muscle is divided with an electric cautery and the ends retract. No attempt is made to reapproximate muscle when closing the wound.

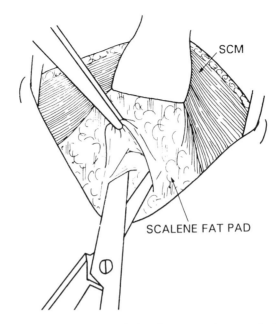

Fig. 10-1E.   Scalene fat pad is dissected bluntly over lateral edge of anterior scalene muscle. It is retracted medially and laterally with Richardson retractors.

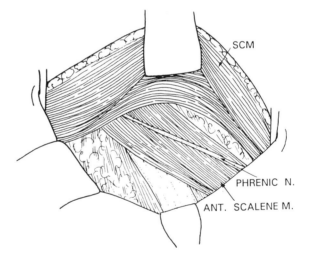

Fig. 10-1F.   Anterior scalene muscle is carefully cleaned of connective tissue and phrenic nerve is identified on its surface. The nerve usually runs from lateral to medial as it approaches the clavicle. Phrenic nerve is freed on its lateral side only. Lifting SCM upwards pulls the phrenic away from anterior scalene without touching the nerve.

lateral side only. By lifting the SCM muscle and medial portion of the fat pad with a small Richardson retractor, the phrenic nerve can be elevated without touching the nerve. No suture is placed around the nerve because it can lead to nerve injury. The phrenic nerve is never touched with a retractor because even minimal retraction can cause temporary diaphragmatic palsy.

Dividing the Anterior Scalene Muscle (Fig. 10-1G, H)

The phrenic nerve is easily spared when it lies on the medial edge of the anterior scalene muscle, but is in jeopardy when it lies on the lateral edge. In the latter case, the phrenic is best left alone while the anterior scalene is carefully dissected medial to the nerve or is pulled as far lateral as possible with an umbilical tape. To pass the tape, a right angle hemostat is passed in the plane below the muscle and immediately above the plexus. Because defining this plane can be difficult, three or four repeat passes are often made, each successive passage including a few more muscle fibers than the previous one. When the phrenic nerve lies in the middle or on the lateral side of the anterior scalene, it is included with the muscle in the first pass, then excluded by a second pass under nerve but superficial to muscle.

The anterior scalene is divided as close to its first rib insertion as is safe. The subclavian artery lies behind the muscle but it can lie low, near the rib, or high, 3 or 4 cm above the rib. If its precise location has not been identified prior to sectioning the muscle, the deepest muscle fibers must be divided carefully to avoid injuring the artery. Occasionally a right angle hemostat is used to separate muscle fibers from the artery. However, caution must be used because the point of the instrument can damage the artery. Accessory phrenic nerves (incidence, about 13%) usually run on the lateral side of the anterior scalene and are easily injured.

Should significant venous bleeding occur when dissecting below the clavicle,

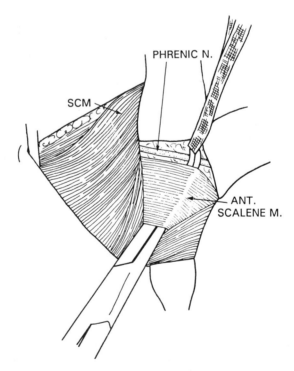

Fig. 10-1G.   Umbilical tape is passed around anterior scalene muscle by dissecting the plane immediately superficial to C-5, C-6, and C-7. This permits lateral traction, pulling the muscle away from phrenic nerve.

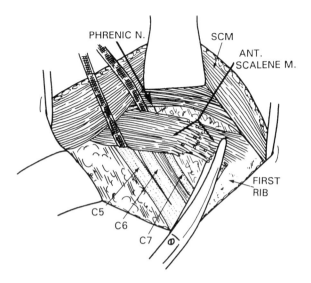

Fig. 10-1H.   Anterior scalene is divided as close to first rib as safety permits. After cutting a few muscle fibers, the scissors pulls those fibers upwards to expose the next layer of muscle fibers below. Subclavian artery lies immediately below anterior scalene.

the subclavian vein may have been injured. If it cannot be repaired easily, bleeding is controlled by tamponading the vein against the clavicle with a retractor while scalenectomy and first rib resection are completed. The subclavian vein is then exposed through a new, infraclavicular incision and an assistant's finger controls the bleeding while the surgeon repairs the vein from the supraclavicular incision.

Dividing the Upper End of the Anterior Scalene Muscle (Fig. 10-1I)

At this point in the operation, the surgeon is usually standing so he/she can look caudad, down toward the first rib. The surgeon's position should now change to look cephalad for the remainder of the scalenectomy.

After the anterior scalene has been divided at the first rib, the muscle is held by its divided end and lifted upwards so the adhesions of the muscle to the C-5, C-6, and C-7 nerves and to the middle scalene muscle can be freed. The upper end of the anterior scalene muscle is divided as close to the transverse processes as possible, taking care to avoid injury to the phrenic nerve and the nerves of the brachial plexus. Sometimes it is safer to remove the muscle in fragments.

Completing Anterior Scalenectomy (Fig. 10-1J)

After removing the anterior scalene, the C-5 and C-6 nerves are usually observed forming the superior trunk of the plexus and C-7 lies alone. All loose muscle fibers are removed from the surface of the nerves without disturbing the nerve sheaths. In some patients, the most medial fibers of the middle scalene muscle are found medial to C-7, above the subclavian artery. Those medial fibers can be removed through that plane. Bleeding from small veins is common and is

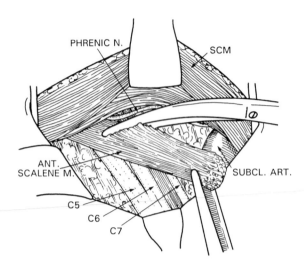

Fig. 10-1I. Origin of anterior scalene is divided as high as possible, near the transverse processes. The phrenic nerve and nerves of the brachial plexus are continually observed and protected. Muscle fibers that cannot be reached without stretching the nerves are left behind.

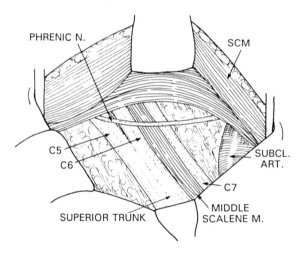

Fig. 10-1J. Anterior scalenectomy is complete. The field includes the phrenic nerve; C-5 and C-6, which have usually fused forming the upper trunk of the brachial plexus; portions of middle scalene lying between C-6 and C-7; and sometimes the subclavian artery in the lower field.

controlled either by mosquito hemostats left on vessels for a few minutes and then removed or by a bipolar cautery. Using an open electric cautery in this area carries the risk of a spark permanently injuring nearby nerves.

Beginning Middle Scalenectomy (Fig. 10-1K)

The main portion of the middle scalene muscle is approached by first gently mobilizing C-5 and C-6 laterally and medially over the length of the field. This will prevent stretching the nerves when the middle scalene is excised. The suprascapu-

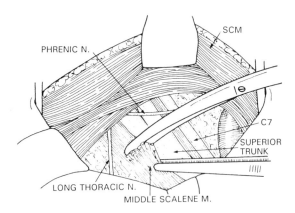

Fig. 10-1K.   After extensively mobilizing C-5 and C-6 on both lateral and medial sides, middle scalene muscle is excised, a few fibers at a time. Long thoracic nerve is sought in belly of middle scalene and spared. Only muscle fibers medial to long thoracic need be excised.

lar nerve, going to the supraspinatus muscle, is usually seen in the lower portion of the field. Traction on this nerve may cause postoperative pain over the scapula.

Middle scalene fibers are found posterior, lateral, and medial to C-5, C-6, C-7, and C-8. Middle scalenectomy is begun by dividing a few fibers at a time. A heavy, smooth, and wide forceps is used to grasp a few muscle bundles. If the shoulder jumps when the muscle is squeezed, the forceps bite probably includes a portion of the long thoracic nerve. The nerve should be isolated before that bite of muscle is cut. Usually, only a single branch of the C-5, C-6, and C-7 contributions to the long thoracic nerve is found in the belly of the middle scalene muscle but occasionally a second nerve is identified. The position of the long thoracic nerve varies, but it is usually found behind the C-5 nerve root.

The middle scalene is divided down to the neck of the first rib, often 2 to 3 cm below C-5. As much as possible of the bulk of the muscle is removed. If a cervical rib is present, it is found in the midst of the middle scalene muscle and excised. The fibers lying behind the plexus can be removed with the aid of a right angle clamp until C-8 is seen clearly.

Excising Middle Scalene Muscle (Fig. 10-1L)

In many cases, the medial portion of the middle scalene muscle is easier to remove through the space between C-6 and C-7. This space is closer to the muscle fibers and using it reduces the amount of stretching on C-5 and C-6. It is unnecessary to remove the middle scalene muscle fibers lying lateral to the long thoracic nerve as these also lie lateral to the first rib.

At this point, anterior and middle scalenectomy is complete. If first rib resection is not to be performed, the operation terminates here. A closed suction drain is left in the wound, a single suture approximates the scalene fat pad, and the wound is closed with subcutaneous and subcuticular absorbable sutures.

If first rib removal is to be done, the steps for supraclavicular first rib resection are shown in Figure 10-2, A through G.

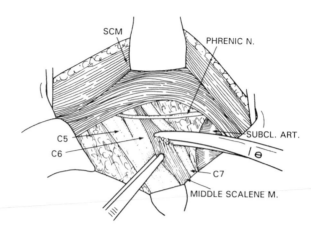

Fig. 10-1L.   The plane between C-6 and C-7 is also used to remove medial portions of middle scalene muscle.

Brachial Plexus Neurolysis for Recurrence After Scalenectomy

Neurolysis is performed through the same supraclavicular approach that was used for the earlier scalenectomy. Skin flaps are elevated and the lateral edge of SCM is mobilized and retracted medially. The scalene fat pad may be loose or may be scarred and tight from the previous operation. The fat pad is gently spread until the nerves of the brachial plexus come into view. Assuming a complete anterior scalenectomy was performed previously, there should be no muscle interposed between fat pad and nerves.

Dissection begins laterally, where C-5 and C-6 are often fused as the superior trunk of the plexus. A fine curved hemostat and pediatric right angle hemostat are excellent instruments with which to free scar tissue from nerve. The anterior surfaces of C-5, C-6, and C-7 are freed first. The phrenic nerve is buried in scar tissue and difficult to identify. It is assumed that the phrenic nerve lies medially, and no attempt is made to dissect it from the scar tissue for fear of injuring it. Obviously, if the phrenic nerve is seen, it is mobilized enough to protect it. As dissection of the brachial plexus proceeds from lateral to medial, if the phrenic nerve has not been identified, vertical running fibers are tested with a nerve stimulator to see if they are the phrenic nerve. Once C-7 has been freed, the operation does not proceed further medially in the plane anterior to the brachial plexus.

After freeing C-5, C-6, and C-7, the dissection moves lateral and deep to C-5, looking for the neck of the first rib, if it is still evident by x-ray. This rib segment is dissected free and excised. A Raney neurosurgical rongeur, a duck bill rongeur, and an Urschell first rib rongeur are used, as needed, to remove the posterior remnant of the rib, back to its articulation with the transverse process. Safe exposure of the neck of the rib usually requires mobilizing the lateral edge of C-5 and C-6 to their full extent so they can be gently pushed medially and not damaged.

Scar tissue is next removed from behind C-5, C-6, and C-7, the area of the middle scalene muscle. Any portion of the muscle that has remained from previous surgery is also removed. The long thoracic nerve is in this area, deep to C-5, in the unresected portions of the middle scalene muscle. This nerve is usually identified and preserved. However, if the long thoracic nerve is not easily identified, additional efforts to find it are not made routinely.

Scar tissue around C-8 is encountered medial and posterior to C-7. It is removed if it can be done with good vision and without stretching C-5, C-6, or C-7. If these nerves will be stretched in the attempt to see C-8, the procedure is terminated without dissecting C-8. When a wide space exists between C-6 and C-7 (Fig. 10-1L), this plane can be used to free C-8 instead of the plane lateral to C-5. The wound is closed in the same manner as the original scalenectomy wound. A suction drain is left below the plexus, the scalene fat pad is approximated over the nerves, and skin is closed with a running subcuticular suture.

First Rib Resection

There are six routes through which the first rib can be removed: posterior, transaxillary, supraclavicular, infraclavicular, transthoracic, or through the bed of the resected clavicle. The location of the clavicle is the reason for so many choices. Resecting the clavicle is the easiest approach to the first rib, but the clavicle's removal can result in significant cosmetic defects over the chest wall. Therefore, other routes have been developed: superior, inferior, posterior, or lateral to the clavicle in order to avoid its removal.

The fact that there are several choices usually means that no single one is ideal in all cases. This is certainly true for first rib resection because the relationship between clavicle and first rib is quite variable. When exposure through one route is extremely difficult, an alternative approach may prove easier. For example, a first rib that lies well above the clavicle may be very difficult to remove from the transaxillary approach but very easy to remove through a supraclavicular approach. Likewise, when the clavicle lies well above the rib, it may be difficult to remove the rib supraclavicularly but quite easy through a transaxillary or infraclavicular approach. Unfortunately, there is no way, preoperatively, to know with certainty which route will be easiest.

Procedures Common to All Techniques of First Rib Resection

Although there are several approaches for first rib resection, wound closure, drainage requirements, and postoperative care are the same. Once the rib has been resected, the anesthesiologist is asked to expand the lung. This will help identify holes in the pleura as well as force out of the pleural space any air that entered through the hole. When the pleura is intact, the lung is seen moving directly beneath the parietal pleura. A small tube, 3–5 mm in diameter with multiple holes, is left in the bed of the resected rib and brought out the corner of the wound or through a separate small stab wound. The drain is connected to closed suction and the tube sutured to the skin to prevent its accidental removal. If the pleura has been opened, no attempt is made to suture it closed because the pleura tears so easily. A straight catheter, 18–20 French, can be left in the pleural space and brought out the corner of the wound. After the wound has been sutured closed, air is aspirated through it and the tube removed. The closed suction drain remains in the wound for 12 to 48 hours. It can remove blood as well as residual air trapped in the wound or pleural space.

A chest tube (20–36 French) is not used unless the lung has been injured (which is extremely rare). A portable sitting chest x-ray is obtained within one hour of surgery. Pneumothorax of under 20% is left alone while one greater than 30% is needle aspirated through the third anterior interspace. A chest tube is rarely needed. Its indications are these: failure of the lung to expand after aspiration; reaccumulation of air following aspiration; or a significant hemothorax. Open drains, such as Penrose type, are never used because a pneumothorax can develop if a small hole is left in the pleura.

Supraclavicular Approach (Fig. 10-2, A through G)

Supraclavicular rib resection is sometimes called anterior first rib resection to differentiate it from rib resection through the posterior or transaxillary approach. However, the term anterior first rib resection is ambiguous because there are two anterior approaches: supraclavicular and infraclavicular. Since the term anterior does not differentiate between the two, the terms supra- or infraclavicular should be used for clarity.

Prior to supraclavicular first rib resection, the anterior and middle scalene muscles are removed as described in the preceding section and Figure 10-1, A through L.

Beginning Rib Resection (Fig. 10-2A)

Once scalenectomy is complete, removal of the rib begins by freeing the medial and lateral intercostal muscle attachments with an Overholt No. 1 rib elevator (Fig. 10-2A; see Figure 10-3A for instruments). The right-angled tip of this instrument encircles the lateral edge of the first rib and the elevator is passed anteriorly and posteriorly until all muscle attachments are divided. The right-angled tip is then carefully inserted over the medial edge of the rib, which is freed in a similar fashion. An index finger passes above the rib, from posterior to anterior, and muscle attachments to the top of the rib are freed. In performing this maneuver, it is important to keep the fingernail against the rib and be aware of the cords of the brachial plexus lying above the finger.

A suction tip is used to gently retract C-5 and C-6 and a Raney rongeur transects the neck of the first rib in several small bites. Injury to C-5, C-6, or C-7 is most likely to occur during this step if the nerve roots are retracted too vigorously.

Smoothing the Posterior Rib Stump (Fig. 10-2B)

After the posterior rib has been transected, the posterior remnant of the rib is resected until the line of rib removal is flush with the transverse process. Because C-8 and T-1 nerve roots often touch the neck of the rib in this area, the jaws of the rongeur must be visualized during this maneuver. If visualization is poor, it is best to leave this small posterior stump of rib rather than risk nerve injury.

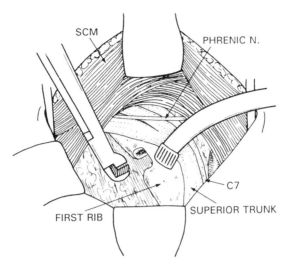

Fig. 10-2A. After medial and lateral edges of first rib have been freed with an Overholt No. 1 elevator, suction tip gently retracts nerves as Raney rongeur transects neck of first rib in a few small bites.

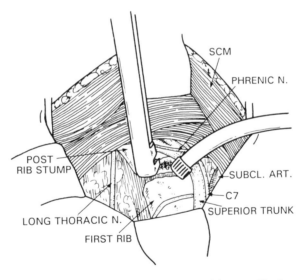

Fig. 10-2B. After rib is totally divided, the posterior stump is smoothed and shortened back to transverse process with Raney rongeur.

Arterial bleeding is sometimes encountered just beneath the neck of the rib and is controlled with a metal clip or a bipolar cautery. The transverse cervical or subscapular artery and vein may lie at this level in the belly of the middle scalene muscle (these arteries may also run above or below the anterior scalene muscle). When seen, the arteries are divided and ligated. If significant bleeding occurs when the middle scalene muscle is divided, the cause is usually an injury to one of these vessels. Bleeding is controlled by finger pressure, the use of a small tipped oral suction, and careful isolation of the bleeding vessel. Once the proximal end of the vessel is ligated, the distal end should be sought and also ligated to avoid postoperative bleeding.

Freeing the Rib From Pleura (Fig. 10-2C)

The remainder of the rib is mobilized by index finger dissection beginning posterior to the rib. The right-angled end of the first rib elevator lifts the medial corner of the rib to widen the space for the finger. Moving from posterior to anterior, the rib is freed from the pleura. In this manner, the finger can free the rib to below the subclavian artery. If brisk bleeding occurs at this stage, it is usually a torn transverse cervical or suprascapular artery or vein. It should be handled as described above.

Tearing Intercostal Muscle Fibers (Fig. 10-2D)

The intercostal muscle fibers are torn by forceful pulling of the index finger just lateral to the edge of the rib. In muscular patients, this maneuver is difficult. If a few fibers resist strongly, they can be left for the moment. They will be easier to divide after the anterior rib end has been transected.

Transecting the Rib (Fig. 10-2E)

Complete mobilization of the anterior end of the first rib is accomplished by inserting an index finger around the medial edge of the rib anterior and inferior to the subclavian artery. From this position, the finger can sweep the underside of the rib to free it from the pleura up to the costochondral junction. Prior to inserting a finger in this area, the subclavian artery should be seen and mobilized, if necessary, to avoid stretching or injuring it.

When the rib is free of all attachments, the anterior portion is divided medial and inferior to the subclavian artery with an angled, duckbill rongeur. Because the clavicle lies anterior and superior to the front of the first rib, this step can be dif-

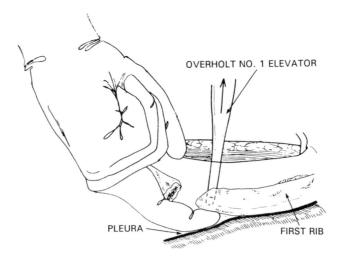

Fig. 10-2C.   Overholt No. 1 elevator lifts the posterior corner of divided rib as index finger frees pleura from posterior surface of rib. Keeping finger against rib at all times usually avoids entering pleural space.

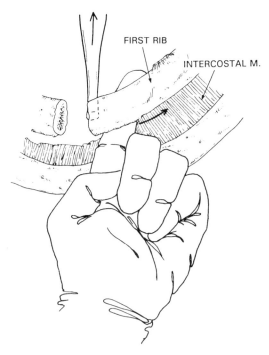

Fig. 10-2D. Finger dissection continues by tearing intercostal muscles from their attachment to lateral edge and underside of rib. Upper surface of rib is also freed of all attachments.

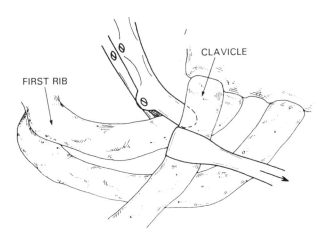

Fig. 10-2E. Field of exposure is changed. Narrow Richardson retractor (4–5 cm long) elevates clavicle, protecting subclavian vein and exposing anterior rib. Finger dissection completes freeing underside of anterior rib from pleura by passing finger below subclavian artery under rib. Artery is freed from rib if necessary. Duckbill rongeur is used to transect anterior rib as medial as possible, which is usually about 2 cm from the costochondral junction. Anterior rib is smoothed with Urschel first rib rongeur.

ficult. A one-and-a-half-inch long, narrow Richardson retractor, positioned below the subclavian vein and clavicle, is used to pull these structures upward, both for exposure and to protect the vein. The angled rongeur is positioned under direct vision, but the cutting tip frequently cannot be seen. Additional exposure can sometimes be achieved by pulling the ipsilateral shoulder upwards, off the table, to raise the clavicle anteriorly. When exposure is still too difficult, an infraclavicular incision can be made and the anterior part of the rib removed through the second incision. The infraclavicular incision is described in the section that follows.

It rarely is possible to remove the medial 1–2 cm of the first rib through the supraclavicular route because this part of the rib is usually unreachable safely through this approach. However, experience has shown that this portion of the rib can be left behind without sequelae. It is usually at least 1 cm away from the nearest nerve of the brachial plexus.

Removing the Rib (Fig. 10-2F)

Once the rib has been divided posteriorly and anteriorly, it is removed by traction on the posterior end. Occasionally, the rib can be delivered anteriorly and removed from below the subclavian artery. However, delivery of the anterior end should be abandoned in favor of the posterior end if any traction is necessary, because traction on the anterior end can damage the subclavian artery. As the rib is delivered into the wound, any remaining muscle attachments are torn or cut.

Closing the Wound (Fig. 10-2G)

After positioning a suction drain beneath the plexus above the pleura, the fat pad is approximated, the platysma muscle reunited, and the skin closed with a subcuticular absorbable suture. The end of this running suture is tied to one of the ends of a subcutaneous suture so that the knot is buried inside the wound.[1]

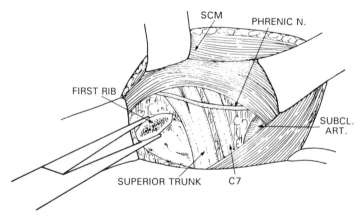

Fig. 10-2F.   Once anterior end is divided, rib is delivered into wound with a Kocher clamp posteriorly, from under plexus. Occasionally the rib is removed anteriorly, but this route is less safe for fear of injuring subclavian artery.

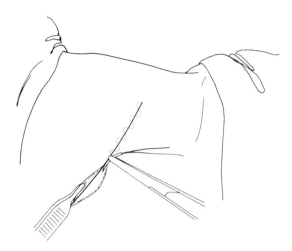

Fig. 10-2G. Wound closure begins by placing suction drain below plexus and approximating scalene fat pad with a single suture. Platysma muscle is approximated with three or four sutures and the skin closed with running subcuticular absorbable suture.

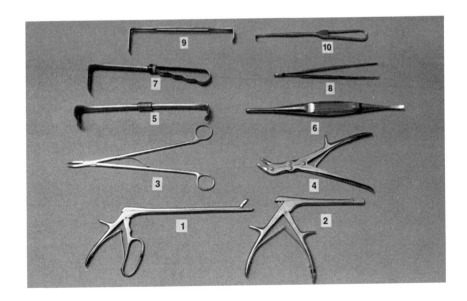

Fig. 10-3A. Instruments used for supraclavicular scalenectomy and first rib resection. 1: Urschel first rib rongeur—used for trimming the anterior stump of the rib below the clavicle. Also used in transaxillary rib resection to trim and shorten the posterior stump. 2: Raney neurosurgical rongeur. 3: Medium size hemoclip applier. 4: Duckbill orthopedic rongeur. 5: Small double-ended Richardson retractor. 6: Overholt No. 1 first rib elevator. 7: Four to five cm long, thin Richardson retractor. 8: Nine-inch-long, wide, smooth forceps for grasping muscle without tearing it. 9: Army-navy retractor. 10: Vein retractor. (Fig. 10-3 continues on next page).

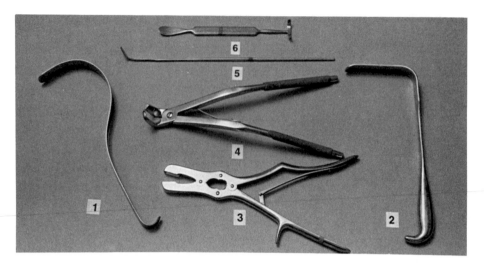

Fig. 10-3B.   Additional instruments used for transaxillary first rib resection. **1:** Narrow Deaver retractor. **2:** Simon-Heaney vaginal retractor for lifting pectoral muscles. The tip should be positioned over the second rib. **3:** Sauerbruch rib rongeur. **4:** Roos right-angled rib cutter. **5:** Roos plexus retractor. **6:** Periosteal elevator (this is a Matson, but many others will do).

Infraclavicular Approach[2] *(Fig. 10-4, A through I)*

Making the Incision *(Fig. 10-4A)*

A 10–15 cm skin incision is made about 4 cm below the center of the clavicle (Fig. 10-4A). The medial edge is 4–5 cm from the midline. The fascia over the pectoralis major muscle is opened and the muscle is split in the direction of its fibers. Ideally, the avascular plane between the sternal and clavicular heads of origin of the pectoralis major muscle is opened. However, if this plane cannot be found, any plane running parallel to the muscle fibers can be used. With retractors spreading the pectoralis major muscle, finger dissection is used to identify the lateral edge of the first rib.

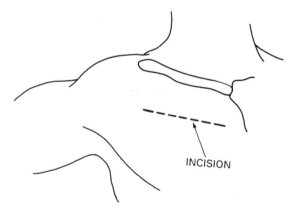

INCISION

Fig. 10-4A.   Subclavicular rib resection begins with a 10–15 cm skin incision 4 cm below the clavicle. Subcutaneous tissue is divided and pectoralis major muscle split in the direction of its fibers.

Dividing Intercostal Ribs (Fig. 10-4B)

The intercostal muscles below the rib are divided, with the scissors kept as close to the rib as possible (Fig. 10-4B).

Freeing the Rib From the Pleura (Fig. 10-4C)

A No. 1 Overholt periosteal elevator is used to free the underside of the rib from the pleura. The plane beneath the rib is opened from the lateral to the medial side of the rib. With the right angle pointing upward, the right-angled end of the elevator is advanced under the rib until it engages the medial edge of the rib. The elevator is passed medially and laterally beneath the rib, cleaning the medial edge of the rib and freeing more of the intercostals on the lateral edge.

Transecting the Anterior Scalene Muscle (Fig. 10-4D)

The anterior scalene muscle is encountered on the upper medial edge of the rib and transected. The subclavian vein will be noted to lie just anterior to the muscle,

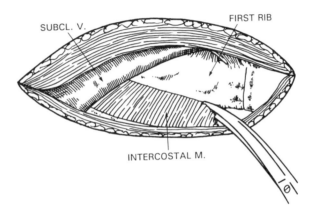

Fig. 10-4B.   Intercostal muscles are divided below inferolateral edge of first rib.

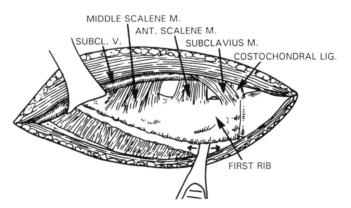

Fig. 10-4C.   First the smooth end of the No. 1 Overholt rib elevator is used to carefully free rib from pleura; then right-angled end of elevator is passed under rib to engage medial edge and free remaining pleural attachments with a back and forth movement of the elevator.

the subclavian artery posterior to it, and C-8 and T-1 nerves near the artery. These structures may be gently retracted upward with a finger or retractor.

Dividing the Middle Scalene Muscle (Fig. 10-4E)

The middle scalene muscle is divided on top of the rib and more intercostal muscles are divided.

Dividing the Costochondral Ligament (Fig. 10-4F)

The costochondral ligament is divided. Sharp dissection with a knife is often more precise than a scissors in this tight corner.

Dividing and Removing the Rib (Fig. 10-4G, H)

The rib is divided with a rib shears at the costochondral junction, or as close to it as possible. The end of the rib is grasped with a firm instrument, and the rib

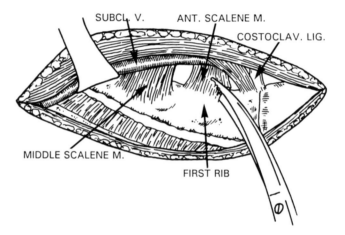

Fig. 10-4D.   Anterior scalene muscle is transected as far away from rib as possible. Subclavian vein is retracted upwards.

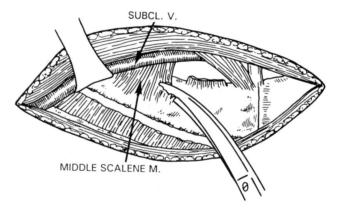

Fig. 10-4E.   Middle scalene muscle is divided on upper surface of rib. Its attachment is about 3 cm long. Remaining intercostal muscles are also divided keeping scissors close to rib to avoid injuring long thoracic nerve, which is seldom seen through this approach.

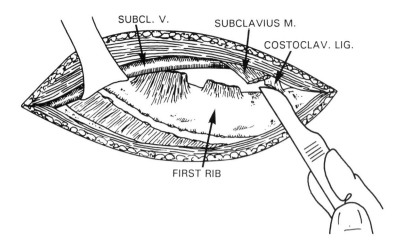

Fig. 10-4F.   Subclavius muscle and costoclavicular ligament are sharply divided at costochondral junction. Subclavian vein must be visualized and avoided.

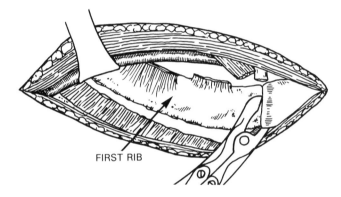

Fig. 10-4G.   Rib is divided with bone cutter or rongeur at costochondral junction. In cases of venous obstruction, a portion of cartilage may also be removed if necessary to decompress vein.

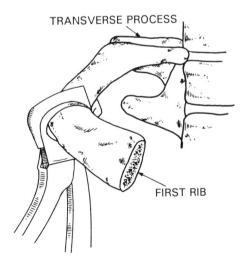

Fig. 10-4H.   Posterior end of rib is transected as far posteriorly as is safe. This usually leaves a 2–3 cm posterior stump behind.

pulled caudad. The remaining intercostal muscles on the lateral edge of the rib are divided, 1–2 cm at a time.

The posterior extent of the dissection varies from patient to patient depending upon the exposure provided by the position of the clavicle. Manipulating the shoulder and elevating the arm may improve the depth of exposure. The rib is transected posteriorly as far back as safety will permit. The tip of the shears must be visualized to be sure no nerve is entrapped in the tip. Once the rib is removed, additional posterior rib can be removed with a rongeur. A ribbon retractor can be used to depress the pleura. It is usually difficult to safely remove the posterior 2–3 cm of rib through this approach. However, experience has shown (in spite of admonishments to the contrary) that leaving a posterior stump of this length is usually not a problem.

Closing the Incision (Fig. 10-41)

Once the rib has been removed, the anterior end at the costal cartilage is smoothed. In patients with histories of hand swelling or venous obstruction, and when the subclavian vein appears to be pinched by the costoclavicular ligament, the ligament is divided. A portion of the cartilage may also be removed if it appears to be compressing the vein. The incision is closed with subcutaneous and subcuticular sutures. It is unnecessary to reapproximate the pectoralis muscle.

Combined Supra- and Infraclavicular Approach

Combining supra- and infraclavicular exposure may be the safest way to remove the entire first rib from the transverse process to the costochondral junction. The reason is that the supraclavicular approach provides excellent exposure of the neck of the rib back to the transverse process, but poor exposure of the anterior end of the rib. Conversely, the infraclavicular approach provides ideal exposure of the costochondral junction, but poor exposure of the neck of the rib. Combining the two incisions provides the best feature of each incision. In addition, the supraclavicular approach permits complete removal of the anterior and middle

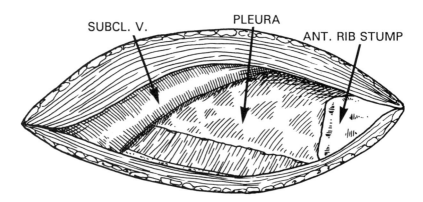

Fig. 10-41.   Rib resection is complete. Pleural surface is exposed. Incision is closed with subcutaneous and subcuticular sutures. It is unnecessary to reapproximate pectoralis major muscle.

scalene muscles, something that cannot be done through either the infraclavicular or transaxillary approach.

The combined approach should begin with the supraclavicular skin incision, anterior and middle scalenectomy, and division of the first rib as described under the supraclavicular approach (Figs. 10-1, A through L and 10-2, A through D). If the first rib can be divided safely below the subclavian artery, anterior to the passage of the brachial plexus (Fig. 10-2E), nothing further need be done. However, if dividing the rib anteriorly cannot be done safely, the infraclavicular incision is made either below the clavicle or by extending the medial corner of the supraclavicular incision vertically, over the sternum.*

The anterior part of the rib is then exposed as described in the previous section (Fig. 10-4, B and C) and the anterior end of the first rib is divided at the costochondral junction with good exposure (Fig. 10-4, F and G). The rib can easily be removed through either the infraclavicular or supraclavicular incision.

Transaxillary Approach[3] (Fig. 10-5, A through J)

Positioning the Patient (Fig. 10-5A)

Following intratracheal anesthesia, the patient is positioned so that the side to be operated upon is elevated to 60 degrees if the surgeon elects to stand during the operation or to 30 degrees if the surgeon prefers to sit. The ipsilateral hand and arm are suspended with wide adhesive tape on an IV pole; skin preparation includes the arm, elbow, and midforearm; the IV pole and arm are covered individually with sterile drapes so the arm can be held or manipulated during the procedure.

A 9–12 cm transverse incision is made in the axilla 1 cm below the hairline. Incisions below the hairline heal better than those in the hairline.

Dividing the Subcutaneous Tissue (Fig. 10-5B)

The subcutaneous tissue is divided until the chest wall and pectoralis major muscle is seen. The second intercostal brachial cutaneous nerve is often encountered at this point as it exits the chest wall, passes across the axilla, and proceeds toward the arm. Injury to this nerve is common. The nerve may be preserved and retracted. However, there is risk of painful paresthesia in the inner arm if retraction damages the nerve extensively. The alternative, and sometimes the best choice, is to divide the nerve and accept anesthesia in the area.

The pectoralis major muscle is freed for several inches along its lateral border and the pectoralis minor muscle is similarly freed by blunt dissection against the chest wall without actually exposing the muscle. A long, thin Simon-Heaney vaginal retractor is placed under the two pectoral muscles together, with the tip of the retractor lying over the second rib.

Dividing the Intercostal Muscles (Fig. 10-5C)

The first rib is identified and freed on its lateral edge by cutting the intercostal muscles near the rib.

---

* Suggested by Dr. Edouard Kieffer, Paris, France.

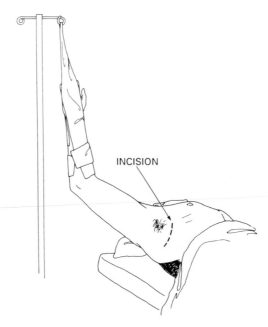

Fig. 10-5A.   Position showing 30-degree elevation of chest and arm suspended from IV pole, held there by wide adhesive tape. A sand bag over foot of IV pole will stabilize it. An assistant lifts arm when needed, but can rest the arm through much of the procedure. Incision is 9–12 cm just below the hairline.

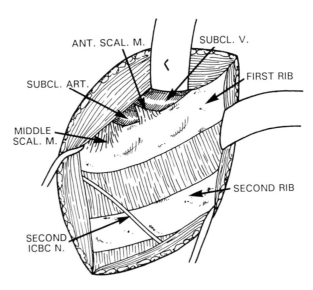

Fig. 10-5B.   Exposure of second and first ribs after retracting pectoral muscles with Simon-Heaney retractor. Second intercostal brachial cutaneous nerve crosses lower part of field and is preserved if possible. Subclavian vein is seen at upper end while subclavian artery is usually not seen yet.

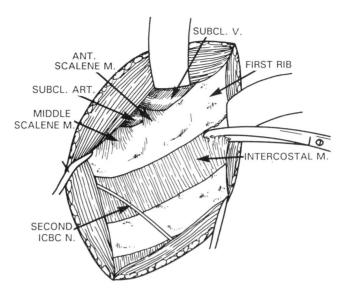

Fig. 10-5C.   Division of intercostal muscles below the first rib.

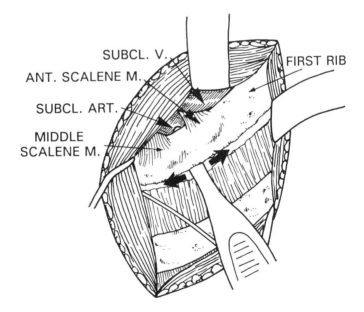

Fig. 10-5D.   Rib with periosteum is freed from pleura with No. 1 Overholt rib elevator. Initially, the smooth end of elevator finds the plane of dissection below the rib. The right angled end is then inserted until it engages the inner rib edge. Moving the elevator below the rib in both directions frees rib from pleura over distance of 6–9 cm.

Freeing the Rib From the Pleura (Fig. 10-5D)

Once an extraperiosteal plane is opened below the rib, a No. 1 Overholt periosteal elevator is used to free the rib from the pleura. A scissors is used to cut the more lateral intercostals, the scissors being kept close to the rib to avoid cutting the long thoracic nerve that passes downward, over the edge of the rib, and often close to the rib.

Dividing the Anterior Scalene Muscle (Fig. 10-5E)

The anterior scalene muscle is identified at its tubercle where it attaches to the first rib. This muscle is surrounded with a right angle hemostat and divided as far away from the rib as possible so that 1–2 cm of muscle remains attached to the rib.

Dividing the Middle Scalene Muscle (Fig. 10-5F)

The middle scalene muscle, attaching to the top of the rib, is divided near the rib with a scissors or periosteal elevator.

Dividing the Posterior End of the Rib (Fig. 10-5G)

The posterior end of the rib is now divided with a right angle rib cutter, which is slid as far posteriorly as possible while making sure that C-8 and T-1 nerve roots are not caught in the jaws of the rongeur (Fig. 10-5G). A Roos plexus retractor (Fig. 10-3B) has been designed to assist in gently pushing the plexus away from the rongeur at this stage of the procedure. When the posterior end of the rib has been divided, it may be possible to avulse the anterior end of the rib by simply pulling the posterior end of the rib forward. If the anterior end cannot be avulsed, a bone cutter is used to cut the rib as far anteriorly as possible. The subclavian vein should be

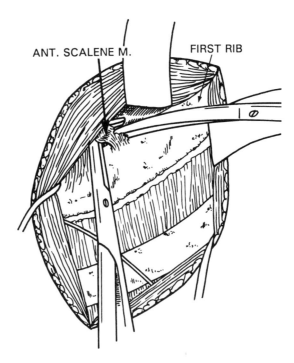

ANT. SCALENE M.   FIRST RIB

Fig. 10-5E.   Right angle clamp is passed around anterior scalene muscle and muscle is divided as far from the rib as possible to remove as much muscle as possible.

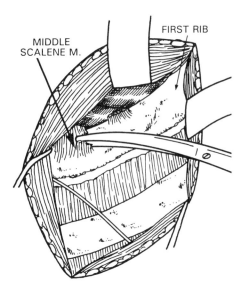

Fig. 10-5F.   Middle scalene muscle is divided with scissors or periosteal elevator. Remaining intercostal muscle fibers are also divided keeping scissors close to rib to avoid long thoracic nerve.

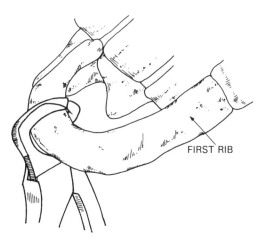

Fig. 10-5G.   Neck of rib is transected with right angled rib cutter. Good exposure is obtained by assistant elevating arm and by gently retracting plexus with carefully held Deaver retractor or Roos plexus retractor.

observed at this point to make sure it is not injured by the bone cutter. The main segment of rib is removed.

Dividing the Anterior Section of the Rib (Fig. 10-5H)

The anterior section of the rib is now divided with a bone cutter or rongeur. The anterior stump is trimmed with a rongeur by taking small bites of bone up to the costochondral junction, which is recognized by its smooth shiny surface.

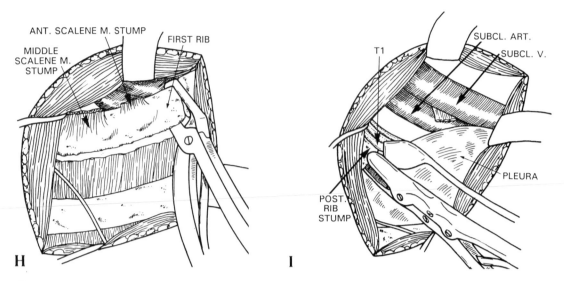

Fig. 10-5H.   Anterior rib is transected close to costochondral junction with rib cutter or rongeur, whichever will be safest. Subclavian vein may lie just above inner corner of rib and must be spared. After rib is removed, anterior stump is trimmed and smoothed back to cartilage.

Fig. 10-5I.   Posterior rib stump is shortened with Sauerbruch (boxcar) or Urschel first rib rongeur. The Urschel rongeur has the advantage of not blocking the field of vision. The Roos plexus retractor protects C-8 and T-1. Rib is removed to as close to transverse process as safety permits.

Shortening the Posterior Rib Stump (Fig. 10-5I)

The posterior remnant of rib is shortened with a Sauerbruch, Urschel, or duckbill rongeur to as close to the transverse process as possible. However, this can be a dangerous maneuver because the cords of the plexus lie close to and often on top of the posterior end of the rib. The Roos plexus retractor is used to protect the nerves at this point in the operation. If the posterior rib cannot be removed safely, it should not be removed.

Closing the Wound (Fig. 10-5J)

The wound is closed with closed drainage, 3 or 4 subcutaneous sutures, and approximating the skin with a running, absorbable subcuticular stitch (Fig. 10-5J).

Posterior Approach

Following intratracheal anesthesia, the patient is placed in the lateral decubitus position with the ipsilateral knee flexed and the ipsilateral arm abducted. A high posterior thoracoplasty incision is used running midway between the spine and medial border of the scapula. The incision begins 2–3 cm above the spine of the scapula and extends downward, curving 2–4 cm laterally around the angle of the scapula. The latissimus dorsi muscle below the incision is transected. By finger dissection, the plane beneath the scapula and serratus anterior muscle is mobilized and the highest rib identified, which is usually the second rib.

The serratus anterior muscle is divided near the ribs and the scapula retracted

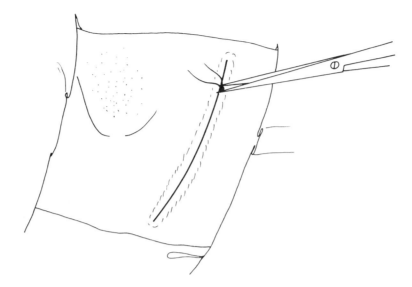

Fig. 10-5J.   Closed suction drain is positioned near rib bed and subcutaneous and subcuticular layers are closed.

upwards and laterally. The rhomboid major muscle is divided, and the lateral border of the paraspinal muscles are mobilized and retracted medially. The posterior scalene muscle can be seen inserting on the second rib. It is divided to permit better exposure of the first rib.

Finger dissection is used to identify the neck of the first rib, which is cleaned with periosteal elevators extraperiosteally. By dissecting from posterior to anterior, the middle scalene muscle on top of the rib is divided, the intercostal muscles on the lateral edge are sectioned, and the anterior scalene muscle is finally divided. Remaining attachments to the rib can be freed by finger dissection. The rib is transected posteriorly at the transverse process with a rib shears. The rib is then divided as far anterior as possible with gentle retraction on the neurovascular bundle to protect it.

Transthoracic Approach[4]

Following intratracheal anesthesia, the patient is placed supine with the operated side elevated about 30 degrees. An anterolateral thoracotomy approach is used through an incision in the submammary groove. The pectoralis major and minor muscles are retracted medially but their lateral edges can be divided if necessary for greater exposure. The intercostal muscles of the second or third interspace are divided and the pleural space entered. The apex of the lung is depressed to expose the first rib, which is dissected from the sternal to the posterior ends.

The anterior end of the rib is divided at the costochondral junction and the ligaments, anterior and middle scalene muscles, and intercostal muscles are systematically divided close to the rib. Countertraction on the rib helps identify the dissection plane as the subclavian vein and artery are gently pushed away when they come into view. When the entire rib has been freed, the posterior end is divided as close to the transverse process as possible. One or two chest tubes are left to drain the apex and base of the pleural space and the wound is closed in layers.

Dorsal Sympathectomy

Dorsal sympathectomy is an infrequently performed operation because the results of sympathectomy for pain relief and improved blood flow to the hand are often only partially successful and they tend to deteriorate in the first few years after surgery. For this reason, surgery is regarded as a "last resort" procedure when all other nonoperative measures have been unsuccessful. Probably the best results are in patients operated upon for hyperhidrosis.

In the 1950s, techniques for direct arterial repair and replacement became available for aneurysms and occlusions of the subclavian and axillary arteries. The results of these operations are far superior to those of dorsal sympathectomy for ischemia of the hand. As a result, sympathectomy for ischemia is considered only when direct repair is not possible or has failed.

Indications

Dorsal sympathectomy is performed for pain, ischemia, or hyperhidrosis of the upper extremity. The symptoms should be persistent for at least a few months, conservative measures should have been tried and failed, and the symptoms should be severe enough that the patient is willing to undergo an operation that may be unsuccessful. In addition, patients should demonstrate temporary improvement following a sympathetic block with either lidocaine injection of the stellate ganglion or an injection of tolazoline hydrochloride (Priscoline) directly into the brachial artery.

The specific indications are

1. Pain in the hand or arm that cannot be relieved by medication. The underlying causes include reflex sympathetic dystrophy (RSD), causalgia, Raynaud's phenomenon associated with collagen vascular disease, or extreme sensitivity to cold.

2. Digital gangrene or severe ischemic digital necrosis from small vessel or diffuse arterial disease. Such arterial disease can be seen in thromboangiitis obliterans (Beurger's disease), severe arteriosclerosis, and collagen vascular disease. Digital necrosis also may be due to multiple small emboli dislodged from subclavian artery aneurysms and mural thrombosis.

3. Hyperhidrosis (excessive sweating).

Extent of Sympathectomy

There is no consensus today regarding how much of the sympathetic chain must be removed to achieve complete ablation of sympathetic activity in the upper extremity. The options range from removal of the lower half of the cervical chain, plus the first 3–4 inches of the thoracic chain, to removal of just the second thoracic ganglia with all of its rami and intricate communicating branches. Lemmons has emphasized the importance of the second thoracic ganglia as well as alternate pathways for sympathetic fibers that include branches from the second spinal intercostal nerve.[5] He suggests that the frequent failures of dorsal sympathectomy may be because those alternative pathways cannot be divided by the standard forms of transthoracic sympathectomy. For that reason, he advocates removal of not only the second and third thoracic ganglia, but also segments of the intercostal nerves and dorsal and ventral nerve roots.[5] That extensive dissection can only be performed through a posterior approach and does not include the stellate ganglion.

Because normally no sympathetic fibers pass from the cervical sympathetic trunk to the upper extremity, it is unnecessary to remove this portion of the sympathetic system. This applies to the stellate ganglion as well. The stellate is the fusion of the lower cervical and upper thoracic ganglia. Its removal is well known to produce a Horner's syndrome. Since the nerve fibers that go to the eye and eyelid arise from the lower cervical ganglion, it was proposed by Palumbo that a Horner's syndrome could be avoided by removing only the lower quarter of the stellate ganglion when performing a dorsal sympathectomy.[6] In our experience with this technique, Horner's syndrome occurred in the majority of patients. To avoid this, excision of the dorsal chain is currently begun just below the stellate ganglion. The clinical results have been just as good as when the lower portion of the stellate had been removed and Horner's syndrome usually has been avoided. Removal of the first thoracic ganglia does not seem to be important.

Choice of Surgical Approach

Dorsal sympathectomy can be performed through several approaches: supraclavicular, transaxillary intrapleural, transaxillary extrapleural, transthoracic, and posterior. The supraclavicular incision used for cervical rib resection can also be employed for dorsal sympathectomy. Exposure is difficult through this route, but morbidity usually is minimal. Transthoracic sympathectomy through the third interspace via an anterolateral incision provides the best exposure,[6] but postthoracotomy chest pain was severe in three of Kirtley's patients.[7]

The transaxillary approach can be used either intrapleurally or extrapleurally. The second interspace is entered in the intrathoracic variation.[8] The exposure is excellent, but postoperative morbidity is the same as with any other thoracotomy. Extrapleural transaxillary sympathectomy has been described by Roos.[9] It requires first rib excision for exposure, but can be quite effective.

The posterior approach of Smithwich,[10] later expanded by Lemmens,[5] includes removal of the second and third sympathetic ganglia along with the intercostal nerves, dorsal and ventral roots, spinal ganglia of thoracic segments two and three, and all tissue that lies between T-1 and T-4, including intercostal muscles and nerves. However, this approach has been associated with considerable postoperative neuralgia in a significant number of patients.[7]

Supraclavicular Dorsal Sympathectomy

This approach is the same as that for anterior scalenectomy (Fig. 10-1, A through I). Following removal of the anterior scalene muscle, the subclavian artery is mobilized and sometimes isolated with a plastic tape. The sympathetic chain lies posterior to the proximal subclavian artery against the transverse processes of the lower cervical and thoracic vertebrae. It is difficult to locate through this approach. The landmark is the stellate ganglion, a firm, irregularly shaped elliptical body, about 2 cm long and 0.4 cm wide. It is found by palpating the tissue just medial to the transverse process of C-7 at the point where the dorsal spine curves sharply posteriorly. The route to the ganglion depends upon the position of the subclavian artery in relationship to the clavicle. A plane either anterior or posterior to the proximal subclavian artery will be appropriate in individual cases.

A fiberoptic light on the head of the surgeon is very helpful at this stage of the procedure, because the field of vision becomes quite narrow as the retropleural space is entered. Once the stellate ganglion has been identified, the pleura is mobilized by blunt finger dissection away from the thoracic vertebrae and the neck of the ribs. A thin malleable retractor holds the pleura and lung away from the spine. The sympathetic chain is divided between clips placed just below the stellate ganglion; the thoracic end of the chain is grasped with a long hemostat.

The chain is freed caudally by sharp and blunt dissection, reaching as deeply into the posterior mediastinum as possible, usually to about the fourth interspace. Countertraction on the chain by tensing the hemostat is essential. The rami entering the second and third sympathetic ganglia are clipped and divided. The lowest accessible part of the chain is also clipped, the chain divided and removed. A small closed suction drain is left in the wound, as is done following scalenectomy. Not all surgeons place metal clips on divided nerves and their branches. Roos avoids these clips, feeling that crushing the nerve endings with metal clips accounts for postoperative neuralgia.[9]

The pleura is seldom opened, but an upright chest x-ray is obtained postoperatively to exclude a pneumothorax. If present, it is evacuated through the suction drain or by a thoracentesis needle (plastic, size 14 or 16, inserted in the anterior second interspace). A chest tube is rarely needed.

Phrenic nerve damage can occur during this operation by traction against the nerve in gaining exposure. The nerve should be visualized and avoided each time a retractor is inserted.

Extrapleural Transaxillary Dorsal Sympathectomy

The transaxillary extrapleural route requires removal of the first rib in order to achieve adequate exposure. Therefore, it is applicable only in those patients who have indications for both first rib resection and dorsal sympathectomy. After removing the first rib through the transaxillary approach (Fig. 10-5, A through I), dorsal sympathectomy is performed by bluntly dissecting the pleura away from the necks of the upper four or five ribs. The stellate ganglion is identified by palpating the transverse processes of T-1 and C-7 at the junction of the cervical and dorsal spine where there is an acute posterior curve. The ends of the rami and chain are clipped and divided. The chain is removed from just below the stellate to about the fourth rib.

Intrapleural or Transthoracic Dorsal Sympathectomy

Entering the pleural space provides the best exposure for dorsal sympathectomy and can be performed by thoracotomy through either the third interspace in a straight lateral position or through the second or third interspace in an anterolateral position. The lateral approach through the axilla is illustrated in Figure 10-6, A through E.

Positioning the Patient (Fig. 10-6A)

A lateral thoracotomy position is used with the arm suspended as shown. A 10–12 cm incision is made 2–3 cm below the hairline in the axilla.

Splitting the Serratus Anterior (Fig. 10-6B)

Serratus anterior muscle is split in the direction of its fibers. Long thoracic nerve lying anteriorly and thoracodorsal nerve lying posteriorly are preserved.

Mobilizing the Rib (Fig. 10-6C)

After retracting serratus anterior muscle, the intercostal muscles below the third rib are divided and the rib is mobilized extraperiosteally with a rib elevator.

Opening the Pleura (Fig. 10-6D)

The pleura is opened in the rib bed and the upper lobe of the lung is depressed.

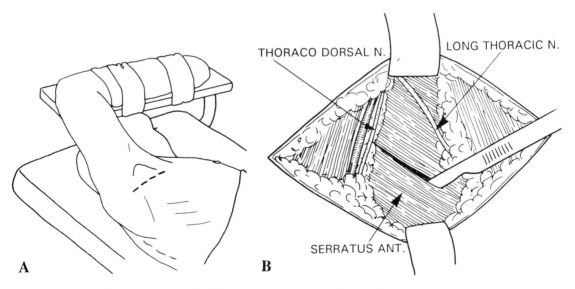

THORACO DORSAL N. LONG THORACIC N.

SERRATUS ANT.

A   B

Fig. 10-6A.   Table position with 10–12 cm incision 2–3 cm below hairline.

Fig. 10-6B.   Serratus anterior is split.

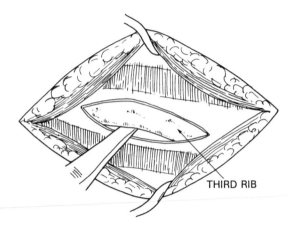

Fig. 10-6C.   Third rib is mobilized.

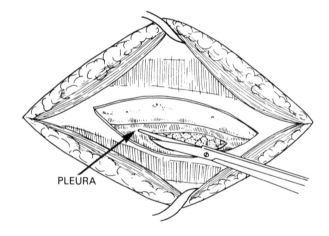

Fig. 10-6D.   Pleura is opened.

Removing the Sympathetic Chain (Fig. 10-6E)

Posteriorly, the parietal pleura is opened near the transverse processes of the upper vertebrae. By blunt dissection, the sympathetic chain is identified by locating the second or third thoracic ganglia. The chain is removed from just below the stellate ganglion to the fourth or fifth rib.

Although this approach provides the best exposure for dorsal sympathectomy, the morbidity of a thoracotomy is a high price to pay. The same long-term results are achievable with less patient discomfort by the other routes.

Posterior Dorsal Sympathectomy

This procedure is performed in a prone position through a paravertebral incision from the first to the sixth ribs. The muscles below the incision are divided until the necks of the second and third ribs are reached. Sections 3–4 cm long are excised from each rib, the pleura freed and retracted laterally, and the transverse

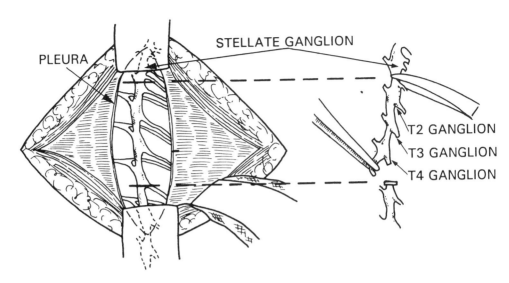

Fig. 10-6E.   Pleura is opened over the sympathetic chain. Stellate ganglion is identified and chain divided just below it. T-2 through T-4 ganglia are removed.

processes identified. The chain is found ventral to the processes, clipped and removed from the second to the fourth rib. This excision includes the second thoracic ganglion, which is the essential source of sympathetic fibers to the upper extremity. Postoperative recovery is usually uneventful.

References

1. Sanders RJ. Subcuticular skin closure: description of technique. J Dermatol Surg 1975; 1:61–64.
2. Gol A, Patrick DW, McNeel DP. Relief of costoclavicular syndrome by infraclavicular removal of first rib. J Neurosurg 1968; 28:81–84.
3. Roos DB. Transaxillary approach for first rib resection to relieve thoracic outlet syndrome. Ann Surg 1966; 163:354–358.
4. Pretre R, Spiliopoulos A, Megevand R. Transthoracic approach in the thoracic outlet syndrome: an alternate operative route for removal of the first rib. Surgery 1989; 106:856–860.
5. Lemmens HAJ. Thoracodorsal sympathectomy en bloc. Vasc Surg 1979; 13:331–335.
6. Palumbo LT. New surgical approach for upper thoracic sympathectomy: a method to avoid Horner's syndrome. Arch Surg 1958; 76:807–810.
7. Kirtley JA, Riddell DH, Stoney WS, Wright JK. Cervicothoracic sympathectomy in neurovascular abnormalities of the upper extremities: experiences in 76 patients with 104 sympathectomies. Ann Surg 1967; 165:869–879.
8. Kleinert HE, Cook FW, Kutz JE. Neurovascular disorders of the upper extremity: treated by transaxillary sympathectomy. Arch Surg 1965; 90:612–616.
9. Roos DB. Transaxillary thoracic outlet decompression and sympathectomy. In: Bergan JJ, Yao JST, eds. Techniques in arterial surgery; Philadelphia: WB Saunders Co. 1990:305–316.
10. Smithwick RH. The problem of producing complete and lasting sympathetic denervation of the upper extremity by preganglionic section. Ann Surg 1940; 112:1085–1100.

11
Postoperative Management and Complications

Richard J. Sanders
Angelica Voelkel

Postoperative Care and Physical Therapy

Preoperative Preparation

When possible, postoperative care begins prior to thoracic outlet syndrome (TOS) surgery by explaining to the patient the postoperative rehabilitation program and the expectations for the postoperative period:

1. Numbness and tingling in the hand will usually improve within 24 hours of surgery if the operation proves to be successful. If paresthesia has not improved by then, it seldom improves with time. However, the plastic drainage tube that will be left in the wound for 24 hours will sometimes lie against the plexus and cause temporary paresthesia that disappears when the drain is removed.

2. Increased pain from surgery is common in the neck, chest, and along the inner border of the scapula; it can last 4–8 weeks.

3. Reduced range of motion of the arm is common for 1–3 weeks postoperatively.

4. Postoperative hospitalization is 1–2 days following scalenectomy and 2–3 days when the first rib has been resected through transaxillary, supraclavicular, or infraclavicular routes. Rib resection via the posterior approach may require 3–5 days of hospitalization postoperatively.

5. Convalescence after hospital discharge takes about 4–6 weeks following scalenectomy and a few weeks longer following first rib resection.

6. The time off work depends upon the type of job to which the patient will return. For nonstrenuous jobs, such as those that involve mostly desk-sitting, patients may be ready to return to work in as little as 1–2 weeks. For heavy work or jobs requiring use of the upper extremities for a good part of the day, including continuous keyboard operations, the time off work may be anywhere from 3–4 weeks to 12 weeks. Some patients who do very heavy labor may never be able to return to heavy-duty work again because it brings back their upper extremity symptoms.

When possible, patients are seen by a physical therapist who reviews with the patient the postoperative exercise program and gives the patient a written copy of the program with descriptions and pictures of the exercises. The preoperative discussion includes an explanation of the transcutaneous nerve stimulator (TNS), exercises, and possible modalities.

Day of Surgery

In recent years a TNS unit has been routinely positioned on the patient in the recovery room following surgery. The electrodes are placed along the medial border of the scapula because this is frequently the most painful area postoperatively. The electrodes may be repositioned to other more painful areas as the patient desires.

Postoperative Management

Postoperatively, the healing process starts in the first week as scar tissue begins to form. This is best laid down in an anatomical, physiological pattern, compatible with a full range of motion. To prevent postoperative contracture of the scar tissue, range of motion exercises should begin the first few days after surgery and continue until normality is reached (Table 11–1). The exercises should be performed for a few minutes at least twice a day for the first 3–7 days. After the first week, progressive resistive exercises with increasing weight, one-half to five pounds, are added. After 3 weeks, exercises continue as needed.

The most important exercise postoperatively is neck stretching to help reduce tightening of the scar tissue that will form around the plexus. Other areas that may require exercising are the shoulder and scapula. The choice of exercises (see Chapter 9, Appendix) include the following:

1. Neck exercises:
    Lateral side bending
    Oblique stretching
    Rotation
    Flexion/extension
    Chin tucks

2. Shoulder exercises:
    Pendulum exercises (Codman)
    Stretching onto a flat surface
    Climbing a wall with the fingers
    Broomstick exercises
    Levator scapula stretching

3. Scapula exercises:
    Protraction/Retraction
    Elevate shoulders to touch ears
    Corner exercises

Postoperative exercises are begun in the hospital under the guidance of a physical therapist. A written protocol, individualized for each patient, is sent home with the patient (Tables 11–1 and 11–2). In some patients, no further therapy is needed, but in others, particularly those with other diagnoses, postoperative physical therapy will improve long term results.

Follow-up

Repeat visits with the therapist and the surgeon at regular intervals (weekly to monthly for the first 3 months) to monitor progress are recommended. The purpose is to detect recurrent symptoms soon after their appearance so that conservative programs and medication adjustments can be instituted early enough to prevent progression.

Table 11–1. **Postoperative Thoracic Outlet Exercises**[a]

Do these exercises _____ times a day.
Do _____ repetitions of each exercise.

Neck Flexion/Extension
Slowly roll chin toward chest to feel gentle stretch of the muscles behind the neck and upper back. Hold for _____ seconds and slowly roll head back to neutral.

Neck Rotation/Oblique Stretching
Keeping chin level, turn head so that your chin comes toward your shoulder. Do not lift or lower chin. Hold for _____ seconds. Repeat lifting chin for oblique rotation. Hold for _____ seconds.

Neck Sidebending
Keeping chin level and face forward, slowly bring your ear toward your shoulder until you feel a gentle stretch in the top of your shoulder and the side of your neck.

Chin Tuck
Gently push chin backward as far as you are comfortably able. Let your neck relax forward. Try to maintain this posture as long as possible and repeat.

Wall Climbing
Stand facing a wall about two feet away. Place your fingers on the wall and walk them up the wall moving your body as close to the wall as able. Lower hand and let your neck relax. Try to maintain this posture as long as possible.

Stand sideways to wall about two feet away. Place fingers on wall and walk fingers up wall as high as possible moving closer to the wall as needed. Lower slowly.

Call if you have any questions: Phone number is: _____

Signed: _____, Therapist.

[a] The exercises were assembled with the assistance of the physical therapists at Rose Medical Center, Presbyterian Hospital, Aurora Presbyterian Hospital, and Veterans Administration Hospital, Denver, Colorado.

Table 11–2. **Postoperative Home Instructions**

1. Activity:		No lifting over 15 pounds; No scrubbing or tugging; gradually increase activities as tolerated, including makeup and hair care.
2. Driving:		You may try to drive a car; avoid a standard shift for 2–3 weeks after surgery.
3. Occupation:		The time off work depends upon how much use of the arm your job entails.
4. Exercises:		Do exercises daily as instructed in hospital.
5. Wound care:		You may shower two days after surgery; Do not scrub over incision for first 2 weeks after surgery; pat wound dry.
6. Pain:		Heating pad or ice pack can be tried to relieve pain around shoulder blade. If indicated TNS unit can be used. A pillow under the affected arm when sitting, lying, or driving may help.
7. Medication:		As directed by physician

Call your surgeon's office if you have questions about any of these instructions.

Postoperative Complications

Prevention and Management

The complications of TOS surgery include injury to the structures of the neurovascular bundle, injury to adjacent nerves and thoracic duct, and the introduction of air or fluid into the pleural space. Table 11–3 lists the complications in our experience in over 800 primary and recurrent TOS operations. Interestingly, the complications following reoperations were no more frequent than those following primary operations.

Day of Hospital Discharge

A rough idea of postoperative morbidity can be gleaned from noting how soon after surgery patients were discharged from the hospital. Table 11–4 tabulates the day of hospital discharge for the different surgical procedures. Operations involving rib resection required another day or two for recovery in the hospital as compared to operations in which the first rib was left intact.

Nerve Injuries

Vessel injury can usually be repaired with good functional results; this is not true for nerve injuries. Once a nerve has been stretched, time is the only factor for healing. Antiinflammatory drugs or steroids may help reduce swelling in the nerve and nerve sheath as well as in the operative area. Postoperative stretching of the arm should be avoided to prevent stretching the injured nerve. The symptoms of sensory loss can be treated with drugs that reduce nerve irritation, such as antiseizure medication (Dilantin, Tegretol).

Nerves that are torn or cut can be reapproximated if the ends are found. However, there exists no data at this time as to the effectiveness of these repairs.

Table 11–3. Surgical Complications: 1964 to 1989

	Transaxillary 1st Rib Resection (n = 113)[a]	Anterior Middle Scalenectomy (n = 301)[a]	Supraclavicular 1st Rib Resection (n = 326)[a]	All Recurrent Operations (n = 141)[a]	Total (n = 881)[a]
Plexus injury—Temp[b]	1 (0.9%)	0	7 (2.3%)	1 (0.7%)	9 (1%)
Plexus injury—Perm[b]	2 (1.8%)	0	2 (0.6%)	0	4 (0.4%)
Phrenic paralysis—Temp	1 (1%)	18 (6%)	9 (2.2%)	7 (4.9%)	35 (4%)
Phrenic paralysis—Perm	0	1 (0.3%)	1 (0.3%)	2 (1.4%)	3 (0.3%)
Winged Scapula	2 (1.8%)	0	1 (0.3%)	0	3 (0.3%)
Arterial injury	0	0	1 (0.3%)	0	1 (0.1%)
Venous injury	2 (2%)	1 (0.3%)	4 (1.2%)	1 (0.7%)	8 (0.9%)
Pleura opened, no pneumothorax	34 (30%)	4 (1.3%)	39 (12%)	13 (9.2%)	76 (8.6%)
Pneumothorax requiring tap	10 (9%)	1 (0.4%)	7 (2.1%)	0	18 (2%)
Bleeding over 500 mL	3 (2.7%)	1 (0.3%)	5 (1.5%)	2 (1.3%)	11 (1.2%)

[a]The operations included here are all TOS operation between January, 1964 and December, 1989. These numbers are a little larger than the life tables in Chapter 12, where the time covered was only through December, 1988.
[b]Temp = temporary; Perm = permanent.

The diagnosis of nerve injury is made by electromyogram (EMG) and ulnar nerve conduction velocities (UNCV), which can become positive 2 weeks after nerve injury. Nerve recovery is monitored by the same tests as well as by grading muscle strength. Improvement may progress over a year or more.

Physical therapy is prescribed to maintain muscle tone and range of motion pending the return of motor function, but this is not begun during the first 3 postoperative days. After this time, the usual postoperative protocol is resumed.

Brachial Plexus

The most serious complication of surgical treatment for TOS is injury to the brachial plexus. Although most plexus injuries are temporary, some are permanent. The symptoms are complete or partial paralysis, numbness, and/or pain in the arm and hand. In 1982, Dale canvassed 920 vascular surgeons, all members of the North American Chapter of the International Cardiovascular Society, to determine the incidence and character of brachial plexus injuries during transaxillary rib resection for TOS.[1] Three hundred fifty-one surgeons (38%) responded of whom 259 performed first rib resections. Of these, 52% had seen at least one

Table 11–4. Day of Discharge

Postoperative Day	Scalenectomy (n = 301)	Transaxially 1st Rib Resection (n = 113)	Scalectomy & Supraclavicular Rib Resection (n = 326)	Reops With Rib Resection (n = 45)	Reops Without Rib Resection (n = 96)
1	46%	8%	15%	14%	35%
2	34%	18%	42%	17%	30%
3	16%	41%	35%	52%	22%
4	4%	22%	7%	14%	9%
5	0%	10%	1%	3%	4%
6 or more	0%	1%	0%	0%	0%

neurologic complication among their own patients or among those of associates. These surgeons averaged 10 rib resections a year, twice as many as those who saw no neurologic complications.

There were 273 instances of postoperative plexus injuries among the 134 surgeons who had seen neurologic complications, 102 cases of complete and 171 cases of partial paralysis. Seventy-eight percent of the patients with complete paralysis and 82% of those with partial paralysis enjoyed total recovery; the remaining patients, 52 of 273 (19%), failed to achieve complete return of function. While the total number of operations performed by this large group of surgeons was not stated, the number probably exceeded 5,000, which makes the incidence of permanent paralysis under 1%.

In 1985, Horowitz reported four cases of permanent plexus injury. The worst symptom was prolonged intense pain of a burning quality carrying a diagnosis of reflex sympathetic dystrophy (causalgia). Electrophysiologic and clinical findings suggested severe damage to the lower trunk of the brachial plexus and lesser involvement of another trunk.[2]

The plexus can be injured in several ways. With the transaxillary approach, excessive traction by the assistant holding the arm can stretch the plexus and cause damage. Obviously, it is possible for one of the nerves of the plexus to be cut by a bone rongeur or rib shears. The nerve most susceptible is T-1, which is hidden under the rib when viewed through the axilla. When obtaining exposure of the neck of the rib, the field of exposure is often deep and narrow. To prevent bone shears and rongeurs from cutting nerves, it is usually necessary to retract the lower nerves of the plexus. However, because it is difficult to quantitate the amount of pressure these instruments exert against the nerves, nerve damage can occur from excessive pressure by the same retractors that are preventing the nerves from being cut.

The supraclavicular approach provides better exposure of the neck of the first rib than the transaxillary approach, but plexus injury can still occur through this route. It is often necessary to retract the cords of the plexus medially to expose the rib. Usually, this retracting can be done by using a forceps or suction tip to gently push C-7 and C-8 just enough to insure that they are not in the jaws of the rongeur. However, T-1 lies deep to the rib and is usually not retracted. When dividing the most medial portion of the neck of the rib, tiny bites are taken with minimal opening of the rongeur to prevent the blades from catching a nerve root. If there is concern about T-1, a thin curved elevator or retractor is used to protect it, such as the plexus retractor designed by Roos (see Chapter 10, Fig. 10-3B).

Other investigators who have performed supraclavicular first rib resection have noted temporary brachial plexus palsy in a significant number of patients. Thomas et al., in 1978, reported five of 38 patients (13%)[3] and Reilly and Stoney, in 1988, observed five of 41 patients (12%)[4] with postoperative plexus palsy. Both authors also noted complete recovery in all of their patients. Our experience with postoperative plexus paralysis was nine of 326 patients (3%) undergoing supraclavicular rib resection; seven completely recovered while the two patients who did not recover appeared to have reflex sympathetic dystrophy.

Several surgeons who have reported results of transaxillary first rib resection have also observed occasional cases of damage to the brachial plexus, usually T-1.[5-9] As noted in Dale's survey, these incidents are fairly widespread across the country.

Phrenic Nerve

Because the phrenic nerve lies on the surface of the anterior scalene muscle, it is subject to injury during any supraclavicular operation—scalenotomy, scalenectomy, supraclavicular first rib resection, and brachial plexus neurolysis—near the anterior scalene muscle.

The phrenic nerve is easily bruised and is sensitive to mild traction. Some surgeons suggest encircling the nerve with a suture to help identify it throughout the dissection. That can be helpful but does not guarantee protection. A single tug on the suture can injure the nerve and paralyze the diaphragm. Retracting the phrenic nerve with any one of a variety of instruments can have the same effect. In our experience, preventing phrenic nerve injury is best achieved by retracting the scalene fat pad upward and medially during anterior scalene muscle dissection. The connective tissue on the lateral side of the nerve is sharply divided permitting the nerve to be lifted above the muscle without touching the nerve (see Chapter 10, Fig. 10-1F).

Anatomical variations of the phrenic nerve are probably the most important factor in phrenic nerve injuries. The usual course of the phrenic nerve is across the anterior scalene muscle from lateral to medial as it descends in the neck and enters the mediastinum. It lies superficial to the subclavian artery and behind the subclavian vein. More than 80% of phrenic nerves follow the pattern and they are rarely injured.

On the other hand, a phrenic or accessory phrenic nerve that lies on the lateral side of the anterior scalene muscle is in jeopardy. Thirteen percent of phrenic nerves have two branches, one running medial and the other lateral, along the anterior scalene muscle. Another 3% of phrenic nerves run through the neck on the lateral side of the muscle and remain there when the nerve enters the mediastinum. The lateral-lying nerve is directly in the path of dissection of the anterior scalene muscle.[10] Either the dissection must be performed in part medial and in part lateral to the nerve, or the nerve must be retracted to permit dissection. The best choice is to dissect on either side of the nerve, leaving the nerve untouched. However, the space for dissection is small and it is easy for the scissors to stretch the nerve causing nerve injury.

The incidence of temporary phrenic paralysis was 6% in our early review, but fell to 2.2% with more experience (Table 11-1). Loh found six instances of phrenic paralysis in 40 cases (12%), three of which lasted more than 4 months.[11] Most of our cases of phrenic nerve paralysis were in patients with a lateral-lying phrenic nerve. Nerve function usually recovered, sometimes within a few weeks but at other times taking several months. Unilateral phrenic paralysis reduces lung capacity about 10–20% and most patients are asymptomatic or have mild dyspnea on extreme exertion. The reason our reported incidence of phrenic paralysis is so high is that we have routinely flouroscoped each patient postoperatively to determine the incidence of this complication. Paralysis of the diaphragm is sometimes missed on inspiration and expiration films; chest fluoroscopy is the most accurate means of diagnosis. Since there is no treatment for phrenic paralysis, its discovery is primarily of academic interest, although it does permit the surgeon to explain to the patient the reason for postoperative exertional dyspnea.

The phrenic nerve is not seen when the transaxillary incision is used and phrenic paralysis is rarely a complication of that approach. However, we did have one occurrence of phrenic paralysis following transaxillary first rib resection, probably from stretching a lateral-lying phrenic nerve when dividing the anterior scalene muscle near the first rib.

Long Thoracic Nerve

The long thoracic nerve is formed by branches of C-5, C-6, and C-7 that traverse the belly of the middle scalene muscle and join together either within or lateral to the muscle to form the long thoracic nerve. The nerve or its branches lie just lateral to the first rib, after exiting from the lateral surface of the middle scalene, and descend toward their insertion in the serratus anterior muscle.

In rib resection by any approach, the long thoracic nerve can be stretched or cut. When performing middle scalenectomy through the supraclavicular approach, the long thoracic nerve is also in jeopardy.

In transaxillary first rib resection, the nerve is usually not visualized. It can be avoided by dividing the middle scalene muscle at its insertion directly on the upper surface of the first rib. If the cutting instrument strays lateral to the rib, the nerve or its components may be injured. Similarly, when dividing the intercostal muscle from the lateral edge of the first rib with a scissors, the tip of the scissors should be minimally opened and the scissors held firmly against the edge of the rib while cutting the muscle. If the scissors moves lateral to the rib, the long thoracic nerve can be damaged.

Middle scalenectomy through the supraclavicular approach usually permits good visualization of the long thoracic nerve or its components. The nerve is found in the belly of the middle scalene muscle moving laterally toward the lateral edge of the first rib. It has no fixed landmark to aid identification. It is found by grasping small bundles of muscle with a forceps and squeezing the muscle. If the long thoracic nerve is caught in the forceps, the shoulder will jump. If the patient has been given medication to produce skeletal muscle paralysis, this sign will be lost. Therefore, the anesthesiologist should discontinue muscle paralysis once tracheal intubation has been performed. After the long thoracic nerve has been identified within the middle scalene muscle, only those portions of middle scalene muscle medial to the nerve are excised. The lateral portions of muscle are left behind.

Long thoracic nerve injury causes the scapula to project away from the posterior chest wall as a result of weakness in the serratus anterior muscle. This winging of the scapula is usually temporary as the injury has probably occurred to a branch rather than the entire nerve. Most patients experience partial or complete recovery. Petersen, Staab, and Brintnall reported four cases of winged scapula in six transaxillary rib resections.[12] All four were temporary and the patients were usually not aware of winging. None experienced permanent loss or disability. In our experience of 881 operations, winging occurred three times and was temporary in each (Table 11–1).

Second Intercostal Brachial Cutaneous Nerve (ICBN)

The second ICBN emerges from the second interspace of the anterior chest wall. It moves laterally over the chest wall, crosses through the lower part of the axilla, and carries sensory fibers from the inner aspect of the arm. It often lies in the middle of the operating field during transaxillary rib resection where it frequently is stretched, torn, or cut. The incidence of damage to this nerve was 35% in our experience[13] and 27% in that of Lepantalo.[14] Anesthesia of the area is the commonest manifestation of this injury. However, an occasional patient has required a neurectomy at a later date to convert hypersensitivity and burning pain to simple numbness, a symptom with which it is easier to live. This complication is only seen with the transaxillary approach.

Recurrent Laryngeal and Vagus Nerves

These nerves are not in the plane of dissection of either the anterior or middle scalene muscles. They lie medial to this area, just lateral to the trachea, deep and medial to the internal jugular vein. In reoperations following scalenectomy, normal anatomical planes can be difficult to identify and dissection can inadvertently be carried in the wrong direction. In one of our early cases of recurrent TOS, the recurrent laryngeal nerve was damaged, probably owing to dissection having been carried too far medially. Injury can be avoided by using the internal jugular vein as a landmark and keeping all dissection lateral to this vein.

Cutaneous Nerves

Areas of postoperative anesthesia, hypesthesia, and hyperesthesia are commonly seen on both sides of incisions in all body areas. Incisions for thoracic outlet surgery are no exceptions. With supraclavicular incisions, it is common to observe small nerves lying on top of the sternocleidomastoid muscle. These are probably supraclavicular nerve branches to the anterior chest wall. When seen, they can often be preserved. However, if they are badly stretched, they should be totally divided because anesthesia is less uncomfortable than hyperesthesia.

Venous Injury

Subclavian vein injury is primarily a complication of rib resection by any route; it is seldom seen with scalenectomy alone. Injury to the subclavian vein is more common than to the subclavian artery because the vein lies closer than the artery to the point where the rib is divided. When dividing the costoclavicular ligament or the anterior end of the rib, it is very easy to cut or tear the subclavian vein. The vein can be protected by a retractor but the instrument can also compromise exposure. Subclavian vein hemorrhage also occurs from avulsion of small venous branches from their insertion points in the subclavian vein.

In reoperations, scar tissue frequently surrounds the subclavian vein, making safe dissection of this vein difficult and injury more likely. We have seen the first rib periosteal elevator tear a hole in the subclavian vein when using it to free the inner edge of the first rib during a reoperation following scalenectomy.

The incidence of subclavian vein injury during first rib resection is small, 1–2% in our experience (Table 11–1), but the sequelae can be serious. Several hundred mL of blood can be lost in just a few seconds and more blood lost during attempts to control the hemorrhage. When the vein is open, deep inspiration, augmenting the negative intrathoracic pressure, can cause aspiration of air into the venous system and subsequent pulmonary air emboli. We are aware of one death that occurred from this complication.

Major venous bleeding can usually be controlled by following this protocol: First, venous bleeding is controlled by direct pressure with a finger and then a small sponge on a long instrument; next, adequate exposure, suction, and light are secured; a fiberoptic headlight is helpful. If the transaxillary route is used, the first rib should be excised while holding pressure on the venous bleeding point; it is usually difficult or impossible to position a needle holder to repair the vein with the first rib in place. In working through the supraclavicular approach, exposing the vein through a separate infraclavicular incision will permit control of the subclavian vein from below the clavicle while it is repaired from above the clavicle.

Once there is adequate exposure, good light, a functioning suction, and the anterior end of the first rib has been excised (transaxillary route), the bleeding point is exposed and attempts are made to grasp the injured area with a vascular forceps. Often the bleeding area is small and can be controlled in this way. A vascular suture is placed adjacent to the forceps and, holding the two ends of the suture together and upwards, the vein is now under good control and the bleeding area can be oversewn.

If the bleeding cannot be controlled by this method, other techniques of vascular repair are employed. Balloon catheters placed through the venous laceration can be inflated to achieve proximal and distal control. Plastic tapes or loops can be passed around the vein for the same purpose, but this may be difficult, especially at the proximal end. Controlling the bleeding with a small, side-biting Satinsky vascular clamp is another approach. Reclamping the vein with a second, slightly larger vascular clamp can then expose enough of the torn vessel wall to permit its repair with fine vascular sutures.

Arterial Injury

Arterial injuries are uncommon. In Dale's survey, there was one case of cardiac arrest from an arterial injury and another that required arterial ligation with later reconstruction.[1] When arterial injury occurs through the transaxillary approach, bleeding is controlled with direct pressure. Good exposure, lighting, and suction are obtained before proceeding further. The methods described previously for controlling bleeding in venous injuries should be used if possible. If it is difficult to control the bleeding point through the axilla, pressure is held on the bleeding area while a supraclavicular incision is made to better expose the subclavian artery. The artery can be surrounded with a plastic loop to secure proximal control. Once that is done, the bleeding point can usually be found and repaired. Often it is a torn branch of the subclavian artery rather than the artery itself.

If the artery has been extensively damaged, or if the artery has become significantly narrowed by repeated suturing, it may be prudent to excise the segment and perform an end-to-end anastomosis or bypass graft. This may be done through a combined supraclavicular and transaxillary approach or sometimes just through the transaxillary incision. Whether or not the supraclavicular approach will be helpful depends upon how high the subclavian artery lies above the clavicle. If the artery lies at the level of the clavicle or lower, a supraclavicular anastomosis may not be feasible. As a last resort, a claviculectomy can be done to secure good exposure. The other alternative is a mediastinotomy for good exposure of the proximal subclavian artery. These extensive procedures are rarely needed but they should be in the armamentarium of the surgeon in the event of uncontrollable hemorrhage.

Pleural Space Air and Fluid

Pneumothorax

Opening the pleura during transaxillary rib resection is quite common and should not be considered a complication unless a postoperative thoracentesis is necessary to evacuate air or fluid. The reported incidence of entering the pleura varies widely. In our experience the pleura was entered in 30% of transaxillary first rib resections and 12% of supraclavicular first rib resections. Needle aspiration and occasionally chest tube insertions were needed in 9% and 2.5%, respectively, for rib resections by each route (Table 11–1). This generally has been a minor and temporary complication.

Obtaining a routine postoperative chest x-ray will usually detect pneumothorax and permit its appropriate management. No treatment is necessary for small pneumothoraces (under 10%, an apical cap); the air will be absorbed within a few days. Larger pneumothoraces, large enough to demonstrate air pushing the lung away from the side of the chest wall, are treated by plastic needle aspiration followed by a repeat chest x-ray. This usually handles the problem because the air entered the pleural space through the incision, not from a hole in the lung. If air reaccumulates, a chest tube is inserted; however, air rarely reaccumulates.

Hemothorax

Once the pleura has been opened, it becomes possible for blood from the operative area to enter the pleural space and produce a hemothorax. In over 400 rib resections, we have seen that occur in three patients, two of whom had histories of bleeding tendencies. They were initially treated with thoracenteses and one required a chest tube later the same day because of reaccumulation. None had further sequelae, but there is always the potential for pleural fibrosis and reduced ventilatory capacity when hemothorax occurs.

The instillation of water or saline into the incision just prior to closing the wound to detect a rent in the pleura is a common practice. However, we have not employed the practice because such a rent in the pleura will not affect the management of the case and, if there should be a sizable pleural defect, the water will disappear into the pleural space causing a hydrothorax.

To avoid postoperative pneumothorax when the pleural space has been entered, the anesthesiologist is asked to expand the lungs just prior to closure, thereby evacuating any air that might have entered the pleural space undetected. The patient is then ventilated with the lung in an expanded position while the incision is closed. This takes only a few minutes and reduces the size of postoperative pneumothoraces. In addition, the routine use of a small (3–5 mm diameter), closed suction drainage tube with several holes will help remove any extra- or intrapleural air in the first few minutes after skin closure. The same drain will also reduce the amount of blood collecting over the nerves of the plexus in the first several hours postoperatively.

Thoracic Duct Injury

In the left neck, the thoracic duct passes through the scalene fat pad to enter the subclavian vein. In our experience, the duct has seldom been seen. However, in a handful of cases, lymph has been seen floating in the wound. When this occurs, efforts are made to identify and ligate the thoracic duct. In one of our cases in which the duct had been ligated, a lymph fistula still developed in the neck. This was managed by exploring the wound and occluding the duct with a metal clip, thereby keeping dissection to a minimum to prevent tearing the duct again.

References

1. Dale A. Thoracic outlet compression syndrome: critique in 1982. Arch Surg 1982; 117:1437–1445.
2. Horowitz SH. Brachial plexus injuries with causalgia resulting from transaxillary rib resection. Arch Surg 1985; 120:1189–1191.
3. Thomas GI, Jones TW, Stavney LS, Manhas DR. Thoracic outlet syndrome. Am Surg 1978; 44:483–495.
4. Reilly LM, Stoney RJ. Supraclavicular approach for thoracic outlet decompression. J Vasc Surg 1988; 8:329–334.
5. Graham GG, Lincoln BM. Anterior resection of first rib for thoracic outlet syndrome. Am J Surg 1973; 126:803–806.
6. Stayman JW. Thoracic outlet syndrome. Surg Clin North Am 1973:667–671.
7. Stanton PE Jr, McClusky DA Jr, Richardson HD, Lamis PA. Thoracic outlet syndrome: a comprehensive evaluation. South Med J 1978; 71:1070–1073.
8. Kelly TR. Thoracic outlet syndrome: current concepts of treatment. Ann Surg 1979; 190:657–662.
9. Wood VE, Twito R, Verska JM. Thoracic outlet syndrome: the results of first rib resection in 100 patients. Orthop Clin North Am 1988; 19:131–146.
10. Sanders RJ, Roos DB. The surgical anatomy of the scalene triangle. Contemp Surg 1989; 35:11–16.
11. Loh CS, Wu AVO, Stevenson IM. Surgical decompression for thoracic outlet syndrome. J R Coll Surg Edin 1989; 34:66–68.
12. Petersen RE, Staab FD, Brintall ES. An evaluation of transaxillary removal of cervical and first rib. J Iowa Med Soc 1971; 61:554–556.
13. Sanders RJ, Monsour JW, Gerber FG, Adams WRA, Thompson N. Scalenectomy versus first rib resection for treatment of the thoracic outlet syndrome. Surgery 1979; 85:109–121.
14. Lepantalo M, Lindgren K-A, Leino E, Lindfors O, vonSmitten K, Nuutinen E, Totterman S. Long term outcome after resection of the first rib for thoracic outlet syndrome. Br J Surg 1989; 76:1255–1256.

12
Results of Treatment and Comments

Richard J. Sanders

The results of surgery for thoracic outlet syndrome (TOS) vary among individual reports, but in general, they are similar. The English-language medical literature has been reviewed extensively and the results of the different surgical approaches for TOS have been summarized in the several tables that follow.

Summary of Results of the Literature

Grading of Results

There is no uniformity in the grading of postoperative results. The standards are all subjective. The most complete evaluations divide results into four categories:

Excellent—Complete relief of all symptoms
Good—Relief of major symptoms but some symptoms persist
Fair—Partial relief but some major symptoms persist
Poor—No improvement

In spite of the fact that many reports do not define degrees of success or do so in different ways, it is still possible to assign some broad definitions to all of these reports so that comparisons can be made. The following classification is used in describing the cases from the literature:

Good Result—Relief of all or most major symptoms; the patient feels the operation was a success (excellent and good results are combined).
Fair Result—Relief of some symptoms but persistence of other major symptoms; the patient feels the operation was worthwhile in spite of incomplete improvement.
Poor Result—No improvement; the patient feels the operation was a failure.

Length of Follow-up

It is recognized that the results of TOS surgery deteriorate with time regardless of which operation is performed. This is not evident from most of the reports in the literature that tend to state the results over a time range that extends from a few months to a few years, but where the actual number of patients followed for a few years is not stated. When our own cases were expressed this way, the majority of follow-ups were under one year. Even when the operation was performed many years ago, the actual last contact may have been just a short time postoperatively. It cannot be assumed that since the patient has not contacted the surgeon for a long time that the patient is asymptomatic. In general, most reports should be regarded as stating short-term success, that is, for the first few months following surgery, unless the publication indicates the specific length of time of the follow-up information.

Long-term results are best expressed with the life-table method[1] that we have used to record our own results in the tables that follow (Tables 12–11 through 12–16). These results extend to 10–15 years postoperatively. A disadvantage of the life-table method is that it recognizes only one degree of success; excellent, good, and fair results cannot be separated in the graphs (although they can be separately listed in tables). This is not a major problem as the advantages of the life-table method far outweigh the disadvantages. In using the life-table method, the definitions of results are as follows:

Success—Improvement from surgery, including excellent, good, and fair relief of symptoms. The patient feels the operation was worthwhile.

Failure—No improvement or so little improvement that the patient feels the operation was not worthwhile.

Statistics

Chi-square analysis was used to test for statistical significance. In many situations, although there were differences that appear to be great, they did not reach the statistical value of less than 0.05, probably because the numbers of subjects were not large enough.

Scalenotomy and Scalenectomy

Operations on the scalene muscles include anterior scalenotomy—cutting the muscle without removing it; anterior scalenectomy—excising the muscle; and combined anterior and middle scalenectomy—excising both muscles. Eight reports on scalenotomy totaling 241 operations had an average failure rate of 31%. The range of individual reports is large, from 7% to 60% failure (Table 12–1). In

Table 12–1. **Results of Anterior Scalenotomy**

Author	Year	No. Oper- ations	Good No.	Good %	Fair No.	Fair %	Failed No.	Failed %	Length of Follow-up
Annersten[2]	1947	19	17	89%			2	11%	14 for 2–10 months 5 for 24–96 months
Holden et al.[3]	1951	28	22	79%	4	14%	2	7%	Under 36 months
Raff et al.[4]	1955	17	8	47%			9	53%	Not stated
Shenkin, Somach[5]	1963	28	14	50%			14	50%	36–150 months
deBruin[6]	1966	106	55	52%	19	18%	32	30%	Not stated
Urschel et al.[7]	1971	23	6	26%	9	39%	8	35%	84–294 months
Narakas et al.[8]	1986	10	4	40%			6	60%	Not stated
Takagi et al.[9]	1987	10	8	80%			2	20%	12–96 months
TOTALS		241	134	56%	32	13%	75	31%	
RANGES		241		26–89%		0–39%		7–60%	

comparison, six reports of scalenectomy totalling 338 cases had an average failure rate of 12% with a range of 0–25% (Table 12–2). Although there is a difference in failure rates of 31% versus 12%, this difference was not statistically significant ($P = 1.6$).

Although simple division of the anterior scalene muscle has had some success, a number of people have observed reconstitution of this muscle at a later date with the reproduction of symptoms. We have operated upon a few patients with histories of having had a scalenotomy who at surgery had a normal-appearing, intact anterior scalene muscle. Enough poor results from anterior scalenotomy have been recorded to at least replace division of the muscle with its excision. Technically, scalenectomy is not much more difficult than scalenotomy and the complications are no different. Because of the potential for fewer recurrences, scalenectomy would logically seem to be a superior procedure to scalenotomy, even though the difference of 31% vs. 12% failures was not statistically significant.

In patients with cervical ribs, both scalenotomy and scalenectomy have been done *without* resecting the cervical rib. (The reason for not removing the rib goes back to Adson's experiences in the 1920s and 1930s when he found that scalenectomy alone was adequate to relieve symptoms in many patients with cervical ribs and it avoided brachial plexus injury, which was frequently seen following cervical rib resection in the early 1900s). In these cases, there were no instances of subclavian artery aneurysm or obstruction. The results in both series were excellent (Table 12–3).

Middle scalenectomy, added to anterior scalenectomy, has only twice been reported. One report is by Cikrit et al.[15] in the group of scalenectomies in Table 12–2, and the other is our series of 286 scalenectomies (Table 12–12), which included the middle as well as the anterior scalene muscle (most of the patients in this group were first reported in 1979[16]).

Anterior and middle scalenotomy are an integral part of every first rib resection because detachment of these muscles is essential to removing the first rib.

Table 12–2. **Results of Anterior Scalenectomy**

Author	Year	No. Oper- ations	Good		Fair		Failed		Length of Follow-up
			No.	%	No.	%	No.	%	
Adson[10]	1947	53	43	84%	3	6%	7	13%	12–240 months
Stowell[11]	1956	154	123	84%	14	9%	17	7%	12–72 months
Woods[12]	1978	90	68	75%	10	11%	12	14%	84 months average
Gu et al.[13]	1988	12	7	58%	2	17%	3	25%	24–180 months
Loh et al.[14]	1989	14	11	59%	3	21%	0	0%	4–72 months
Cikrit et al.[a, 15]	1989	15	14	93%			1	7%	36 months average
TOTALS		338	266	79%	32	9%	40	12%	
RANGES		338		58–93%		0–21%		0–25%	

[a] Both anterior and middle scalenectomy.

Table 12–3. **Results of Scalenectomy or Scalenotomy in Patients With Cervical Ribs, Without Cervical Rib Resection**

Author	Year	No. Operations	Good No.	Good %	Fair	Failed No.	Failed %	Length of Follow-up
Adson[a, 10]	1947	63	57	90%	0	6	10%	12–240 months
Shenkin Somach[b, 5]	1963	15	15	100%	0	0		36–150 months
TOTALS		78	72	93%	0	6	7%	

[a] Scalenectomy.
[b] Scalenotomy.

Anatomical studies of the brachial plexus and scalene muscles have demonstrated the close relationship of C-7 and C-8 to the middle scalene muscle. C-7 is often totally surrounded and sometimes encased by middle scalene muscle fibers. Congenital bands and ligaments, particularly ligaments running from the transverse process of C-7 to the first rib, usually run in the belly of the middle scalene, close to C-7 and C-8.

Although no study has been published comparing the results of anterior scalenectomy with those of combined anterior and middle scalenectomy, knowing the many anatomical variations and anomalies involving the middle scalene muscles[17,18] suggests that middle scalenectomy along with anterior scalenectomy should be carried out when scalenectomy is performed. The one exception to this conclusion would be the case of upper plexus involvement only, for which anterior scalenectomy will probably suffice.

First Rib Resection—All Approaches

Five different routes have been described to remove the first rib: transaxillary, supraclavicular, infraclavicular, posterior, and transpleural. Each approach has its advantages and proponents.

Transaxillary Approach

An incision in the axilla has been the most popular route for first rib resection since its introduction by Roos in 1966. Between 1968 and 1989, over 3,000 of these operations have been recorded in 21 separate reports.[*] The good results varied widely between authors, from 37% to 100%, averaging 83% (Table 12–4). Failures ranged from 0% to 41%, averaging 12%. Differences can be attributed, at least in part, to short follow-up and to a lack of standardization of definitions of success and failure. Demonstrating the importance of length of follow-up is the report of Lepantalo, who in 1989 noted that the number of asymptomatic patients fell from 52% one month postoperatively to 37% when the minimum follow-up was 30 months.[36]

---

[*] In Tables 12–1 to 12–9 a few publications were excluded because the statistics in the manuscripts were unclear or because their numbers were too small.

Table 12–4. Results of Transaxillary First Rib Resection

Author	Year	No. Oper- ations	Good No.	Good %	Fair No.	Fair %	Failed No.	Failed %	Length of Follow-up
Sanders et al.[19]	1968	69	62	90%			7	10%	4–36 months
Roeder et al.[20]	1973	26	24	92%	1	4%	1	4%	6–42 months
Hoofer, Burnett[21]	1973	135	135	100%			0		Not stated
Dale[22]	1975	49	46	94%			3	6%	1–96 months
Kremer, Ahlquist[23]	1975	48	41	86%			7	14%	6 months minimum
McGough et al.[24]	1979	113	90	80%	15	13%	8	7%	6–60 months
Youmans, Smiley[25]	1980	258	193	75%	42	16%	23	9%	3–96 months (avg. = 34 months)
Roos[26]	1982	1,315	1,210	92%			105	8%	Presumed 3–180 months
Batt et al.[27]	1983	94	76	80%			18	20%	
Sallstrom, Gjores[28]	1983	72	58[a]	81%	9	12%	5	7%	Average 30 months
Heughan[29]	1984	44	33	75%			11	25%	Not stated
Qvarfordt et al.[30]	1984	97	77	79%			20	21%	4–48 months
Narakas et al.[8]	1986	43	33	77%			10	23%	Not stated
Takagi et al.[9]	1987	48	38	79%			10	21%	12–96 months
Davies, Mes- serschmidt[31]	1988	115	103	89%			12	11%	6–180 months
Selke, Kelly[32]	1988	460	363	79%	64	14%	33	7%	6–240 months
Stanton et al.[33]	1988	87	74	85%	4	4%	10	11%	12–144
Wood et al.[34]	1988	54	48	89%	5	9%	1	2%	6 month minimum
Cikrit et al.[15]	1989	30	19	63%			11	37%	Average 36 months
Lindgren et al.[35]	1989	175	103	59%			72	41%	24 months
Lepantalo et al.[36]	1989	112	56	52%	27	25%	29	23%	1 month
Lepantalo et al.[36]	1989	84[b]	31	37%[b]		?		?	Minimum 30 months
TOTALS		3,444	2,882	83%	169	5%	396	12%	
RANGES		3,444		37–100%		0–14%		0–41%	

[a] Three cases had late recurrence, yet are classified by authors as success.
[b] Not included in summary: duplicates above entry and lacks no. of total improved.

Supraclavicular Approach

Supraclavicular rib resection has been reported in a total of 715 cases by six investigators, the largest experiences being those of Hempel in 1981[37] and Thomas in 1983.[17] Good results averaged 83% with a range of 59% to 91%; failures averaged 4% with a narrow range, 3–13% (Table 12–5).

Infraclavicular Approach

The infraclavicular, sometimes called the "anterior," approach has not been used as often as the other routes. Only 44 cases have been reported, with good results averaging 82% and with a failure rate of 9% (Table 12–6).

Table 12–5. Results of Supraclavicular First Rib Resection (includes Anterior and Middle Scalenectomy)

Author	Year	No. Oper- ations	Good		Fair		Failed		Length of Follow-up
			No.	%	No.	%	No.	%	
Graham, Lincoln[38]	1973	78	71	91%	4	5%	3	4%	4–84 months
Thompson, Hernandez[39]	1979	15	13	87%			2	13%	Not stated
Hempel et al.[37]	1981	433	366	84%	55	13%	12	3%	Not stated
Thomas et al.[17]	1983	128	106	83%	17	13%	5	4%	Not stated
Reilly, Stoney[18]	1988	39	23	59%	13	33%	3	8%	1–30 months
Loh et al.[14]	1989	22	15	68%	5	23%	2	9%	4–72 months
TOTALS		715	594	83%	94	13%	27	4%	
RANGES		715		59–91%		5–33%		3–13%	

Table 12–6. Results of Infraclavicular First Rib Resection

Author	Year	No. Oper- ations	Good		Fair		Failed		Length of Follow-up
			No.	%	No.	%	No.	%	
Brodsky, Gol[40]	1970	22	20	91%			2	9%	Not stated
Murphy et al.[41]	1980	22	16	73%	4	18%	2	9%	Not stated
TOTALS		44	36	82%	4	9%	4	9%	

Posterior Approach

Five reports of the posterior thoracoplasty approach were available from 1962 to the early 1970s. The total of 175 cases had a success rate averaging 86% and a failure rate averaging 5%, with relatively small ranges (Table 12–7).

Transpleural Approach

First rib resection through the chest has only recently been reported in France by Pretre.[45] His results, using a life-table method, show a 75% success rate and a 25% failure rate among 18 cases (Table 12–8).

Combined Transaxillary and Supraclavicular Approach

By performing a scalenectomy through the neck and a rib resection through the axilla, Qvarfordt et al. achieved 99% good results with a 1% failure rate. However, the follow-up is relatively short[30] (Table 12–9). Following their study, the authors changed their approach to the combined operation by performing both scalenectomy and rib resection via the supraclavicular approach and abandoning the transaxillary route.[18]

Table 12–7. Results of Posterior First Rib Resection

Author	Year	No. Operations	Good No.	Good %	Fair No.	Fair %	Failed No.	Failed %	Length of Follow-up
Clagett[42]	1962	12	10	83%			2	17%	Not stated
McBurney, Howard[43]	1966	9	7	78%	2	22%	0		Few months
Lango et al.[44]	1970	37	27	73%	7	19%	3	8%	5–200 months
Roeder et al.[20]	1973	11	9	82%	1	9%	1	9%	6–42 months
Johnson[45]	1974	106	98	92%	6[a]	6%	2	2%	1–20 years
TOTALS		175	151	86%	16	9%	8	5%	
RANGES		175		73–92%		6–22%		2–17%	

[a] One case reoperated upon after 5 years for recurrence is classified as improved.

Table 12–8. Results of Transpleural First Rib Resection

Author	Year	No. Operations	Good	Fair	Failed	Length of Follow-up
Pretre et al.[46]	1989	18	75%		25%	36 month life-table

Table 12–9. Results of Combined Transaxillary First Rib Resection With Anterior and Middle Scalenectomy

Author	Year	No. Operations	Good No.	Good %	Fair	Failed No.	Failed %	Length of Follow-up
Qvarfordt et al.[29]	1984	94	93	99%		1	1%	4–48 months

Accuracy of Reports

Tables 12–1 through 12–9 are summarized in Table 12–10. The results of most of the operations are in the same range, except for scalenotomy and transpleural rib resection. It should also be recognized that some inaccuracies in reporting can occur. For example, in at least two studies, the investigators noted that cases listed in their tables as improved were later operated upon for recurrence, yet those cases still retained their listing as benefiting from their initial operation.[29, 45] Such patients are more accurately described as late failures. Carroll and Hurst also noted three cases of carpal tunnel syndrome in patients who were initially reported to have had good results following TOS surgery but in whom, according to the patients, the symptoms had not changed until after their carpal tunnel operations.[47]

Life-Table Method—Author's Data

In 1968 we reported our initial 69 cases of TOS treated by transaxillary first rib resection with short follow-ups of 4–36 months. The results are included in Table 12–4 and are similar to those of other authors in that table, 90% improved. In the next decade, as the life-table method became popular, we began collecting

Table 12–10. Summary of Results of All Operations for TOS[a]

Technique	No. Operations	Good	Fair	Failed
Anterior scalenotomy	241	57%	13%	30%
Anterior scalenectomy	338	79%	9%	12%
Transaxillary 1st rib resection	3,444	83%	5%	12%
Supraclavicular 1st rib resection	715	83%	13%	4%
Infraclavicular 1st rib resection	44	82%	9%	9%
Posterior 1st rib resection	175	86%	9%	5%
Transpleural 1st rib resection	18	75%		25%
Combined transax & scalenec	94	99%		1%

[a] This table summarizes the bottom lines of Tables 12–1 through 12–9, omitting 12–3.

our data and storing it in a computer database to provide more reliable longitudinal assessment. We also changed our operative approach to TOS based upon our ongoing observations. The data was first published using life tables in 1979 with a 5-year follow-up[16] and again in 1989 with a 10–15-year follow-up.[48]

The data for four operations is presented here: transaxillary first rib resection in Table 12–11; anterior and middle scalenectomy in Table 12–12; anterior and middle scalenectomy with supraclavicular first rib resection in Table 12–13; and anterior and middle scalenectomy plus supra- and infraclavicular first rib resection in Table 12–14. The data cover a 25-year period, from 1964 to 1988. The cases were not randomized but were performed in three time periods: transaxillary first rib resection from 1964 to 1972; anterior and middle scalenectomy from 1972 to 1980; and anterior and middle scalenectomy plus supraclavicular first rib resection

Table 12–11.   Transaxillary First Rib Resection—Life Table[a]

Time (months)	No. Operations at Risk[b]	Results Excellent	Good	Fair	Fail	ReOp[c]	Failed in Period	Cumulative Success Rate	Lost	Inadequate Follow-up[d]
1–3	112	41	55	6	8	2	10/112 = 9%	91%	0	0
4–6	102	26	43	5	0	6	6/91 = 6.6%	85%	22	0
7–9	74	24	38	3	1	3	4/70 = 5.7%	80%	5	0
10–12	65	20	37	4	0	0	0	80%	4	0
13–24	61	20	34	2	0	4	4/60 = 6.7%	75%	1	0
25–36	56	19	24	2	0	1	1/51 = 2%	73%	10	0
37–60	45	17	21	3	0	1	1/43 = 2.3%	71%	3	0
61–120	41	9	16	4	0	2	2/36 = 5.5%	68%	10	0
121–180	29	1	10	1	0	1	1/20 = 5%	64%	15	19
TOTALS					9	20	29/112 = 26%			

[a] Life table formula—Failure in an interval $= \dfrac{\text{No. failed}}{\text{No. at beginning} - \frac{1}{2} \text{ withdrawals}}$.

[b] Number of operations at beginning of time interval.

[c] Reop = reoperation.

[d] Inadequate follow-up, or not followed long enough.

Table 12–12.   Scalenectomy—Life Table[a]

Time (months)	No. Operations at Risk[b]	Results				Reop[c]	Failed in Period	Cumulative Success Rate	Lost	Inadequate Follow-up[d]
		Excellent	Good	Fair	Fail					
1–3	286	68	175	23	16	4	20/286 = 7%	93%	0	0
4–6	266	50	151	14	12	13	25/253 = 10%	84%	23	3
7–9	215	44	140	19	0	3	3/210 = 1.4%	83%	9	0
10–12	203	41	125	18	2	3	5/196 = 2.6%	80%	10	4
13–24	184	35	106	16	4	6	10/175 = 5.7%	76%	13	4
25–36	157	28	80	7	1	5	6/139 = 4.3%	73%	30	6
37–60	115	25	67	3	2	3	5/107 = 4.7%	69%	9	6
61–120	95	21	50	5	0	1	1/86 = 1%	68%	18	0
121–180	76	11	27	2	1	1	2/59 = 3.4%	66%	15	19
TOTALS				38	39		77/286 = 27%			

[a] Life table formula—Failure in an interval $= \dfrac{\text{No. failed}}{\text{No. at beginning} - \frac{1}{2} \text{ withdrawals}}$.

[b] Number of operations at beginning of time interval.

[c] Reop = reoperation.

[d] Inadequate follow-up, or not followed long enough.

Table 12–13.   Supraclavicular First Rib Resection and Scalenectomy—Life Table[a]

Time (months)	No. Operations at Risk[b]	Results				Reop[c]	Failed in Period	Cumulative Success Rate	Lost	Inadequate Follow-up[d]
		Excellent	Good	Fair	Fail					
1–3	249	52	158	19	19	1	20/249 = 8%	92%	0	0
4–6	229	44	137	20	4	4	8/219 = 3.7%	89%	13	7
7–9	201	41	125	23	5	0	5/197 = 2.5%	86%	5	0
10–12	189	38	115	23	0	1	1/183 = 0.5%	86%	6	6
13–24	176	35	94	17	11	5	16/161 = 10%	77%	7	7
25–36	146	28	74	12	5	2	7/134 = 5.2%	73%	11	14
37–60	114	22	57	8	5	1	6/104 = 5.8%	69%	4	17
61–120	87	15	31	4	0	0	0	69%	4	33
121–180	50	0	2	0	0	0	0	69%	0	48
TOTALS				49	14		63/249 = 25%			

[a] Life table formula—Failure in an interval $= \dfrac{\text{No. failed}}{\text{No. at beginning} - \frac{1}{2} \text{ withdrawals}}$.

[b] Number of operations at beginning of time interval.

[c] Reop = reoperation.

[d] Inadequate follow-up, or not followed long enough.

Table 12–14.   **Supra- and Infraclavicular First Rib Resection and Scalenectomy—Life Table[a]**

Time (months)	No. Operations at Risk[b]	Results				Reop[c]	Failed in Period	Cumulative Success Rate	Lost	Inadequate Follow-up[d]
		Excellent	Good	Fair	Fail					
1–3	45	7	35	1	2	0	2/45 = 4%	96%	0	0
4–6	43	5	29	3	1	0	1/41 = 2%	94%	2	3
7–9	37	2	28	5	0	0	0	94%	2	0
10–12	35	2	24	3	1	0	1/33 = 3%	91%	4	1
13–24	29	2	21	3	2	1	3/29 = 10%	82%	0	0
25–36	26	1	17	3	0	0	0	82%	2	3
37–60	21	1	11	2	0	1	1/18 = 5.5%	78%	6	0
61–120	14	0	9	0	0	0	0	78%	3	2
121–180	9	0	0	0	0	0	0	78%	0	9
TOTALS				6	2		8/45 = 18%			

[a] Life table formula—Failure in an interval $= \dfrac{\text{No. failed}}{\text{No. at beginning} - \frac{1}{2}\text{ withdrawals}}$.

[b] Number of operations at beginning of time interval.

[c] Reop = reoperation.

[d] Inadequate follow-up, or not followed long enough.

from 1980 to 1988. A small number of cases of supraclavicular first rib resection had an infraclavicular incision added to aid in removing the anterior part of the first rib. These cases are listed separately, since it first appeared that their results would be superior to those of the other operations, but with time, the difference has not been statistically significant. Therefore, in Table 12–15, the combined results of the supraclavicular approach, with and without an infraclavicular extension, are presented. The graph in Figure 12-1 shows that the short- and long-term results of the three operations are virtually identical.

Fair Results

In the life-table method, the fair results are counted as successes, just like good and excellent results. However, the tables permit identification of the number of fair results.

A "fair" result indicates only partial improvement. Some of the symptoms in the extremity were relieved, usually the paresthesia and arm pain, but other symptoms persisted and were significant factors in interfering with the patient's work, recreation, sleep, or daily living activities. In these cases, the diagnosis of TOS was probably correct. Failure to achieve more improvement was due to one of two factors: Either associated diagnoses accounted for the patient's continued discomfort or, following initial good relief of symptoms, enough scar tissue accumulated around the plexus to irritate or partially compress some of the nerve trunks. Fair results comprised 2–12% of the results at various time intervals in Tables 12–11 to 12–15.

Table 12–15.   **All Supra- and Infraclavicular First Rib Resections With Scalenectomy—Life Table[a] (Combined Tables 12–13 and 12–14)**

Time (months)	No. Operations at Risk[b]	Results				Reop[c]	Failed in Period	Cumulative Success Rate	Lost	Inadequate Follow-up[d]
		Excellent	Good	Fair	Fail					
1–3	294	59	193	20	21	1	22/294 = 7.5%	93%	0	0
4–6	272	49	166	23	5	4	9/260 = 3.5%	89%	15	10
7–9	238	43	153	28	5	0	5/235 = 2%	87%	2	0
10–12	224	40	139	26	1	1	2/216 = 1%	86%	10	7
13–24	205	37	115	20	13	6	19/198 = 10%	78%	7	7
25–36	172	29	91	15	5	2	7/134 = 5.2%	76%	13	17
37–60	135	23	68	10	5	2	7/122 = 5.7%	71%	10	17
61–120	101	15	40	4	0	0	0	71%	7	35
121–180	59	0	2	0	0	0	0	71%	0	57
TOTALS				55	16		71/294 = 24%			

[a] Life table formula—Failure in an interval = $\dfrac{\text{No. failed}}{\text{No. at beginning} - \frac{1}{2}\text{ withdrawals}}$.

[b] No. ops at risk = number of operations at beginning of time interval.

[c] Reop = reoperation.

[d] Inadequate follow-up, or not followed long enough.

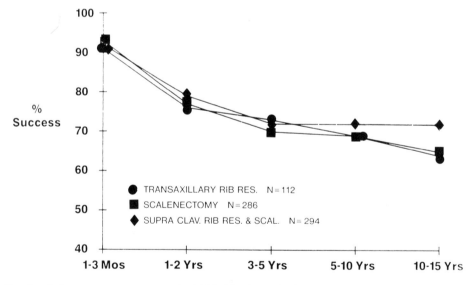

Fig. 12–1.   Results of three primary operations for TOS. Numbers of subjects are in Tables 12–11, 12–12, 12–15, and 12–18.

It is debatable whether or not "fair" results should be classified with successes or failures. They have been included here with successes because in each case the patient stated that the operation provided enough improvement to undergo surgery again for the same amount of relief. Patients who would not consider surgery again for the amount of improvement they received were classified as failures.

Life-Table Method vs. Standard Method

The life-table data is summarized in Table 12–16 to permit all of the procedures to be compared. In addition, the results are expressed for each operation using the standard method of dividing the total number of failures by the total number of operations over the entire length of time of the study. With follow-ups that went to 15 years, the life-table method indicates a success rate 5–9% lower than the conventional method. This also permits comparing these results to the other cases in the literature, bearing in mind that the follow-up period in these cases is longer than most of the other reported series.

When the life-table method is used, late failures reduce the cumulative success rate by a greater percentage than early failures because failure is expressed as a ratio in which the denominator is the number of cases at risk in that time interval. Since the number at risk steadily falls at each time interval by the total of the number failed, lost, and not followed to the end of the interval, the denominator steadily falls. This is the explanation for the 10–15-year success rate being lower by the life-table method than by the standard method (Table 12–16).

Time of Failure

The time that failure occurred was remarkably similar for each of the three operative approaches. By 6 months, 55% (16 of 29) of the failures following transaxillary first rib resection were evident; for scalenectomy, the 6-month figure was 58% (45 of 77); and for supraclavicular first rib resection, the 6-month figure was 44% (31 of 71). By 2 years, the percentage of failures for the three procedures was 83%, 82%, and 80%, respectively (Tables 12–11, 12–12, and 12–15). The remaining 17–20% of the failures occurred more than 2 years postoperatively.

Table 12–16. **Results—Comparison of Life-Table and Standard Methods**

| | Life-Table Method[a] | | | | | | | | | Standard Method[b] | | |
| | 1–3 months | | 1–2 years | | 3–5 years | | 5–10 years | | 10–15 years | | 1–180 months | | |
Operation[c]	%	No.	%	No.	%	No.	%	No.	%	No.	Fail No.	Fail %	Success %
1. Transax RR	91%	112	75%	61	71%	45	68%	41	64%	29	77	27%	73%
2. Scalenec	93%	286	76%	184	69%	115	68%	95	66%	76	39	26%	74%
3. Supracl RR	92%	249	77%	176	69%	114	69%	87	69%	50	63	25%	75%
4. Supracl and Infracl RR	96%	45	82%	29	78%	21	78%	14	78%	9	8	18%	82%
5. Comb 3 and 4	93%	294	78%	205	71	135	71	101	71	59	70	24%	76%

[a] Successful results, which includes excellent, good, and fair results.
[b] Standard method is dividing total number of failures by total number operated upon. The denominator in each case is the same number of operations as in the 1–3 month column.
[c] Transax RR = transaxillary first rib resection; Scalenec = anterior and middle scalenectomy; Supracl RR = supraclavicular first rib resection with anterior and middle scalenectomy; Supracl and Infracl RR = supra- and infraclavicular first rib resection with anterior and middle scalenectomy; Comb 3 and 4 = combined lines 3 and 4 (both variations of supraclavicular first rib resection).

First Rib Resection vs. Scalenectomy

In describing the reasons for discarding scalenectomy in favor of first rib resection, many investigators have selected the reports of Raaf,[4] Urschell,[7] and Clagett,[42] to stress the point that scalenotomy is a poor operation. However, when all of the articles on scalenotomy, scalenectomy, and first rib resection are reviewed and compared together, the differences between the operations are not as great as is sometimes depicted. This is particularly true as the initial high success rates from first rib resection have deteriorated with time and the reports of more observers now indicate less glowing improvement rates than the early 90% successes that first appeared (Table 12–4). Illustrating this are the last two series in this table, which were reported from Scandinavia in 1989 and contain the highest failure rate, 41%. In both instances, the follow-up was a minimum of 2 years.[35, 36]

Two comparisons are worth noting. From the literature, the reported failure rate of anterior scalenectomy compared to transaxillary first rib resection is very similar (Table 12–10); From the results we have reported with the life-table method, the short- and long-term results of scalenectomy compared to either transaxillary or supraclavicular first rib resection are virtually identical (Tables 12–11, 12–12, and 12–15 and Fig. 12-1).

Another interesting study also failed to find any difference in outcome between scalenectomy and first rib resection. In a subgroup of 38 patients with bilateral symptoms, anterior and middle scalenectomy was performed on one side and first rib resection on the other. Rib resections were transaxillary in six and supraclavicular in 32. The results between the two sides were identical in 27 (71%); better with rib resection in six (16%); and better with scalenectomy in five (13%) (Table 12–17). Furthermore, the improvement of one operation over the other was only one grade of success in 8 of the 11 patients who did not have identical results (excellent vs. good; good vs. fair). Their was a major difference between the two sides in only three of the 38 patients (Table 12–17).

These observations raise the obvious question concerning the role of the normal first rib in neurogenic TOS if the same amount of improvement that is seen following rib resection can be achieved by scalenectomy without rib resection. The question is particularly pertinent when scalenectomy is not accompanied by the same risks of nerve injury and postoperative morbidity as rib resection.

The answer to this question is that the first rib, in all but a small number of cases, is merely an attachment point for the scalene muscles; rib resection is

Table 12–17. **Bilateral Operations: Scalenectomy One Side; Rib Resection Other Side**

Result	No. Patients	Better by 1 Grade[a]	Better by 2 Grades[a]
Identical, both sides	27		
Rib resection better	6	4	2
Scalenectomy better	5	4	1
TOTALS	38	8	3

[a] Grade = grades are excellent, good, and fair.

effective probably because the scalene muscles must be cut (anterior and middle scalenotomy) in order to excise the rib; and removal of the first rib itself is incidental. The first rib serves as a point to which postoperative scar tissue can attach and reproduce plexus compression. However, even when the rib is removed, thereby eliminating the attachment point, the incidence of recurrence due to postoperative scarring is the same as when the rib is not removed (Tables 12–11 to 12–16). Therefore, the role of the first rib and the benefits derived from its removal in patients with neurogenic TOS has yet to be demonstrated.

Reoperation and Primary vs. Secondary Success

The effect of reoperation on the initial operation is determined by comparing primary and secondary success rates in a manner similar to the comparison of primary and secondary vascular graft patency.[49] The primary success rate is defined as the percentage of success of each initial operation (patient-side), using the life-table method; any patient-side requiring reoperation is regarded as a failure. Secondary success is the combined success rate of each primary operation plus the success rate of each reoperation. In secondary success, each patient-side is counted only once, and the success or failure of that patient-side determined by the current status of the last operative procedure. For example, a patient who had a primary scalenectomy and later required a first rib resection as a reoperation for recurrence, would be regarded as a primary failure but a secondary success of the scalenectomy as long as the symptoms were improved. The secondary success rates for transaxillary first rib resection, scalenectomy, and supraclavicular rib resection with scalenectomy are presented in Table 12–18 and Figure 12-2. The secondary success rates for transaxillary first rib resection and for scalenectomy were statistically significantly higher than the primary success rates for each operation. The difference between primary and secondary success for supraclavicular first rib resection with scalenectomy was not statistically significantly different, probably because very few of the patients in this group were reoperated upon when their primary operation failed.

Table 12–18. **Life-Table Results of Primary Operation and Effect of Reoperation**

Operation	I or II Success[a]	No. Operations	1–3 months %	No.[b]	1–2 years %	No.	3–5 years %	No.	5–10 years %	No.	10–15 years %	No.
Transax rib	I	112	91%	112	74%	61	71%	45	68%	41	64%	29
	II	112	92%	112	90%	71	90%	62	86%	55	86%	47
Scalenectomy[c]	I	286	93%	286	76%	184	69%	115	68%	95	66%	76
	II	286	94%	286	87%	202	84%	139	84%	115	82%	93
SC rib and scalenec[d]	I	294	93%	294	78%	205	71%	135	71%	101	71%	59
	II	294	93%	294	82%	208	74%	141	74%	106	74%	61

[a] I = Primary success—successful result from first operation; no further operations; II = secondary success—includes all cases with primary success plus those in whom the initial operation failed but subsequent reoperations succeeded.
[b] Number of cases at risk at beginning of that time interval.
[c] Anterior and middle scalenectomy.
[d] Supraclavicular first rib resection and anterior and middle scalenectomy.

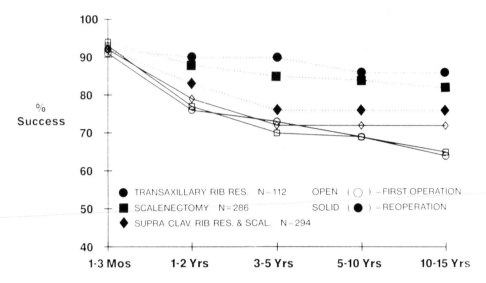

Fig. 12-2.   The influence of reoperation on the success rates of initial operations for TOS. The initial success rates (open symbols) of 3 different operations for TOS were virtually identical ($P > 0.05$ at all time periods for all comparisons). Reoperation improved the success rate for primary first rib resection from 69% to 86% at the 5–10-year time period; for scalenectomy from 69% to 84% over the same time period. These differences are reflected in the secondary success rates (solid circles). The difference between primary and secondary success rates for each of these two operations was statistically significant for all time intervals beyond six months ($P < 0.05$ to two years and $P < 0.01$ after two years). Also statistically significant was the difference between the secondary success rate of rib resection or scalenectomy compared to the primary success rate of the combined operation ($P < 0.05$ for all time intervals after 9 months). Only 6% of the patients who initially received the combined operation were reoperated upon (solid diamond), so there is little possibility, statistically, for significant secondary success in this group ($P > 0.05$ at all time intervals). Numbers of subjects are in Tables 12–11, 12–12, 12–15, and 12–18. For secondary success, each patient-side is counted only once, and the success or failure of that patient-side determined by the current status of the last operative procedure.

Staging the Operative Treatment

Because combining scalenectomy with rib resection in one operation failed to reduce the failure rate of either operation alone (Table 12–18, Fig. 12-2), performing both operations simultaneously has little advantage. Statistically, performing only one procedure at a time seems preferable as it permits raising the success rate about 15% by performing the other operation as a reoperation in the event of recurrence.

Variables

Influence of Physical Examination on Results

Two findings on physical examination have been present in almost 90% of TOS patients who underwent operation: tenderness over the scalene muscles in the supraclavicular area and reproduction of the patient's symptoms with the arms abducted to 90 degrees in external rotation (90-degree AER position). A third physical finding, reduction of the radial pulse with the arms in the 90-degree AER position, often referred to as the modified Adson maneuver, has been present in about 30% of our patients. The presence or absence of each of these physical findings is matched against the failure rate of surgery for 687 primary operations in Table 12–19. The number of failures was not statistically significantly different for each of the physical findings.

This raises the question of how important these physical findings are and what their role is in diagnosis. At the present time, the answer is a poor one: These are the only physical findings that fit the clinical picture and we use them because there are no others. However, they should not be regarded as absolutely essential in making the diagnosis.

Similar correlations were tested by Lepantalo et al. and it was found that neither vascular laboratory studies, functional angiography, electromyography (EMG), positional pulse cut off, nor the 90-degree AER test were helpful in predicting which patients with clinical diagnoses of TOS would benefit from surgery.[36] However, their study did find that first rib resection was more often unsuccessful in patients whose preoperative symptoms were associated with neck pain or were worse at night than in patients in whom these complaints were absent.

Influence of Etiology on Results

The different etiologies of TOS are listed in Table 12–20 and correlated with the numbers of failures for each etiology. In the separation of different types of trauma, there are two categories related to the work place: work accidents and work-related symptoms that could also be called "chronic trauma." Only five cases are listed as having an etiology of a cervical or rudimentary first rib. There were many more instances of osseous abnormalities in this series, but in all of the others, there was also a history of trauma immediately preceding the onset of symptoms. Therefore, those cases are classified under etiology "trauma." Table 12–20 indicates that general neck trauma and auto accidents correlated with 20–26% failures, whereas work-related symptoms and accidents had a failure rate of over 40% (differences not statistically significant; $P \geq 0.05$ for all comparisons).

Table 12–19. **Influence of Physical Findings on Results of 687 Primary Operations (Variable Factors)**

Physical Exam	Variation	No. Operations	No. Failed	% Failed
Supraclavicular	Present	621	162	26%
Tenderness	Absent	66	14	21%
Duplication of Symptoms at 90 AER[a]	Present	628	163	26%
	Absent	46	11	21%
	Unknown	13	2	15%
Pulse Change at 90 AER[a]	Decrease	196	49	25%
	Unchanged	491	127	26%

[a] 90 AER = arms abducted to 90 degrees in external rotation.

Table 12–20.   Influence of Etiology on Results

Etiology	No. Operations	Failures							
		1–3 months		1–6 months		1–24 months		1–180 months	
		No.	%	No.	%	No.	%	No.	%
Trauma (unspecified)	308	20	6%	38	12%	55	18%	62	20%
Cerv Rib or Rud 1st Rib[a]	5	0		0		0		0	
Auto Accident—Rear-ended	112	5	4%	13	12%	24	21%	29	26%
Auto Accident—Not Rear-ended	89	6	7%	9	10%	15	17%	23	26%
Unknown	71	7	10%	12	17%	17	24%	21	30%
Work Accident	78	9	12%	13	17%	23	29%	32	41%
Work-related (No accident)[b]	14	2	14%	4	29%	6	43%	6	43%
TOTALS	677	49	7%	89	13%	140	21%	173	26%

[a] Cervical rib or rudimentary first rib.
[b] Patients who developed symptoms on a job requiring extensive use of their arms and/or hands, but had no accident.

Despite this, others have shown that etiology, and particularly work habits, may matter. In studies by Youmans and Smiley[25] and by Lepantalo et al.,[36] patients whose symptoms developed in relationship to their jobs did not have as good results as those patients whose injuries were not job-related. The relationship between certain types of occupations and cervico-brachial or TOS symptoms has been studied by a few investigators who have pointed out that jobs requiring repetitive motions, such as assembly line jobs, keyboard operating, and cash register clerking have a much higher incidence of shoulder, arm, and hand symptoms than people in other occupations.[50–52] Precisely how these occupations cause the symptoms has not been learned with certainty, but constant stress and stretch on shoulder or neck muscles is a probable mechanism. If these muscles include the scalenes, the opportunity for brachial plexus compression has been established.

A discouraging observation among TOS patients from these same occupational areas is that even when there is good relief of symptoms following surgery, the patients frequently develop recurrent symptoms when they return to their previous occupations. Changing jobs to ones requiring less continuous use of the arms and shoulders in elevated positions is needed. These observations have been true both for patients suffering acute neck injuries at work as well as for those who developed symptoms on the job in the absence of an acute injury. Including both the failures and "fair" results in these patients, more than half have been unable to return to their previous jobs. Another characteristic of this group of patients is that many of them have had several nerve decompression operations, including carpal tunnel and ulnar nerve releases. A good explanation for that observation has yet to be provided.

Upper Plexus vs. Lower Plexus

TOS can present with symptoms of paresthesia in the fourth and fifth fingers (lower plexus); first three fingers (upper plexus); all five fingers (both plexuses); or no paresthesia at all. In Table 12–21, the successful results of each operation are

Table 12–21. Results of Primary Operations: Upper Plexus vs. Lower Plexus

Ops[a]	Lower Plexus Numbness 4 & 5 fingers			Upper Plexus Numbness 1–3 fingers			Both Plexus Numbness All 5 fingers			No Numbness			Totals		
	No. ops	Success No.	%	No. ops	Success No.	%	No. ops	Success No.	%	No. ops	Success No.	%	No. ops	Success No.	%
Transax Rib[b]	20	15	75%	20	14	70%	58	44	76%	14	11	79%	112	84	75%
Scalenec[c]	77	56	73%	33	25	76%	147	105	71%	29	23	79%	286	209	73%
Supracl Rib & Scalenec[d]	90	79	88%	41	23	56%	137	100	73%	26	21	79%	294	223	76%
TOTALS	187	150	80%	94	62	66%	342	249	73%	69	55	80%	692	516	75%

[a] Ops = operations.

[b] Transax Rib = transaxillary first rib resection.

[c] Scalenec = anterior and middle scalenectomy with brachial plexus neurolysis.

[d] Supracl Rib & Scalenec = supraclavicular first rib resection with anterior and middle scalenectomy. This includes 45 cases in which an infraclavular incision was also used.

compared to the different clinical presentations. Although differences exist between the various operations and presentations, none is statistically significant.

It has been suggested that the clinical presentation in the form of upper or lower plexus symptoms is an appropriate criterion to help select the surgical approach in TOS: Because the upper plexus lies beneath the anterior scalene muscle, anterior scalenectomy has been recommended for upper plexus symptoms; similarly, since the lower plexus runs close to the first rib, first rib resection has been recommended for lower plexus symptoms; and when symptoms from both plexuses are present, both operations, scalenectomy and first rib resection, are recommended.[26] However, the findings of Table 12–21 do not support such a strategy. Scalenectomy was as effective for lower plexus symptoms as was rib resection; rib resection had as good results as scalenectomy for upper plexus symptoms.

Mention should be made of the fact that scalenectomy in these patients included both the anterior and middle scalene muscles. It is possible that the reason this type of scalenectomy achieved as good a result as rib resection for lower plexus symptoms is that removal of the middle scalene muscle effectively decompressed C-7 and C-8, which was sufficient to relieve the lower plexus symptoms.

References

1. Colton T. Statistics in medicine. Boston; Little Brown & Co., 1975:237–250.
2. Annersten S. Studies on the scalenus anticus syndrome. Acta Surg Scand 1947; 95:419–439.
3. Holden WD, Murphy JA, Portmann AF. Scalene anticus syndrome: unusual diagnostic and therapeutic aspects. Am J Surg 1951; 81:411–416.
4. Raaf J. Surgery for cervical rib and scalenus anticus syndrome. J Am Med Assoc 1955; 157:219–223.
5. Shenkin HA, Somach FM. Scalenotomy in patients with and without cervical ribs. Arch Surg 1963; 87:30–34.

6. deBruin TR. Costoclavicular space enlargement. Eight methods for relief of neuro-vascular compression. Int Surg 1966; 46:340–360.

7. Urschel HC, Razzuk MA, Wood RE, Parekh M, Paulson DL. Objective diagnosis (ulnar nerve conduction velocity) and current therapy of the thoracic outlet syndrome. Ann Thorac Surg 1971; 12:608–620.

8. Narakas A, Bonnard C, Egloff DV. The cervico-thoracic outlet syndrome. Ann Chir Main 1986; 5:185–207.

9. Takagi K, Yamaga M, Morisawa K, Kitagawa T. Management of thoracic outlet syndrome. Arch Orthop Trauma Surg 1987; 106:78–81.

10. Adson AW. Surgical treatment for symptoms produced by cervical ribs and the scalenus anticus muscle. Surg Gynecol Obstet 1947; 85:687–700.

11. Stowell A. The scalenus anticus syndrome. J Int Coll Surg 1956; 26:711–717.

12. Woods WW. Thoracic outlet syndrome. West J Med 1978; 128:9–12.

13. Gu YD, Wu M, Zheng Y, et al. Combined supra-infraclavicular approach for excision of the first rib in the treatment of the thoracic outlet syndrome. Chung Hua Wai Ko Tsa Chih 1984; 22:692–693.

14. Loh CS, Wu AVO, Stevenson IM. Surgical decompression for thoracic outlet syndrome. J R Coll Surg Edin 1989; 34:66–68.

15. Cikrit DF, Haefner R, Nichols WK, Silver D. Transaxillary or supraclavicular decompression for the thoracic outlet syndrome: a comparison of the risks and benefits. Amer Surgeon 1989; 55:347–352.

16. Sanders RJ, Monsour JW, Gerber FG, Adams WRA, Thompson N. Scalenectomy versus first rib resection for treatment of the thoracic outlet syndrome. Surgery 1979; 85:109–121.

17. Thomas GI, Jones TW, Stavney LS, Manhas DR. The middle scalene muscle and its contribution to the TOS. Am J Surg 1983; 145:589–592.

18. Reilly LM, Stoney RJ. Supraclavicular approach for thoracic outlet decompression. J Vasc Surg 1988; 8:329–334.

19. Sanders RJ, Monsour JW, Baer SB. Transaxillary first rib resection for the thoracic outlet syndrome. Arch Surg 1968; 97:1014–1023.

20. Roeder DK, Mills M, McHale JJ, Shepard BM, Ashworth HE. First rib resection in the treatment of thoracic outlet syndrome. Transaxillary and posterior thoracoplasty approaches. Ann Surg 1973; 178:49–52.

21. Hoofer WD, Burnett AD. Thoracic outlet relief. J Kansas Med Soc 1973; 74:329–331, 352.

22. Dale WA. Management of thoracic outlet syndrome. Ann Surg 1975; 181:575–585.

23. Kremer RM, Ahlquist RE Jr. Thoracic outlet compression syndrome. Am J Surg 1975; 130:612–616.

24. McGough EC, Pearce MB, Byrne JP. Management of thoracic outlet syndrome. J Ther Card Med 1979; 77:169–174.

25. Youmans CR Jr, Smiley RH. Thoracic outlet syndrome with negative Adson's and hyperabduction maneuvers. Vasc Surg 1980; 14:318–329.

26. Roos DB. The place for scalenectomy and first rib resection in thoracic outlet syndrome. Surg 1982; 92:1077–1085.

27. Batt M, Griffet J, Scotti L, LeBas P. Le syndrome de la traversee cervico-brachiale. A proposde 112 cas: vers une attitude tactique plus nuancee. J Chir Paris 1983; 120:687–691.

28. Sallstrom J, Gjores JE. Surgical treatment of the thoracic outlet syndrome. Acta Chir Scand 1983; 149:555–560.

29. Heughan C. Thoracic outlet syndrome. Can J Surg 1984; 27:35–36.

30. Qvarfordt PG, Ehrenfeld WK, Stoney RJ. Supraclavicular radical scalenectomy and transaxillary first rib resection for the thoracic outlet syndrome. A combined approach. Am J Surg 1984; 148:111–116.

31. Davies AL, Messerschmidt W. Thoracic outlet syndrome: a therapeutic approach based on 115 consecutive cases. Del Med J 1988; 60:307.

32. Sellke FW, Kelly TR. Thoracic outlet syndrome. Am J Surg 1988; 154:56.

33. Stanton PE Jr, Vo NM, Haley T, Shannon J, Evans J. Thoracic outlet syndrome: a comprehensive evaluation. Am Surg 1988; 54:129–133.

34. Wood VE, Twito R, Verska JM. Thoracic outlet syndrome: the results of first rib resection in 100 patients. Orthop Clin North Am 1988; 19:131–146.

35. Lindgren SHS, Ribbe EB, Norgren LEH. Two year follow-up of patients operated on for thoracic outlet syndrome. Effects on sick-leave incidence. Eur J Vasc Surg 1989; 3:411–415.

36. Lepantalo M, Lindgren A, Leino E, Lindfors O, vonSmitten, Nuutinen E, Totterman S. Long term outcome after resection of the first rib for thoracic outlet syndrome. Br J Surg 1989; 76:1255–1256.

37. Hempel GK, Rucher AH Jr, Wheeler CG, Hunt DG, Bukhari HI. Supraclavicular resection of the first rib for thoracic outlet syndrome. Am J Surg 1981; 141:213–215.

38. Graham GG, Lincoln BM. Anterior resection of first rib for thoracic outlet syndrome. Am J Surg 1973; 126:803–806.

39. Thompson JB, Hernandez IA. The thoracic outlet syndrome: a second look. Am J Surg 1979; 138:251–253.

40. Brodsky AE, Gol A. Costoclavicular syndrome: relief by infraclavicular removal of first rib. South Med J 1970; 63:50–58.

41. Murphy TO, Clinton AP, Kanar EA, McAlexander RA. Subclavicular approach to first rib resection. Am J Surg 1980; 139:634–636.

42. Clagett OT. Presidential address: research and prosearch. J Thorac Cardiovasc Surg 1962; 44:153–166.

43. McBurney RP, Howard H. Resection of the first rib for thoracic outlet compression: report of nine cases. Am Surgeon 1966; 32:165–169.

44. Longo MF, Clagett OT, Fairbairn JF. Surgical treatment of thoracic outlet syndrome. Ann Surg 1971; 171:538–542.

45. Johnson CR. Treatment of TOS by removal of first rib and related entrapments through posterolateral approach: a 22 year approach. J Thorac Cardiovasc Surg 1974; 68:536–545.

46. Pretre R, Spiliopoulos A, Megevand R. Transthoracic approach in the thoracic outlet syndrome: an alternate operative route for removal of the first rib. Surgery 1989; 106:856–860.

47. Carroll RE, Hurst LC. The relationship of thoracic outlet syndrome and carpal tunnel syndrome. Clin Orthop 1982; 164:149–153.

48. Sanders RJ, Pearce WH. The treatment of thoracic outlet syndrome: a comparison of different operations. J Vasc Surg 1989; 10:626–634.

49. Bandyk DF, Kaebnick HW, Stewart GW, Towne JB. Durability of the in situ saphenous vein arterial bypass: a comparison of primary and secondary patency. J Vasc Surg 1987; 5:256–268.

50. Hagberg M, Wegman DH. Prevalence rates and odds ratios of shoulder neck diseases in different occupational groups. Br J Indust Med 1987; 44:602–610.

51. Sallstrom J, Schmidt H. Cervicobrachial disorders in certain occupations, with special reference to compression in the thoracic outlet. Am J Ind Med 1984; 6:45–52.

52. Mandel S: Neurologic syndromes from repetitive trauma at work. Postgrad Med 1987; 82:87–92.

13
Recurrent Thoracic Outlet Syndrome

Richard J. Sanders
Craig E. Haug

Recurrence implies that a patient experienced temporary improvement following surgery for thoracic outlet syndrome (TOS) before symptoms recurred. The length of time of improvement may be a few weeks to several years. Persistent or continuing symptoms indicates that the patient experienced no improvement for even a short time following surgery. Both conditions will be discussed in this chapter.

Etiology

Recurrent symptoms develop in 15–20% of patients who have received operations for TOS. Although the etiology of recurrence is not known with certainty, theories to explain the possible causes have developed from observations made during surgery for recurrence. The almost constant finding at reoperations for TOS is the presence of scar tissue around the nerves of the plexus. Scar tissue forms regardless of the previous approach or whether or not the first rib was removed. Scar tissue lies not only around the entire neurovascular bundle, but also around the individual nerves comprising the plexus. Presumably it is the maturation and contraction of this scar tissue that produces brachial plexus compression.

A history of neck trauma is present in over 25% of the cases of recurrent TOS, with the incidence being over 40% when recurrence develops more than 2 years after the first operation.[1] Precisely how trauma causes the already existing scar tissue to suddenly elicit symptoms when no symptoms existed previously is unknown. However, it can be postulated that stretching the scar tissue occurs first, followed by edema, a few new fibroblasts, and the subsequent development of tighter scar tissue that now compresses the nerves of the plexus enough to cause symptoms.

Recurrence following first rib resection invariably is associated with reattachment of the insertion of the anterior and middle scalenes to the subclavian artery, the top of the plexus, and often to the bed of the first rib and Sibson's fascia over the apex of the pleura. This probably occurs in almost all cases of transaxillary first rib resection because it is impossible to remove the scalenes through the axilla. The divided scalene muscle insertions have no place to go other than a few millimeters cephalad, up into the neck, and reattach to adjacent structures. It is to prevent this phenomenon of reattachment that some surgeons have advocated complete scalenectomy along with rib resection.[2-4] Unfortunately, even that has not prevented recurrences or reduced the recurrence rate.[4]

Retention of a long posterior rib stump has been observed in many cases of recurrence following transaxillary first rib resection. Perhaps because it is an objective finding that is easy to recognize on x-ray, some surgeons postulate that it is a common cause of recurrence (Fig. 13-1).[5-7] Supporting that view are the observations of Youmans and Smiley, who in their early experiences with the transaxillary approach left long posterior stumps. They reoperated on 12 of these cases for continued or recurrent symptoms, invariably ulnar nerve, and 11 of the 12 had excellent results.[8]

However, retention of a long posterior rib stump is difficult to prove as a cause of recurrence and the fact that the same recurrence rate has been seen following

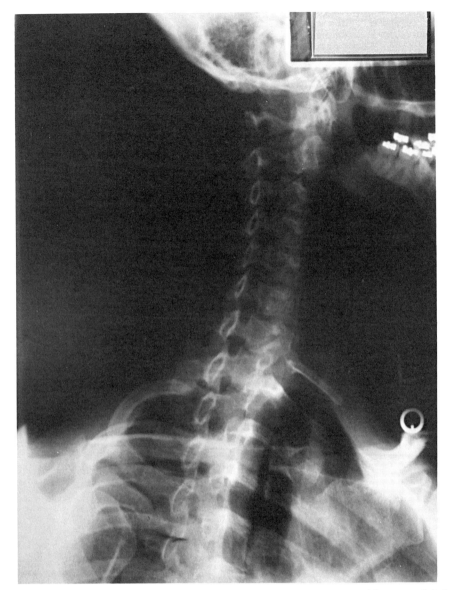

Fig. 13-1.   Three-cm-long posterior first rib stump in patient with recurrent TOS. Excision of this piece of rib did not result in any significant symptomatic improvement.

supraclavicular rib resection, a technique that seldom leaves a posterior stump at all, raises doubts as to the significance of a long posterior stump as the *main* cause of recurrence. Although the posterior rib stump is a nearby structure to which post-operative scar tissue can anchor, the scar tissue would probably attach to another nearby structure if the stump were not there.

From a practical point of view, it seems best to leave as short a posterior stump as possible without risking injury to the T-1 nerve root. It is better to leave a long stump and risk recurrence, which can be managed by reoperations through another route, than to damage a nerve root that cannot be repaired.

Time of Recurrence

Although recurrence can occur weeks, months, or even years after operations to decompress the thoracic outlet area, most recur in the first few months following surgery. As noted in Chapter 12, over 50% of recurrences are seen within 6 months of surgery and 80% within 2 years. This pattern is true regardless of the type of operation performed.

Diagnosis

Clinical Picture

The clinical presentation of recurrent TOS is often similar to the initial presentation, prior to the first operation. Therefore, the diagnosis of recurrent TOS is often easier to establish than is the initial diagnosis of TOS.

Symptoms

The symptoms of recurrent TOS are the same as those of primary TOS. They include paresthesia in the fingers, hand, or arm; pain in the upper extremity, shoulder, neck, and sometimes above or along the medial edge of the scapula; arm weakness; occipital headaches; and aggravation of the symptoms with the arms elevated. Chest pain, facial pain, hand swelling, and color changes are seen in a few patients, but are less frequent. Paresthesia is most common in all five fingers, but it is often worse in the fourth and fifth fingers. A deviation from the original symptoms that is occasionally seen in recurrence is a shift of the areas of involvement from lower plexus (fourth and fifth fingers) to upper plexus (first three fingers) by virtue of the anterior scalene muscle attaching to and compressing the C-5, C-6, and C-7 nerves postoperatively (Table 13–1).

Physical Examination

The findings on physical examination are also similar to the findings that existed prior to the initial operation. Supraclavicular tenderness over the scalene muscle area and duplication of symptoms with the arms abducted to 90 degrees in external rotation (90-degree AER position) are the most consistent findings. Also common are a positive Tinel's sign over the involved brachial plexus and reproduction of symptoms by pressing over the plexus for 20 to 30 seconds. Reduction of the radial pulse in the 90-degree AER position or with the classical Adson maneuver occurs in less than one-third of the cases (Table 13–2).

Other common findings on physical examination include a reduction in range of motion of the neck and the development of neck tightness or pain on the affected side when tilting the head to the contralateral side. This maneuver is performed by having the patient try to touch their ear to their shoulder, which normally causes no discomfort. Neurologic examination may reveal a reduction in sensation to light touch in the involved fingers, usually the fourth and fifth, or the

Table 13–1. **Symptoms in 141 Cases of Recurrent TOS**

	Reoperation Performed				
	Transax 1st Rib[a]	Supracl 1st Rib[b]	Ant & Mid Scalenec[c]	Neurolysis	Total
Number of cases	29	16	59	37	141
Total numbness and tingling	89%	94%	84%	74%	82%
All 5 fingers	54%	47%	37%	30%	39%
Fourth and fifth fingers	25%	35%	35%	30%	31%
First to third fingers	11%	12%	12%	14%	13%
Neck pain	57%	88%	75%	70%	73%
Arm pain	71%	65%	83%	49%	71%
Shoulder pain	39%	65%	67%	68%	62%
Occipital headaches	50%	71%	41%	38%	41%
Arm weakness	36%	35%	43%	24%	33%
Chest pain	11%	24%	20%	22%	18%
Facial pain	4%	0%	8%	0%	4%
Hand swelling	4%	0%	2%	0%	1%
Color changes	0%	0%	2%	0%	1%

[a]Transax 1st Rib = transaxillary first rib resection.
[b]Supracl 1st Rib = supraclavicular first rib resection.
[c]Ant & Mid Scalenec = anterior and middle scalenectomy.

Table 13–2. **Physical Findings in 141 Cases of Recurrent TOS**

	Reoperation Performed				
	Transax 1st Rib[a]	Supracl 1st Rib[b]	Ant & Mid Scalenec[c]	Neurolysis	Total
Number of cases	29	16	59	37	141
Supraclavicular tenderness	57%[d]	88%	90%	84%	81%
Reproduction of symptoms in 90-degree AER position[e]	89%	88%	84%	80%	84%
Pulse decrease in AER position[e]	14%	18%	15%	16%	16%

[a]Transax 1st Rib = transaxillary first rib resection.
[b]Supracl 1st Rib = supraclavicular first rib resection.
[c]Ant & Mid Scalenec = anterior and middle scalenectomy.
[d]Although this figure is significantly lower than that for the other three operations, the reason may be that these patients were operated upon in the earlier years of our experience when this feature of the physical examination was not routinely performed.
[e]90-degree AER = arm abducted to 90 degrees in external rotation (see Fig. 6-2A).

hand. Weakness in grip may be demonstrated by having the patient squeeze a dynamometer with each hand.

Diagnostic Tests

The tests used to diagnose recurrence are the same as for primary TOS. Unfortunately, the poor credibility of these tests is also no different the second time than it was the first time.

Scalene Block

The scalene muscle block, as described in Chapter 7, is particularly helpful if the scalene muscles have not been removed at a previous operation. Improvement in physical findings following the block, particularly increased ease and range of motion of the neck and fewer symptoms with the arms in the 90-degree AER position, is a positive response to the block. Such a positive response supports the diagnosis of recurrent TOS; a poor response does not eliminate the diagnosis, but makes it less likely. As discussed in Chapter 7, if the block is negative, other criteria must be used to establish a diagnosis of recurrent TOS before surgery is considered.

A similar kind of block can also be employed in patients who have already had their scalene muscles removed. In such people, the needle is inserted into the area where the scalene muscles had been and where there is point tenderness in the neck. This area now contains scar tissue, which lies just over the plexus. If the patient experiences shooting pain down the arm when the needle is being advanced, it is touching the plexus and the needle is repositioned nearby. It is possible to produce a brachial plexus block in performing the "scalene area block." If that occurs, the results of the block must be ignored. However, with practice, a brachial plexus block will occur in less than 10–20%. There have been no complications from the block in over 20 years.

Neurophysiologic Diagnostic Studies

Electromyelograms (EMG), ulnar nerve conduction velocities (UNCV), somatosensory evoked potentials (SSEP), and F-wave velocities support the diagnosis of TOS when positive, although positive results are nonspecific; normal studies do not eliminate the diagnosis. These studies are of greater help in diagnosing other more distal forms of nerve compression at the elbow and wrist.

X-rays

Views of the neck, including oblique films, will detect osseous abnormalities that may have been overlooked prior to previous operations, such as small cervical ribs or abnormal first ribs, and they may demonstrate gross cervical spine abnormalities, such as "slipped discs" and cervical arthritis. Computerized axial tomography (CAT scans), myelography, and magnetic resonance imaging (MRI) offer more sophisticated and more reliable diagnostic tools for detecting disease in the cervical spine, particularly ruptured or bulging cervical discs and cervical spine stenosis (see Chapter 8, where these tests are described more fully.)

Angiography and Noninvasive Vascular Laboratory Studies

Studies to detect arterial or venous compression should be done only if there are appropriate vascular symptoms. Hand swelling is an indication for venography. Localized digital ischemia, suggestions of peripheral emboli, reduced arm blood pressure or subclavian bruits at rest are all indications for subclavian arteriography as is the presence of an osseous abnormality. However, vascular involvement is seldom seen with recurrent TOS, even less frequently than in primary TOS.

Differential and Associated Diagnoses

The differential diagnosis includes several conditions that may either be associated with recurrent TOS or must be differentiated from it. These include diffuse muscular inflammation of the shoulder girdle and upper extremity muscles, fibromyositis or myofascitis, biceps/rotator cuff tendinitis, cervical disc disease, cervical arthritis, carpal tunnel syndrome, ulnar nerve entrapment, and primary brachial plexus injury (see Chapter 8).

The presence of another diagnosis does not exclude the diagnosis of recurrent TOS. Many patients have more than one diagnosis, which makes the detection of recurrent TOS more difficult. Primary plexus injury is sometimes a diagnosis made by exclusion when there is no neurological improvement following surgery for TOS and all other areas of nerve compression (wrist, elbow, spine) have been ruled out.

Treatment

Persistence vs. Recurrence

Immediate failure (persistent symptoms) must be differentiated from recurrence. Persistence means the symptoms did not improve for even a short period following surgery whereas recurrence indicates that there was improvement for some length of time, be it only a few weeks.

The cause of immediate failure could be that surgery was not adequate, that another diagnosis predominated, or that the diagnosis of TOS was incorrect. With recurrence, the diagnosis of TOS was correct but something happened around the brachial plexus to again cause nerve compression.

Managing Persistent Symptoms

At times it is difficult to determine the reason for persistent symptoms but efforts should be made to do so, as future treatment depends to some extent upon the cause. Patients experiencing immediate failure usually will not benefit from reoperation. However, there are some exceptions and, depending upon what operation was initially performed, reoperation may be a consideration.

The type of operation initially performed is the first guideline. If the operation included both scalenectomy and first rib resection, the plexus has probably been adequately decompressed and consideration of further surgery in the thoracic outlet area can be abandoned; the problem is not inadequate surgery. If the initial operation was first rib resection, the chances are also good that decompression was adequate, as the anterior and middle scalene muscles, as well as most congenital bands and ligaments, must be divided in order to remove the rib. Rib resection should release the tension from those structures and provide temporary symptomatic relief of at least a few weeks or months.

However, immediate failure following transaxillary rib resection might occasionally be due to scalene muscle anomalies that cannot be released through the axilla. In our experience, two of three reoperated patients in this category also experienced immediate failure of reoperation,[9] but Qvarfordt et al. noted good results from reoperation in all seven of their patients with persistent symptoms.[3]

Patients with persistent symptoms following anterior and middle scalenectomy should be carefully evaluated. If head, neck, and shoulder pain, as well as paresthesia in the hand, were all preoperative symptoms and none improved, first rib resection will probably fail too. However, if the head and neck symptoms were relieved by scalenectomy but the hand and arm symptoms persist, first rib resection may provide improvement in the extremity. Our highest incidence of success with transaxillary rib resection in cases of persistent symptoms has been in this sub-group of patients whose head and neck symptoms were relieved by scalenectomy. The rationale for this is that the head and neck symptoms were due to tight scalene muscles, which were removed, but the extremity symptoms could be due to costoclavicular compression, which requires first rib resection to relieve. On the other hand, it should be noted that costoclavicular compression is seldom the cause of TOS (less than 10% of all TOS cases).

If only the anterior scalene muscle was removed at the initial operation and the symptoms that persist are from the lower plexus, middle scalenectomy might bring improvement. However, should another operation be done to remove the middle scalene muscle, it would be prudent to remove the first rib at the same time. Should the patient not improve following middle scalenectomy without first rib resection, it would be difficult to ask the patient to undergo yet a third operation to finally remove the rib.

Managing Recurrence

Initially, treatment of recurrent TOS, like primary TOS, should be conservative. Conservative treatment includes various modalities of physical therapy, including medication, heat, massage, and ultrasound to the neck and shoulder areas as well as arm strengthening, stretching, and range of motion exercises. Neck traction is seldom helpful and may aggravate symptoms. Patients whose recurrence is due to tight scar tissue around the plexus usually do not respond to conservative therapy. However, if some of the symptoms were due to associated diagnoses, improvement can occur. Patients who do not experience much improvement after a few months of conservative therapy, and in whom symptoms continue to be disabling, are considered candidates for reoperation.

Figure 13-2 is an algorithm of the surgical management of recurrent TOS. The choice depends upon what was performed at previous operations: If the first operation was first rib resection, reoperation should be scalenectomy; if the first operation was scalenectomy, reoperation should be first rib resection. In patients who have already undergone both rib resection and scalenectomy, reoperation is initially a supraclavicular brachial plexus neurolysis. If ulnar nerve compression symptoms persist following supraclavicular neurolysis, transaxillary neurolysis of C-8 and T-1 is performed at a later date.

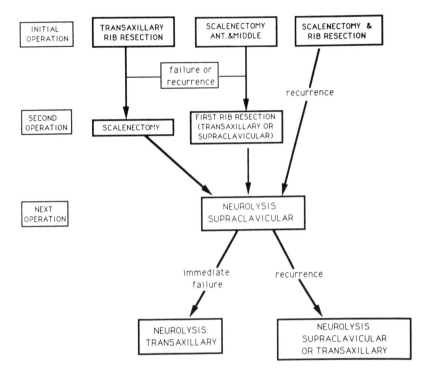

Fig. 13-2. Algorithm for the management of recurrent TOS. (*Reprinted from Sanders RJ, Haug C, Pearce WH. Recurrent thoracic outlet syndrome. J Vasc Surg 1990; 12:390–400. With Permission.*)

If the First Rib Remains

No single surgical approach for recurrence has proved to be superior to any other. The most important criterion in selecting an approach is whether the first rib was removed previously. If not, the operation for recurrence is to remove it through one of several routes.

The *transaxillary route*, introduced by Roos,[10] is often an easy approach through which to remove the first rib because the scalene muscles were detached at scalenectomy. Its advantage is that it is the best approach for removing the anterior portion of the rib, freeing the subclavian vein, and dissecting C-8 and T-1 nerve roots. However, in some cases, adhesions and scar tissue may be present from the earlier procedure, making safe dissection difficult. Particularly prone to injury is the subclavian vein, lying just lateral to the costoclavicular ligament. The vein should only be freed if the patient's preoperative symptoms included hand swelling and cyanosis. These are uncommon complaints, so that subclavian vein compression is seldom present and vein dissection seldom needed. Nerve dissection is indicated for neurologic symptoms in the ulnar nerve distribution. One disadvantage of the transaxillary approach is that C-5, C-6, and C-7 cannot be freed through the axilla.

Supraclavicular first rib resection is performed through the same supraclavicular incision that was used for the previous scalenectomy. Its advantages are several: It is the best approach for performing a neurolysis on the brachial plexus; it is an excellent route through which to visualize and remove the neck of the first rib; and if required, the exposure can easily be extended by adding an infraclavicular incision to provide better visualization of the anterior portion of the rib or to control bleeding from the subclavian vein. A criticism of this route is that the nerves of the plexus are encountered early in the dissection and must be cleaned and mobilized to reach the rib. However, this is not a true disadvantage as neurolysis may be more beneficial than excising the rib.

The *posterior approach* has the advantage of reaching the neck of the rib through a clean field and permitting excellent exposure for removing the posterior rib back to the transverse process. One disadvantage is that postoperative pain from dividing the parascapular muscles is greater than the pain from other approaches. Sessions used the posterior approach in four of his 60 cases of recurrent TOS and all four failed; all improved following reoperation through other routes.[6]

Summary of Choice of Operation

After performing first rib resection as a reoperation through both approaches, we tend to select the transaxillary route if the symptoms are limited to the lower plexus. Also, if the indication for reoperation was improvement of head and neck symptoms but persistent hand and arm symptoms following scalenectomy, the transaxillary approach is appropriate. For upper plexus or diffuse plexus involvement we have used the supraclavicular approach first and, in all but a few cases, it has been successful.

If the First Rib Has Been Removed

Recurrent TOS in patients in whom the first rib has already been removed is treated by supraclavicular neurolysis. If the first operative approach was supraclavicular, the scalene muscles will be gone since this is necessary to do before reaching the rib. If the previous approach was transaxillary, the anterior and middle scalene muscles are found adhering to the brachial plexus, subclavian artery, and pleura. Scalenectomy, both anterior and middle, is performed as well as neurolysis and removal of the posterior rib stump.

Middle Scalenectomy

Middle scalenectomy should routinely be performed when doing supraclavicular exploration for recurrent TOS. Congenital ligaments or bands of scar tissue can lie hidden here, within the muscle belly, and are detectable only by removing the middle scalene muscle.[11, 12] Most patients with recurrent TOS have symptoms of neck pain and headache that are probably muscular symptoms from anterior or middle scalene muscle spasm and tightness rather than neurologic symptoms from plexus compression. For that reason, whenever supraclavicular exploration is done, the middle scalene muscle should be excised along with the anterior scalene. This decompresses C-7 and C-8 and may be the reason scalenectomy is as successful as rib resection in patients with lower plexus symptoms.

Results of Surgical Treatment of Recurrence

Standard Method, Reports From the Literature

Few articles have been written about recurrent TOS, the first appearing in 1979.[9] Table 13–3 summarizes the results of four series that have appeared since then, totalling 469 cases. Definitions of excellent, good, and fair are the same as discussed in Chapter 12. Failure rates, using the standard method of reporting (total number of known failures divided by total number of operations) ranged from 4% to 12%; excellent/good results, 79% to 82%; and fair results, 9% to 14%. The follow-up time in the two largest series was not stated and in the other two was quite short. As discussed in Chapter 12, good results tend to deteriorate with time and the results in this table should be regarded as relatively short term results.

Life-Table Method

Applying the life-table method[13] to the results of reoperations in the same way as was done for primary operations in Chapter 12, significant deterioration of long-term results can be observed. In Table 13–4 and Figure 13-3, the results of 141 reoperations over a 23-year period are summarized. While the initial success rate was 91%, it fell to 72% at 1–2 years; 61% at 3-5 years, and 51% at 5–10 years. There were no statistically significant differences between the four operative procedures performed. The life-tables for each of the four operations are presented in Tables 13–5 to 13–8.

Table 13–4 also expresses these results with the standard method. At the 10–15 year level, the life-table method has about a 10% lower success rate compared to the standard method: 51% versus 61%.

Table 13–3. **Results of Reoperations for TOS**

Author	Year	No. Oper-ations	Excellent/Good		Fair		Failed		Length of Follow-up
			No.	%	No.	%	No.	%	
Sanders[9]	1979	33	26	79%	3	9%	4	12%	12–72 months (minimum = 2 months)
Roos[5]	1984	151	124	82%	21	14%	6	4%	Not stated
Urschel[7]	1986	225	177	79%	32	14%	16	7%	Not stated
Sessions[6]	1989	60		79%		12%		5%	1 month to 144 months Mean = 4 months
TOTALS		469		80%		14%		6%	
RANGES		469		79–82%		9–14%		4–12%	

Table 13–4. Success Rate of Each Reoperative Procedure[a]

| | | Life-Table Method | | | | | | | | | Standard Method[b] | | |
| | | 1–3 months | | 1–2 years | | 3–5 years | | 5–10 years | | 10–15 years | | 1–180 months | | |
Operation[c]	No. Patients	%	No.	%	No.	%	No.	%	No.	%	No.	No. Fail	% Fail	% Success
Transax 1st rib res	29	86%	29	69%	19	57%	13	40%	9	40%	5	13	45%	55%
Supracl rib res & neurolysis	16	94%	16	94%	13	52%	6	52%	5	52%	5	5	31%	69%
Scalenectomy & neurolysis	59	95%	59	71%	39	61%	27	51%	22	51%	16	21	36%	64%
Brach plex neurolysis	37	89%	37	61%	27	54%	16	49%	12	49%	7	16	43%	57%
TOTAL of all reoperations	141	91%	141	72%	98	61%	62	51%	36	51%	33	55	39%	61%

[a]Success includes excellent, good, and fair results.
[b]Standard method is dividing total number of failures by total number operated upon. The denominator in each case is the same number of operations as in the 1–3 month column.
[c]Transax = transaxillary; Supracl = supraclavicular; Brach plex = brachial plexus.

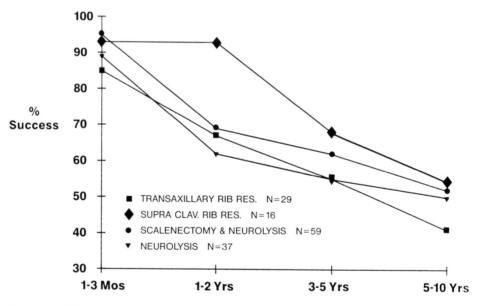

Fig. 13-3.   Success rate following each of four reoperations for TOS. The results are expressed using the life-table method. There was no statistically significant differences between any of the operations ($P > 0.05$).

Surgical Complications Following Reoperations

The surgical complications in 141 reoperations from our own experience are listed in Table 13–9. Nerve injuries to either the brachial plexus or the phrenic nerve were the most serious complications. Phrenic nerve injury occurred only

Table 13–5. Reoperation: Transaxillary First Rib Resection—Life Table[a]

Time (months)	No. Operations at Risk[b]	Results				Reop[c]	Failed in Period	Cumulative Success Rate	Lost	Inadequate Follow-up[d]
		Excellent	Good	Fair	Fail					
1–3	29	4	15	6	4	0	4/29 = 14%	86%	0	0
4–6	25	4	12	5	1	0	1/22 = 4.5%	82%	2	1
7–9	21	4	11	5	0	0	0	82%	1	0
10–12	20	3	10	5	1	0	1/20 = 5%	78%	0	0
13–24	19	3	10	4	2	0	2/18 = 11%	69%	0	0
25–36	17	3	8	2	1	0	1/15 = 6.7%	65%	2	1
37–60	13	2	5	2	0	2	2/18 = 11%	53%	2	0
61–120	9	2	2	1	0	2	2/7 = 29%	38%	1	1
121–180	5	0	1	0	0	0	0	38%	2	2
TOTAL				9	4		13/29 = 45%			

[a] Life table formula—Failure in an interval $= \dfrac{\text{No. failed}}{\text{No. at beginning} - \frac{1}{2} \text{ withdrawals}}$.

[b] Number of operations at beginning of time interval.

[c] Reop = reoperation.

[d] Inadequate follow-up, or not followed long enough.

Table 13–6. Reoperation: Supraclavicular First Rib Resection and Neurolysis—Life Table[a]

Time (months)	No. Operations at Risk[b]	Results				Reop[c]	Failed in Period	Cumulative Success Rate	Lost	Inadequate Follow-up[d]
		Excellent	Good	Fair	Fail					
1–3	16	1	14	0	1	0	1/16 = 6%	94%	0	0
4–6	15	0	12	1	0	0	0	94%	1	1
7–9	13	0	12	1	0	0	0	94%	0	0
10–12	13	0	12	1	0	0	0	94%	0	0
13–24	13	0	9	3	0	0	0	94%	0	3
25–36	12	0	3	3	3	0	3/9 = 33%	63%	0	3
37–60	6	3	2	1	0	0	1/5.5 = 18%	52%	0	0
61–120	5	0	3	2	0	0	0	52%	0	0
121–180	5	0	0	0	0	0	0	52%	0	5
TOTAL				5	0		5/16 = 31%			

[a] Life table formula—Failure in an interval $= \dfrac{\text{No. failed}}{\text{No. at beginning} - \frac{1}{2} \text{ withdrawals}}$.

[b] Number of operations at beginning of time interval.

[c] Reop = reoperation.

[d] Inadequate follow-up, or not followed long enough.

with supraclavicular incisions and most of these were temporary. Entry into the pleural space was more common with first rib resection by either route. The incidence of serious complications following reoperations was no greater and no different than the incidence following primary operations.

Table 13–7. Reoperation: Scalenectomy and Neyrolysis—Life Table[a]

Time (months)	No. Operations at Risk[b]	Results				Reop[c]	Failed in Period	Cumulative Success Rate	Lost	Inadequate Follow-up[d]
		Excellent	Good	Fair	Fail					
1–3	59	7	47	2	3	0	3/59 = 5%	95%	0	0
4–6	56	5	39	2	0	1	1/51 = 2%	93%	4	5
7–9	46	4	32	4	3	1	4/43 = 9.3%	84%	1	0
10–12	40	4	29	6	1	0	1/40 = 2.5%	82%	0	0
13–24	39	2	25	5	3	2	5/35 = 14.3%	71%	0	1
25–36	32	2	23	2	0	2	2/30 = 6.7%	66%	1	0
37–60	27	2	20	0	2	0	2/25 = 8%	61%	0	0
61–120	22	2	12	2	1	2	3/19 = 16%	51%	0	0
121–180	16	1	6	3	0	0	0	51%	4	0
TOTAL				13	8		21/59 = 36%			

[a]Life table formula—Failure in an interval $= \dfrac{\text{No. failed}}{\text{No. at beginning } - \ ^{1}/_{2} \text{ withdrawals}}$.

[b]Number of operations at beginning of time interval.
[c]Reop = reoperation.
[d]Inadequate follow-up, or not followed long enough.

Table 13–8. Reoperation: Brachial Plexus Neurolysis—Life Table[a]

Time (months)	No. Operations at Risk[b]	Results				Reop[c]	Failed in Period	Cumulative Success Rate	Lost	Inadequate Follow-up[d]
		Excellent	Good	Fair	Fail					
1–3	37	8	22	3	2	2	4/37 = 10.8%	89%	0	0
4–6	33	8	17	5	2	0	2/32 = 6%	84%	0	1
7–9	30	8	17	4	0	1	1/30 = 3.3%	81%	0	0
10–12	29	6	17	4	0	0	0	81%	0	0
13–24	27	6	12	3	2	4	6/24 = 25%	61%	0	0
25–36	21	6	9	1	1	1	2/19 = 10.5%	54%	2	1
37–60	16	4	8	0	0	0	0	54%	0	4
61–120	12	0	7	0	0	1	1/10 = 10%	49%	3	1
121–180	7	0	1	0	0	0	0	49%	2	3
TOTAL				7	9		16/37			

[a]Life table formula—Failure in an interval $= \dfrac{\text{No. failed}}{\text{No. at beginning } - \ ^{1}/_{2} \text{ withdrawals}}$.

[b]Number of operations at beginning of time interval.
[c]Reop = reoperation.
[d]Inadequate follow-up, or not followed long enough.

Table 13–9. Complications in 141 Cases of Recurrent TOS

	Operation[a]					
	Transax 1st Rib	Supracl 1st Rib	Ant & Mid Scalenec	Neurolysis	Total	%
Number of cases	29	16	59	37	141	
Brachial plexus palsy, temp[b]	0	0	1	0	1	0.7%
Brachial Plexus palsy, perm	0	0	0	0	0	0%
Phrenic Nerve palsy, temp	0	1	4	2	7	4.9%
Phrenic Nerve palsy, perm	0	0	2	0	2	1.4%
Rec. laryngeal nerve injury	1	0	0	0	1	0.7%
Subclavian vein injury—						0.7%
no sequelae	1	0	0	0	1	
Pleura entered	6(21%)	5(31%)	1(3%)	1(3%)	13	9.2%

[a]Transax 1st rib = transaxillary first rib resection; Supracl 1st rib = supraclavicular first rib resection; Ant & Mid Scalenec = anterior and middle scalenectomy.
[b]Temp = temporary; perm = permanent.

Variables

Trauma

A neck injury was the etiology of recurrence in 39 of the 141 cases (28%). Although it has been our clinical impression that when trauma was the cause of recurrence, the results of reoperation were better than when symptoms recurred spontaneously, our data show no statistical difference between the two groups (Table 13–10 and Fig. 13-4, primary success of 53% versus 49%, respectively). One fact not accounted for in this comparison is that half of the failures in the traumatic group were due to another injury while only a few in the nontraumatic group were due to reinjury. They were successfully operated upon again, and improvement is revealed in the secondary success rate of 81% at 1–2 years, which remained unaltered for the next 10 years. While the secondary success rate for the nontraumatic recurrences increases to only 66%, the differences between the trauma and nontrauma groups did not reach statistical significance (log-rank test). This could be due to the relatively small sample size.

Upper vs. Lower Plexus

On the basis of the location of hand paresthesia, TOS patients can be divided into those with numbness in the fourth and fifth fingers, ulnar nerve distribution; numbness in the first to third fingers, median nerve distribution; numbness in all fingers, combined ulnar and median nerve involvement; and those with no complaints of paresthesia (Table 13–11). The highest success rate, 76%, was in patients with ulnar nerve symptoms compared to success rates of 56%, 56%, and 58% for the other three groups, respectively. However, the differences between these groups were not statistically significant ($P > 0.05$). The results for transaxillary rib resection and for scalenectomy with neurolysis were almost identical in all

Table 13–10.   Influence of Trauma (as Cause of Recurrence) on Primary and Secondary Success Rate

Operation	I or II Success[a]	No. Cases	1–3 months %	No.[b]	1–2 years %	No.	3–5 years %	No.	5–10 years %	No.	10–15 years %	No.
All 4 operations	I	141	93%	141	72%	97	60%	63	51%	48	51%	33
	II	141	93%	141	79%	99	73%	75	72%	60	72%	45
Trauma	I	39	100%	39	70%	28	62%	16	53%	10	53%	5
	II	39	100%	39	81%	29	81%	21	81%	15	81%	11
No trauma	I	102	88%	102	71%	69	58%	47	49%	38	49%	28
	II	102	88%	102	76%	70	68%	54	66%	45	66%	34

[a]I = Primary Success—Improvement rate from each reoperative procedure in 104 patients, 18 bilateral sides. Each of the additional 19 procedures is counted separately; II = Secondary Success. Includes all primary successes plus all those patient-sides that were converted from failure to success by additional reoperations. A patient with one additional reoperation will have had a total of three operations on that side.
[b]Number of cases at risk in that time interval.

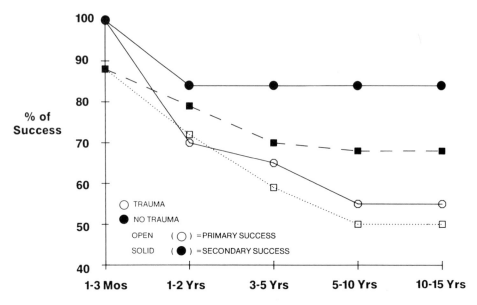

Fig. 13-4.   Influence of trauma as cause of recurrence on primary and secondary success rate. This is a graphic presentation of Table 13–10.

groups except the median nerve group where the numbers were too small for reliable statistical measurements.

It has been suggested that scalenectomy is effective only for upper plexus symptoms because the anterior scalene muscle is in contact primarily with C-5, C-6, and C-7. The corollary to this is that the anterior scalene has no contact with C-8 and T-1; therefore, performing transaxillary neuroplasty or rib resection, rather than scalenectomy, would seem to be the indicated procedure for recurrence with ulnar nerve symptoms. The data in Table 13–11, however, argue against that

Table 13–11. **Results Based on Upper Plexus vs. Lower Plexus Symptoms**

Operation[a]	Ulnar Nerve Numbness 4 & 5 fingers			Median Nerve Numbness 1–3 fingers			Both Ulnar and Median Nerve Numbness All 5 fingers			No Numbness			Totals		
	No. ops	Success No.	%	No. ops	Success No.	%	No. ops	Success No.	%	No. ops	Success No.	%	No. ops	Success No.	%
Transax rib	6	4	67%	4	3	75%	16	9	56%	3	2	67%	29	18	62%
Supracl rib	6	6	100%	2	2	100%	7	2	29%	1	1	100%	16	11	69%
Scalenec	21	15	71%	7	3	43%	21	13	62%	10	7	70%	59	38	64%
Neurolysis	12	9	75%	5	2	40%	10	6	60%	10	4	40%	37	21	57%
TOTALS	45	34	76%	18	10	56%	54	30	56%	24	14	58%	141	88	62%

[a]Transax rib res = transaxillary rib resection; Supracl rib res = supraclavicular first rib resection with brachial plexus neurolysis; Scalenec = scalenectomy with brachial plexus neurolysis; Neurolysis = brachial plexus neurolysis alone, done for patients who previously had received rib resection and scalenectomy.

hypothesis because the success rate for scalenectomy was equal to or better than the success rate for rib resection in treating recurrence with lower plexus symptoms. Perhaps one reason is that scalenectomy in those cases included the middle scalene muscle, which is in contact with C-7 and C-8. That relationship supports the selection of scalenectomy with neurolysis, without transaxillary exploration, as the first operative choice when reoperation is to be performed for recurrence following transaxillary rib resection regardless of the symptom complex.

Prevention

Prevention of postoperative scarring following neurolysis is a problem that has yet to be solved. Covering the nerves with a layer of adipose tissue is a standard neurosurgical maneuver, but its value is unproven. In supraclavicular operations, the scalene fat pad is always replaced on top of the nerves at the conclusion of the procedure, yet this has not prevented recurrence. At reoperation, the fat pad is usually found adherent to the nerves. The instillation of local steroids has been employed in several patients, but this too has not prevented postoperative scarring. Recently, PTFE has been used to cover the plexus to prevent adjacent tissues from attaching to it, although its use does not prevent the nerves from sticking to each other. The long term results are still unknown.[6]

References

1. Sanders RJ, Haug C, Pearce WH. Recurrent thoracic outlet syndrome. J Vasc Surg 1990; 12:390–400.
2. Hempel GK, Rucher AH Jr, Wheeler CG, Hunt DG, Bukhari HI. Supraclavicular resection of the first rib for thoracic outlet syndrome. Am J Surg 1981; 141:213–215.

3. Qvarfordt PG, Ehrenfeld WK, Stoney RJ. Supraclavicular radical scalenectomy and transaxillary first rib resection for the thoracic outlet syndrome: a combined approach. Am J Surg 1984; 148:111–116.

4. Sanders RJ, Pearce WH. The treatment of thoracic outlet syndrome: comparison of different operations. J Vasc Surg 1989; 10:626–634.

5. Roos DB. Recurrent thoracic outlet syndrome after first rib resection. Inter Angio 1984; 3:169–177.

6. Sessions RT. Reoperation for thoracic outlet syndrome. J Cardiovasc Surg 1989; 30:434–444.

7. Urschel HC, Razzuk MA. The failed operation for thoracic outlet syndrome: the difficulty of diagnosis and management. Ann Thorac Surg 1986; 42:523–528.

8. Youmans CR Jr, Smiley RH. Thoracic outlet syndrome with negative Adson's and hyperabduction maneuvers. Vasc Surg 1980; 14:318–329.

9. Sanders RJ, Monsour JW, Gerber WJ. Recurrent thoracic outlet syndrome following first rib resection. Vasc Surg 1979; 13:325–330.

10. Roos DB, Owens JC. Thoracic outlet syndrome. Arch Surg 1966; 93:71–74.

11. Sadler TR Jr. Discussion in Urschel, et al.: Reoperation for recurrent thoracic outlet syndrome. Ann Thorac Surg 1976; 21:24–25.

12. Thomas GI, Jones TW, Stavney LS, Manhas DR. The middle scalene muscle and its contribution to the TOS. Am J Surg 1983; 145:589–592.

13. Colton T. Statistics in medicine. Boston; Little Brown & Co., 1975:237–250.

14
Arterial TOS

Craig E. Haug
Richard J. Sanders

Etiology
Osseous Abnormalities
Pathophysiology of Subclavian Aneurysms and Thrombi

Signs and Symptoms
Thrombosis
Emboli
Vascular vs. Neurologic Symptoms

Diagnosis
Noninvasive Vascular Studies

Treatment
Indications
Review of Surgical Literature
Treatment Options

This chapter is a revision of Sanders RJ, Haug CE. Arterial thoracic outlet syndrome: Report of five cases and of literature. Surg Gynecol Obstet 1991; In Press. With Permission.

Arterial thoracic outlet syndrome (TOS) is compression of the subclavian artery in the region of the scalene triangle and costoclavicular space (thoracic outlet area). The term is applicable only when the artery exhibits dilatation, aneurysm formation, thrombosis, or causes distal emboli. Arterial TOS is uncommon. It occurs in less than 5% of all cases of TOS,[1] and in some series, comprises less than 1% or 2%.[2, 3] Although small in absolute numbers, arterial TOS accounts for a large percentage of the serious disabilities resulting from TOS.

Etiology

Osseous Abnormalities

Most cases of arterial TOS are associated with a bony abnormality, usually a complete cervical rib. Normally the subclavian artery passes from thorax to arm in a smooth curve over the broad surface of the first rib. A cervical rib raises the height of the artery in the neck, increasing the tension and angulation of the inferior arterial wall. Incomplete cervical ribs are usually connected to the first rib by a dense fibrous band that can exert pressure against an arterial wall similar to that imposed by a cervical rib. This arrangement invites stenosis and intimal injury as the normal artery expands with each systole against a sharp, unyielding edge.

Other bony abnormalities, such as rudimentary first ribs, also are associated with TOS. However, even though the incidence of abnormal first ribs approximates that of cervical ribs in the general population, fewer first ribs than cervical ribs have been reported to cause arterial injury. This is probably because they lie lower than cervical ribs and are less likely to deform the artery.

Pathophysiology of Subclavian Aneurysms and Thrombi

Extrinsic arterial compression by osseous or soft tissue abnormalities can cause stenosis, intimal injury, or both. Stenosis is associated with poststenotic dilatation, aneurysms, and mural thrombosis, which, in turn, can produce embolization and arterial occlusion (Fig. 14-1). About half of the patients with arterial complications develop aneurysms (39 of 70 cases in Cormier's large experience[4]); the others develop thrombi from intimal injuries without aneurysm formation.

The precise reasons for aneurysm formation are still unknown. Many theories have been proposed over the past several decades; most have been disproven but some are still valid. Historically, the earliest theories explained aneurysm formation as the result of a weakened arterial wall from spasm or thrombosis of the vasa vasorum. Todd, in 1912,[5] and Telford, in 1930,[6] attributed spasm or thrombosis to sympathetic nerve irritation (trophic theory); Baumgartner, in 1938, suggested that this was due to direct mechanical compression of the vasa vasorum by surrounding structures (mechanical theory).[7] Today it is known that nutrients to the arterial wall also come from the vessel lumen so that the vasa vasorum are not critical.

Halsted and Reid, in 1916, were the first to recognize that poststenotic

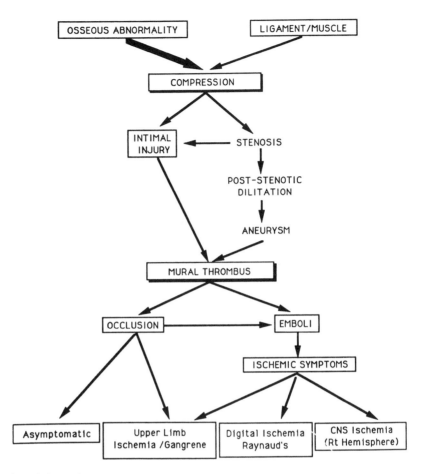

Fig. 14-1.   Algorithm of the pathophysiology of arterial complications in TOS.

dilatation and aneurysm formation could result from arterial stenosis.[8] They observed 27 cases of subclavian artery dilatation associated with cervical ribs and hypothesized the etiology to be cervical rib compression. In a dog model, they produced stenosis in the aorta and demonstrated that aneurysm formation occurred in the poststenotic segment. They speculated that aneurysm was secondary both to lateral forces set up by turbulence and to elevated, prolonged diastolic pressure distal to the stenosis. The theory of increased lateral pressure persisted for many years[9] but could not be supported by direct pressure measurements.[10]

Cavitation, the release of high-energy bubbles, was suggested by Robicsek and associates as a cause of poststenotic dilatation,[10] but it is unlikely that the physical forces required to produce cavitation are present in the human circulatory system.[11]

Arterial stenosis produces turbulence, which has been demonstrated to stimulate high shear stresses in the vessel wall distal to the stenosis.[12, 13] In the presence of atherosclerosis, these increased forces are associated with vessel dilation.[14]

Perhaps the most significant observations of poststenotic dilatation are those that associate it with vessel vibrations. Holman, in 1954, observed in a laboratory model that poststenotic dilatation occurred as a result of hydraulic laws that govern fluid flow in elastic conduits.[9] However, it was Roach, in 1963, who more clearly defined the conditions under which dilatation occurred. Her animal studies demonstrated that poststenotic dilatation developed *only* if associated with an audible thrill or bruit.[15] Further in vitro studies of normal arteries without stenosis demonstrated that vibrations alone, within specific low frequency ranges, caused arterial wall dilatation.[16] Thus it appears that vibrations of the arterial wall may be a significant factor in the development of poststenotic dilatation, and that the vibrations are the product of turbulence set up by arterial stenosis.[17]

Mild poststenotic dilatation is reversible when the cause has been removed. However, beyond a certain point, dilatation is not reversible and aneurysm formation ensues. Neither the precise condition under which this occurs nor the exact pathologic change that makes it irreversible is known. However, it is postulated that aneurysms are the result of permanent elastic tissue alterations that occur when vessels dilate beyond a given point.[15]

Intimal lesions occur at the site of compression, at the stenosis in the subclavian artery, or at the point of impact on the poststenotic arterial wall.[1] Because the artery curves caudad and distal to the stenosis, the point of intimal injury is usually found on the superior surface of the vessel (Fig. 14-2,A and B).

The first recognition that emboli may arise from subclavian artery thrombosis was by Symonds in 1927. He described a case of carotid embolization associated with TOS.[18] Lewis and Pickering, in 1934, were first to record distal embolization, rather than subclavian artery thrombosis alone, as the cause of digital ischemia and gangrene in TOS.[19]

Signs and Symptoms

Thrombosis

In the presence of subclavian artery obstruction there usually is sufficient collateral flow to maintain a viable extremity. People who do not use their arm for vigorous activities may be asymptomatic, whereas others can have intermittent claudication that may not be severe enough to require medical attention.

Emboli

Most patients first present with symptoms of peripheral embolization. Blue digit syndrome and Raynaud's phenomenon are common. Symptoms include the relatively sudden onset of coldness, pain, color changes (pallor or cyanosis), and paresthesia in the hand and fingers. Improved arteriography of the hands and fingers has revealed that many cases of what had been diagnosed as Raynaud's phenomenon were actually microemboli to the digits. These symptoms can progress to digital gangrene as the distal circulation and elbow collaterals are progressively occluded by more emboli and secondary thrombosis.

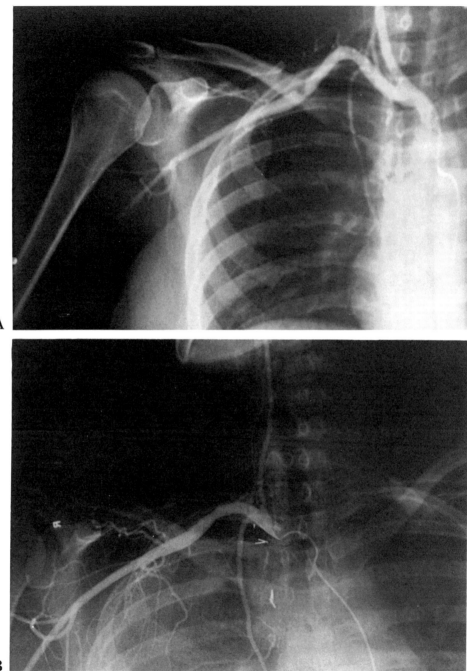

Fig. 14-2.   Conventional x-rays with an intraarterial injection for arteriography in a 32-year-old woman with a right cervical rib, subclavian artery thrombosis, and brachial artery emboli. **A.** Preoperative arteriogram showing mural thrombus on the superior and lateral arterial wall, the site being opposite the point of subclavian artery compression by a cervical rib. **B.** Postoperative arteriogram demonstrating a normal functioning subclavian artery following resection of cervical and first ribs, resection and end-to-end anastomosis of 1.5 cm of subclavian artery, thrombectomy, and dorsal sympathectomy (indicated by metal clips) (Table 14–3, Case 5).

Cerebral emboli are rare, but can occur by retrograde thrombosis. At least 22 cases have been reported.[20, 21]

Vascular vs. Neurologic Symptoms

Stimulation or irritation of the sympathetic nerve fibers that accompany C-8 and T-1 produces peripheral vasoconstriction and symptoms of coldness, color changes, excessive sweating, and on occasion, even ischemic lesions in the fingertips. These mimic symptoms that occur following arterial emboli, but do not occur from transient arterial compression due to positional change. In general, in the absence of peripheral emboli, most "vascular symptoms" or "Raynaud's Phenomenon" are probably due to irritation of the sympathetic nerves rather than to compression of the subclavian artery in the thoracic outlet. As such, they should be regarded as neurologic, rather than vascular, symptoms.

Diagnosis

The diagnosis of arterial TOS can be made objectively as compared to a diagnosis of neurologic TOS, which is usually based on subjective findings. Despite this, the diagnosis of arterial TOS is frequently delayed because poststenotic dilatation, subclavian aneurysm formation, and the development of mural thrombus often are silent. Even when the subclavian artery is totally occluded, the collateral circulation may be so rich that distal pulses remain palpable.

Two useful diagnostic signs that may be present early in the course of the disease are a pulsatile supraclavicular mass and a subclavian bruit with the arm at rest. The presence of a subclavian bruit with positional change is found in many normal people, a fact that renders this sign unreliable for diagnosing TOS in the absence of symptoms. In some patients, a cervical rib is prominent in the supraclavicular area, may be palpated through the skin, and can be confirmed by x-ray.

Often, the first symptoms of arterial TOS are those of ischemia due to embolization. A history of sudden onset of unilateral extremity symptoms in the absence of trauma should raise suspicion of arterial emboli. Depending on the location of emboli, pulses may or may not be altered. The diagnosis is established by complaints consistent with claudication, absent pulses, and digital ischemic changes.

Symptoms of nerve irritation often accompany those of arterial compression as a result of brachial plexus irritation. These symptoms include pain, weakness, and paresthesia in the upper extremity as seen in neurologic TOS.

X-rays of the chest and neck demonstrating cervical ribs (Fig. 14-3) or rudimentary first ribs (Fig. 14-4) should arouse suspicion of arterial TOS. Although the incidence of subclavian aneurysms in all patients with cervical ribs is small, 4%,[8] the major complication, gangrene, is so severe as to warrant aggressive diagnostic studies for even minor symptoms.

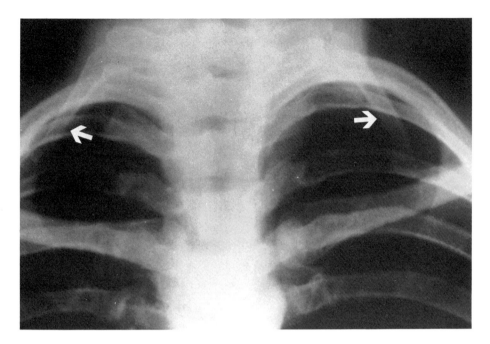

Fig. 14-3.   Bilateral cervical ribs. Photograph by Dr. Herbert Dardik, Englewood, New Jersey.

Noninvasive Vascular Studies

Pulse wave-forms and limb pressures can confirm the findings of physical examination but are unnecessary for establishing a diagnosis and cannot take the place of arteriography. When thrombosis or emboli have been found arteriographically, these noninvasive studies are of value as a baseline for comparison following arterial repair.

Currently, the nature of noninvasive studies is changing. New imaging techniques, such as duplex scanning and magnetic resonance imaging (MRI), may eventually supplant arteriography.

Subclavian arteriography, by direct injection or by intraarterial or intravenous digital subtraction technique, is the definitive diagnostic procedure (Figs. 14-5, 14-6, 14-7). The indications for arteriography are a cervical rib on x-ray plus one of the following:

1. Any ischemic or neurologic extremity symptom
2. A palpable pulsatile supraclavicular mass
3. A subclavian bruit at rest or with positional maneuvers[22]

Positional arteriography is usually unnecessary[23] but should be used if, in the resting position, x-rays are normal.

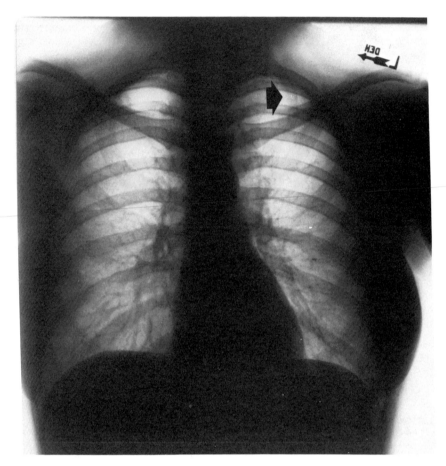

Fig. 14-4.   Rudimentary left first rib. The rib is half as wide as the other ribs. The right first rib was removed previously because of arterial emboli. The subclavian artery was ligated and a vein bypass used to restore circulation (Table 14–3, Case 1).

In the absence of a cervical rib or osseous abnormality, the presence of a bruit or a pulse deficit with positional maneuvers is not an indication for arteriography unless there are symptoms of arterial occlusion. Vasospastic symptoms of coldness, color changes, and mild paresthesia, when occurring alone, usually are due to neurologic rather than arterial causes; they do not warrant arteriography.

Treatment

Indications

In arterial TOS, the goals of therapy are to remove the underlying cause, repair the subclavian artery if indicated, and improve blood flow to the ischemic limb. Treatment is based upon the extent of disease. Four stages of cervical ribs with arterial involvement have been defined by Scher and Vieth. Their guidelines for therapy at each stage are described below[22] and in the algorithm in Figure 14-8.

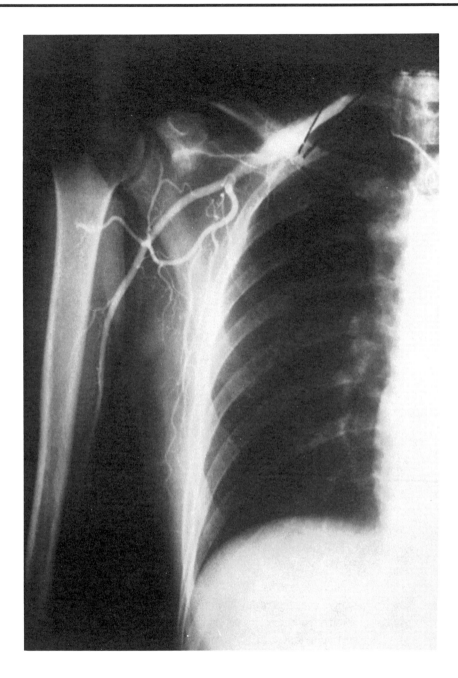

Fig. 14-5.   Conventional arteriogram using retrograde femoral artery catheterization, an intraarterial injection, cut films, and an automatic rapid film changer. This demonstrates a right subclavian aneurysm secondary to a cervical rib. Photograph by Dr. Herbert Dardik, Englewood, New Jersey.

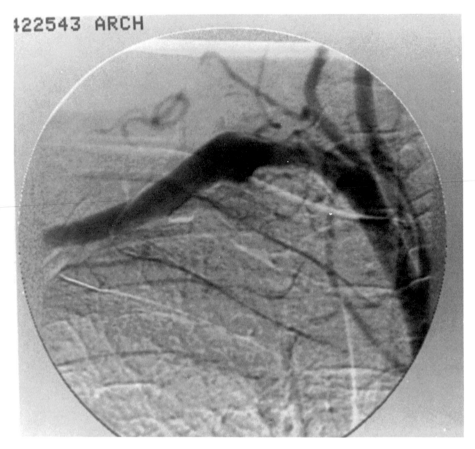

122543 ARCH

Fig. 14-6.   Intraarterial injection for a digital subtraction arteriogram in a woman with a cervical rib and mild paresthesia in her right hand. The osseous structures have been "subtracted" from the film to make the details of the injected areas more prominent. The arteriogram demonstrates an aneurysm that is twice the diameter of the subclavian artery, just borderline size for elective resection. In this case (Table 14–3, Case 2), the aneurysm was resected and the artery reconstructed with an end-to-end anastomosis.

Stage 0: *Cervical ribs with no symptoms and no aneurysm* should be left alone. Neither surgery nor arteriography is indicated. However, a supraclavicular or infraclavicular bruit is an indication for angiography.

Stage 1: *Cervical ribs with minimal stenosis and mild poststenotic dilatation* are treated with arterial decompression by resection of the cervical or abnormal first rib. The artery is left untouched as long as the intima is undamaged.

Stage 2: *Cervical ribs with aneurysms, intimal damage, and mural thrombosis* should be treated with resection of the rib and excision and repair or ligation and bypass of the aneurysm. The precise point at which poststenotic dilatation becomes an aneurysm has not been clearly established, but a rough rule of thumb is to treat as an aneurysm any enlargement that is twice or more the arterial diameter (Fig. 14-6).

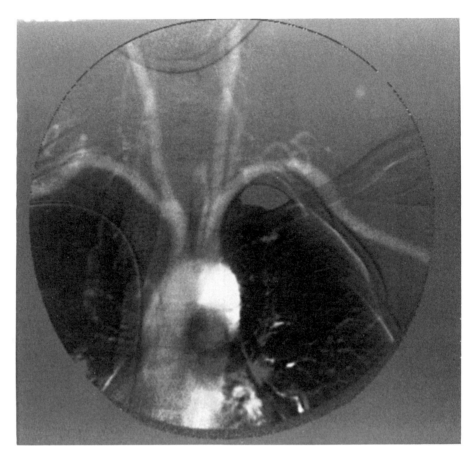

Fig. 14-7.   Intravenous injection for a digital subtraction arteriogram in an asymptomatic 18-year-old woman with bilateral cervical ribs and pulsatile, small supraclavicular masses. The poststenotic dilatations were not large enough to require arterial resection. She was treated by simple bilateral cervical rib excision (Table 14–3, Case 3).

Differentiating Stage 1 from Stage 2 involvement can be difficult. Mild intimal damage, which may be undetectable by arteriography or gross inspection, is capable of forming thrombi. Patients with cervical ribs and *any* vascular symptoms should undergo arteriotomy or resection of the portion of the subclavian artery immediately over and just distal to the cervical rib, regardless of how normal that section of artery appears grossly. This approach is supported by Brown and Charlesworth, who found that only 1 of 8 patients with cervical ribs and vascular symptoms were cured by rib resection alone.[24]

In contrast, Cormier handled this by opening the arteries of all Stage 2 patients and simply closing those in whom no significant abnormalities were found.[25] He had good results in all 14 patients treated in this manner. The development of duplex scanning in the 1990s promises to alter the need to surgically explore normal appearing arteries because duplex scans have the potential to noninvasively detect luminal and intimal changes.

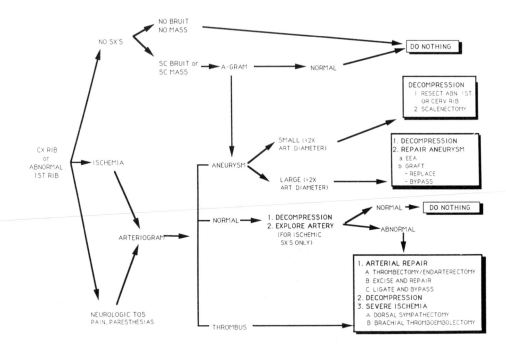

Fig. 14-8.   Algorithm of the treatment options for arterial TOS.

Stage 3: *Cervical ribs with distal emboli* require not only rib resection and subclavian artery repair, but often require distal embolectomy and dorsal sympathectomy to increase peripheral blood flow (Figs. 14-9, A and B, and 14-10, A and B).

Review of Surgical Literature

Arterial TOS is an uncommon condition with little more than 200 cases reported in the English-language literature. An historical review of the management of arterial TOS is a study of the development of vascular surgery. In 1956, Schein reviewed 140 years of medical literature and found 30 patients with arterial thrombosis and cervical ribs.[26] Those were treated in a variety of ways, the most common being excision of the thrombosed artery without repair (seven patients) and excision of the cervical rib and/or scalenotomy (15 patients). Symptomatic improvement was reported in 56% in spite of the fact that arterial continuity was not restored in any of them. Three patients, one of whom died, experienced hemiplegia as a result of proximal propagation of the arterial thrombus from the right subclavian to the right carotid artery. There were two amputations (7%). In his paper, Schein went on to report the first case of a subclavian aneurysm to be successfully treated with an arterial homograft (Table 14–1).

Between 1956 and 1968, there was a change in treatment as techniques were developed to remove thrombi and repair arteries. Excision of the causative bony abnormality, most often a cervical rib, plus excision of soft tissue structures that

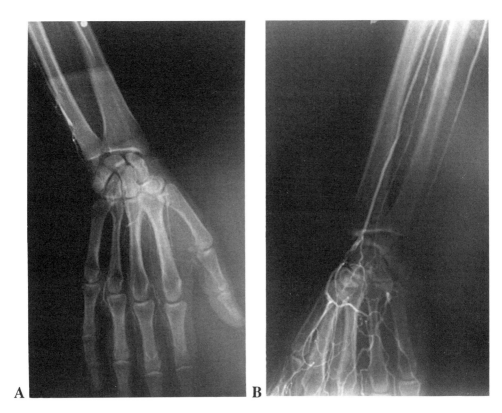

Fig. 14-9.   Distal arteriograms of the same patient in Figure 14-2 (Table 14–3, Case 5). **A.** Ulnar artery embolus with no flow in the radial artery and attenuated, tiny arteries with minimal flow in the palmar arch and digital arteries. **B.** Same hand following a subclavian and brachial artery thromboembolectomy, but not an ulnar artery embolectomy. The embolus in the ulnar artery is still present with collateral flow around it filling the palmar arch and digital arteries.

can produce extrinsic pressure, continued as adjunctive forms of surgical therapy. In addition, direct arterial procedures were performed in 26% of the patients and thrombectomy in another 23%. Combination therapy became the rule: resecting cervical and first ribs, extracting clots from subclavian and brachial arteries, and patching or replacing arteries. Dorsal sympathectomy, as an adjunct to the other procedures, was performed in 39% of the patients. Only a few cases were too advanced to treat as the number of untreated cases fell from 17% to 4% (Table 14–1).

After 1970, refinements and improvements in treatment continued. The incidence of cervical ribs as the primary cause of arterial damage fell from 100% in Schein's review[26] to 80% in the study by Judy,[27] and to 66% in the present review. In recent years, other osseous causes of arterial compression become apparent, such as rudimentary first ribs and fractures of the clavicle or first rib. A few cases of soft tissue compression without osseous abnormalities also began to appear, constituting 12% of the most recent series (Tables 14–1 and 14–2).

Treatment became more complete as surgeons became comfortable with

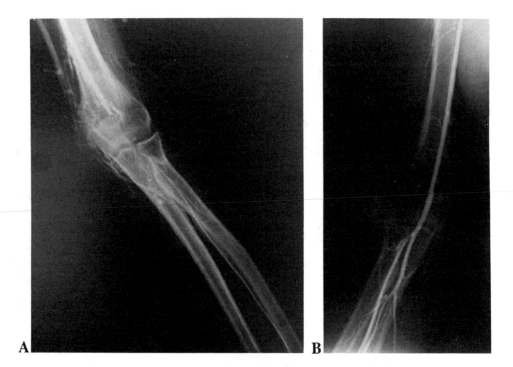

Fig. 14-10.   Brachial arteriogram in the same patient as in Figure 14-2. **A.** Preoperative arteriogram demonstrating brachial artery occlusion by embolus. **B.** Postoperative arteriogram following brachial embolectomy showing a normal artery.

opening, resecting, and reanastomosing or replacing the subclavian artery. The incidence of isolated thrombectomy and embolectomy, which had reached 23% in the 1960s, fell to 2% after 1970. Thrombus removal was usually accompanied by repair or resection of the involved artery. Realization that the subclavian artery was redundant after cervical rib excision encouraged surgeons to resect as much as 2–3 cm of this vessel and reapproximate the ends with vascular anastomoses.

In the most recent series, 26% of the patients were managed with end-to-end anastomosis; in 22%, either a vein or prosthetic graft was required; and in 18%, endarterectomy, local repair, or patch graft was employed. A total of 66% were treated by direct arterial repair. Adjunctive dorsal sympathectomy was performed in 16% (Table 14–1). The details of our five cases are recorded in Table 14–3.

Treatment Options

Choice of Approach

A supraclavicular incision is the approach of choice. In patients with cervical ribs, the subclavian artery usually arches higher than normal because the artery must stretch cephalad to pass over the cervical rib. Through this incision, it is possible to perform resection and end-to-end anastomosis of a portion of the

Table 14–1. Comparison of Three Reviews of Arterial TOS

	Schein, 1885–1955		Judy, 1957–1968		Sanders, 1969–1990	
	No.	%	No.	%	No.	%
Etiology						
Cervical rib	30	100	41	80	91	66
Rudimentary first rib	0	0	3	6	26	19
Fracture clavicle/rib	0	0	4	8	4	3
No bony abnormality	0	0	3	6	16	12
TOTAL	30		51		137	
Treatment						
Extrinsic decompression (rib resection, scalenotomy, claviculectomy)	15	50	20	39	42	31
Resection or ligation of artery (no repair)	7	24	3	6	1	1
End to end anastomosis	0	0	3	6	36	26
Graft (vein or prosthesis)	1	3	5	10	30	22
Repair (often endarterectomy) with or without patch	0	0	5	10	24	18
Thrombectomy/embolectomy	1	3	12	23	3	2
Dorsal sympathectomy, only treatment[a]	1	3	1	2	0	0
No treatment	5	17	2	4	0	0
Dorsal sympathectomy as adjuvant treatment[a]	0	0	20	39	22	16
Claviculectomy as part of treatment					30	22
Results						
Improved	17	56	36	71	108	84
No improvement	9	30	13	25	13	10
Amputation	2	7	2	4	4	3
Stroke (CVA)	2	7	0	0	1	1
Death	1(CVA)	3	0	0	2(CVA)	2

[a]Rx = treatment.

subclavian artery. Alternately, the subclavian artery can be ligated and a bypass graft performed. The supraclavicular incision is quite versatile. It is also a good approach for performing dorsal sympathectomy, resecting a cervical rib, or resecting the first rib. In a minority of cases, a high-lying clavicle can make exposure difficult through the supraclavicular incision. In such instances, an infraclavicular incision can be added or claviculectomy performed (Fig. 14-11).

The infraclavicular approach is through an incision below the clavicle. The pectoralis major muscle is split in the direction of its fibers and the pectoralis minor tendon divided. The distal anastomosis of a bypass graft can be performed through this incision.

Claviculectomy is only occasionally warranted; it is indicated when supraclavicular exposure is inadequate, usually in large people whose arteries lie quite deep. The medial two-thirds of the clavicle can be removed with minimal postoperative deformity, and some advocate total claviculectomy.[39, 40] The clavicle can

Table 14–2. Treatment and Results[a]

Author	Yr	No. pts	Cer Rib	Rud 1st Rib	Fx	No Bny Abn	Ext Dec Only	EEA	Grft	Rep Ptch	Thr/ Emb	+	−	Amp	CVA
			Etiology				Direct Arterial Therapy					Results			
Heyman, Whelan[28]	1970	1	1				1					1			
Judy, Heyman[27]	1972	7	4	1		2	1	1	3	2		2	3	2	
Mathes, Salam[29]	1974	1	1				1						1		
Martin et al.[30]	1976	2	2						2			2			
Banis et al.[31]	1977	5	2	2	1			1	2		2	3	2		
Dorazio et al.[32]	1979	5	3	1		1	5					5			
Etheredge et al.[23]	1979	5	2	3				1	3	1		4	1		
Prior et al.[20]	1979	4	3			1	3				1[b]	2	1		1(1)
Pairolero et al.[33]	1981	6	6				4		2			6			
Lee et al.[34]	1984	2	1			1		2				2			
Scher et al.[22]	1984	15	15				9	2	3		1	14	1		
Al-Hassan et al.[21]	1988	2	2					2				0			2(1)
Brown, Charlesworth[24]	1988	8	8				8					7	1		
Salo et al.[35]	1988	11	6			5	8		3			10	1		
Sullivan et al.[36]	1988	1				1					1[c]	1			
Baumgartner et al.[37]	1989	2		2			2					2			
Cormier et al.[25]	1989	55	32	15	3	5		23	11	21		42[d]	4		
Sanders, Haug[38]	1990	5	4	1			2	2	1			5			
TOTALS		137	91	26	4	16	42	36	30	24	5	108	13	4	3(2)
PERCENT			66%	19%	3%	12%	30%	26%	22%	17%	4%	84%	10%	3%	3%

[a]Cer rib = cervical rib.
Rud 1st rib = rudimentary first rib.
Fx = fracture of clavicle or rib.
No Bny Abn = no bony abnormality.
Ext dec = extrinsic decompression by cervical rib or first rib resection, scalenotomy, or claviculectomy.
EEA = end-to-end anastomosis.

Rep & ptch = repair, endarterectomy, and/or patch graft.
Grft = graft; vein or prosthesis.
Thr/Emb = Thrombectomy, embolectomy, arterotomy.
+ = improvement.
− = no improvement.
Amp = amputation.
CVA = stroke.
( ) = Death.

[b]1 case treated by arterial ligation.
[c]lytic therapy.
[d]no follow up in 9 cases.

Table 14–3. Five New Cases

Age	Sex	Side	Etiology	Symptoms	Treatment	Follow up
1. 24 DK	F	R	Rudimentary 1st Rib	Ischemic, numb, painful, useless hand (x-ray, see Fig. 14-4)	1. 5 years previously: thrombectomy and 1st rib resection 2. 1 year previously: explored for symptoms; nothing done to artery 3. Ligation, vein bypass, dorsal sympathectomy	Much better, minimal symptoms (3 years)
2. 43 PP	F	R	Cervical Rib	Mild tingling (x-ray, see Fig. 14-6)	Cervical rib resection and excision aneurysm with EEA	Asymptomatic (4 years)
3. 23 LV	F	R	Cervical Rib	None. pulsatile supraclav. lump (x-ray, see Fig. 14-7)	Cervical rib resection	Asymptomatic (2 years)
4. 23	F	L	Cervical Rib	None. pulsatile supraclav. lump (x-ray, see Fig. 14-7)	Cervical rib resection	Asymptomatic (2 years)
5. 32 CH	F	R	Cervical Rib	Ischemic, numb, cold painful hand (x-ray, see Figs. 14-2, 14-9, 14-10)	Cervical rib resection, subclavian arterial resection, subclavian thrombectomy, EEA,[a] brachial embolectomy, dorsal sympathectomy	Asymptomatic (2 years)

[a]End-to-end anastomosis.

also be divided and wired together at the end of the procedure. While most authors have reported no complications following claviculectomy, Pairolero reported that in five patients in whom partial claviculectomy was employed, two developed unstable shoulders and one patient required excision of the remaining lateral portion of the clavicle because it was producing intermittent venous obstruction.[32] Since it is possible to work above and below the clavicle to achieve almost every type of reconstruction, claviculectomy for arterial TOS should rarely be necessary. If the clavicle must be divided or partially resected, Pairolero recommends its reconstruction at the end of the operation.

Choice of Vascular Repair

When a thrombus is present or suspected in the subclavian artery, the artery can be opened and examined through a supraclavicular incision. Thrombectomy, endarterectomy, or segmental excision with end-to-end anastomosis can be performed through this single incision. If there is minor aneurysmal dilatation or there is a history of emboli, an arteriotomy should be performed and the intima inspected. If it is normal or has minimal irregularities, the arteriotomy can be closed,

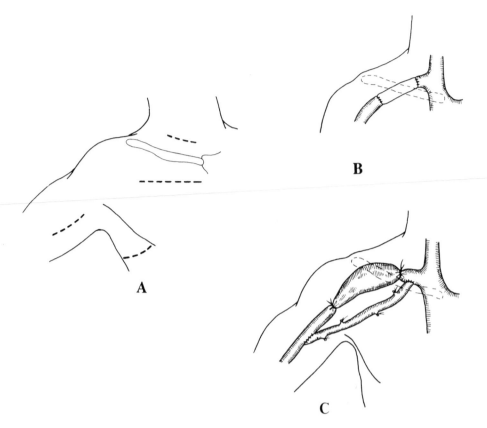

Fig. 14-11.   Surgical options for subclavian artery repair. **A.** Location of four incisions: supraclavicular, infraclavicular, transaxillary, and brachial. **B.** Interposition graft with end-to-end anastomoses requiring both supra- and infraclavicular incisions. **C.** Bypass graft with ligation of aneurysm requiring a
supraclavicular and either a transaxillary or brachial incision.

with large enough bites taken to return the vessel to its normal caliber.[25] If there is
extensive intimal damage, that segment of the artery is resected or replaced.
Duplex scanning has the potential to determine whether or not an artery contains
intimal damage or mural thrombus. When the specificity of this technique has
been ascertained, it may be used to determine the condition of a normal-appearing
artery without performing the arteriotomy.

End-to-end anastomosis following resection of an aneurysm or a damaged
arterial segment is the preferred reconstruction technique, provided there is no
tension on the suture line. A gap of at least 2 cm can be repaired with ease because
following the removal of a cervical rib, the repaired artery drops lower in the neck
and can easily tolerate this shortening without excessive suture line tension.
Interrupted sutures should be used for most if not the entire anastomosis to avoid a
postoperative stricture.

A graft is required for large aneurysms (over 2–3 cm long) or for aneurysms
extending too far below the clavicle where it is difficult to mobilize the distal artery.
The diseased arterial segment is excised if it can be done without damaging the

brachial plexus; it is replaced with an interposition graft. If the plexus is adherent to the artery, or if the artery is hidden by the clavicle, it is best to leave the aneurysm in place, ligate the artery, and sew a bypass graft to the subclavian artery proximally and the axillary artery distally. Autogenous saphenous vein or iliac artery[23] are the preferred graft materials. When these are not easily available, Dacron or PTFE grafts may be used.[41]

In situations in which the proximal subclavian artery is diseased or is technically difficult to expose, the side of the common carotid artery can be used as the site of the proximal anastomosis instead of the subclavian artery. Another alternative is to use the contralateral axillary artery as the inflow site to revascularize the arm.

Distal Thromboembolectomy

Emboli to the brachial artery usually lodge in the antecubital space. Although they can sometimes be removed with balloon catheters through the arteriotomy in the subclavian or axillary artery, a direct arteriotomy in the antecubital space may be the safest approach. It will permit more controlled thromboembolectomy of the radial and ulnar arteries with smaller balloon catheters. Thrombectomy or embolectomy through more distal arteriotomies at the wrist can also be performed, but their success rate is low. Small vessel arteriotomies are closed with a patch of either saphenous vein, autogenous artery, or prosthetic material. When available, a segment of resected subclavian artery may be used.

Dorsal Sympathectomy

The indications for dorsal sympathectomy are digital ischemia with pain and threatened tissue loss due to distal emboli that cannot be removed. It may be used alone or as an adjunct to proximal repairs. The techniques and approaches are discussed in Chapter 10. Few long-term results have been reported.

References

1. Kieffer E, Ruotolo C. Arterial complications of thoracic outlet compression. In: Rutherford RB, ed. Vascular surgery, 3rd ed. Philadelphia: WB Saunders Co., 1989:875–882.
2. Roos DB. Thoracic outlet nerve compression. In: Rutherford RB, ed. Vascular surgery, 3rd ed. Philadelphia: WB Saunders Co., 1989:858–875.
3. Sanders RJ, Pearce WH. The treatment of thoracic outlet syndrome: a comparison of different operations. J Vasc Surg 1989; 10:626–634.
4. Cormier JM, Tabet G. Resultats du traitement chirurgical des complications arterielles des syndromes de la traversee thoraco-brachiale. In: Kieffer E, ed. Les syndromes de la traversee thoraco-brachiale; Paris: AERCV, 1989:169–179.
5. Todd TW. The descent of the shoulder after birth: its significance in the production of pressure-symptoms on the lowest brachial trunk. Anat Anz 1912; 41:385–397.
6. Telford ED, Stopford JSB. The vascular complications of cervical rib. Br J Surg 1930; 18:557–564.
7. Baumgartner A, Clerc A, Macrez C. Sur l'anevrysme arteriel de voisinage et la gangrene ischemique des doigts. Press Med 1938; 46:1665–1667.
8. Halsted WH. An experimental study of circumscribed dilation of an artery imme-

diately distal to a partially occluded band, and its bearing on the dilation of the subclavian artery observed in certain cases of cervical rib. J Exp Med 1916; 24:271–286.

9.   Holman E. The obscure physiology of poststenotic dilatation: its relationship to the development of aneurysms. J Thor Surg 1954; 28:109–133.

10. Robicsek F, Sanger PW, Taylor FH, Magistro R, Fori E. Pathogenesis and significance of post-stenotic dilatation in great vessels. Ann Surg 1958; 147:835–844.

11. Harvey EN. Bubble formation in liquids. In Glasser O, ed. Medical physics, Vol 2; Chicago: Yearbook Publishers, 1950:137–150.

12. Kawaguti M, Hamano A. Numerical study on post-stenotic dilatation. Biorheology 1983; 20:507–518.

13. Ojha M, Johnston KW, Cobbold RSC. Evidence of a possible link between post-stenotic dilatation and wall shear stress. Abs Int Soc Cardiovasc Surg Scientific Meeting 1989; 37:52.

14. Zarins CK, Zatina MA, Giddens DP, Ku DN, Glagov S. Shear stress regulation of artery lumen diameter in experimental atherogenesis. J Vasc Surg 1987; 5:413–420.

15. Roach MR. Changes in arterial distensibility as a cause of poststenotic dilatation. Am J Cardiol 1963; 12:802–815.

16. Roach MR, Melech E. The effect of sonic vibration on isolated human iliac arteries. Can J Physiol Pharmacol 1971; 49:288–291.

17. Dobrin PB. Arterial post-stenotic dilatation. Surg Gynecol Obstet 1991; In press.

18. Symonds CP. Two cases of thrombosis of subclavian artery with contralateral hemiplegia of sudden onset, probably embolic. Brain 1927; 50:259–260.

19. Lewis T, Pickering GW. Observations upon maladies in which the blood supply to the digits ceases intermittently or permanently and upon bilateral gangrene of the digits: observations relevant to so called "Raynaud's Disease." Clin Sci 1934; 1:327–366.

20. Prior AL, Wilson LA, Gosling RG, Yates AK, Russel RWR. Retrograde cerebral embolism. Lancet 1979; 2:1044–1047.

21. Al-Hassan HK, Sattar MA, Eklof B. Embolic brain infarction: a rare complication of thoracic outlet syndrome. A report of two cases. J Cardiovasc Surg 1988; 29:322–325.

22. Scher LA, Veith FJ, Haimovici H, Samson RS, Ascer E, Sushil KG, Sprayregen S. Staging of arterial complications of cervical rib: guidelines for surgical management. Surgery 1984; 95:644–649.

23. Etheredge S, Wilbur B, Stoney RJ. Thoracic outlet syndrome. Am J Surg 1979; 138:175–182.

24. Brown SC, Charlesworth D. Results of excision of a cervical rib in patients with the thoracic outlet syndrome. Br J Surg 1988; 75:431–433.

25. Cormier JM, Amrane M, Ward A, Laurian C, Gigou F. Arterial complications of the thoracic outlet syndrome: fifty-five operative cases. J Vasc Surg 1989; 9:778–787.

26. Schein CJ, Haimovici H, Young H. Recent advances in surgery. Arterial thrombosis associated with cervical ribs: surgical considerations. Surgery 1956; 40:428–443.

27. Judy KL, Heymann RL. Vascular complications of thoracic outlet syndrome. Am J Surg 1972; 123:521–531.

28. Heymann RL, Whelan TJ. Vascular complications of the thoracic outlet syndrome: a case report. Military Med 1970; 135:793–796.

29. Mathes SJ, Salam AA. Subclavian artery aneurysm; sequela of thoracic outlet syndrome. Surgery 1974; 76:506–510.

30. Martin J, Gaspard DJ, Johnston PW, Kohl RD, Dietrick W. Vascular manifestations of the thoracic outlet syndrome. A surgical urgency. Arch Surg 1976; 111:779–782.

31. Banis JC, Rich N, Whelan TJ. Ischemia of the upper extremity due to noncardiac emboli. Am J Surg 1977; 134:131–139.

32. Dorazio RA, Ezzet F. Arterial complications of the thoracic outlet syndrome. Am J Surg 1979; 138:246–250.

33. Pairolero PC, Walls JT, Payne WS, Hollier LH, Fairbairn JF. Subclavian-axillary artery aneurysms. Surgery 1981; 90:757–763.

34. Lee BY, Thoden WR, Madden JL, McCann WJ. Subclavian artery aneurysm secondary to thoracic outlet syndrome. Contemp Surg 1984; 25:19–25.

35. Salo JA, Varstela E, Ketonen P, Ala-Kulja K, Luosto R. Management of vascular complications in thoracic outlet syndrome. Acta Chir Scand 1988; 154:349–352.

36. Sullivan KL, Minken SL, White RI. Treatment of a case of thromboembolism resulting from thoracic outlet syndrome with intraarterial urokinase infusion. J Vasc Surg 1988; 7:568–571.

37. Baumgartner F, Nelson RJ, Robertson JM. The rudimentary first rib: a cause of thoracic outlet syndrome with arterial compromise. Arch Surg 1989; 124:1090–1092.

38. Sanders RJ, Haug CE. Arterial thoracic outlet syndrome: report of five cases and review of literature. Surg Gynecol Obstet. 1991; In Press.

39. Lord JW Jr. Surgical management of shoulder girdle syndromes: new operative procedure for hyperabduction, costoclavicular, cervical rib, and scalenus syndromes. Arch Surg 1953; 60:69–83.

40. Lord JW Jr, Urschel HC Jr. Total claviculectomy. Surgical Rounds 1988; 11:17–27.

41. Gugenheim S, Sanders RJ. Axillary artery rupture caused by shoulder dislocation. Surgery 1984; 95:55–58.

15
Venous TOS

Craig E. Haug
Richard J. Sanders

Primary and Secondary Thrombosis
Nonthrombotic Venous Obstruction
Incidence and Side
Anatomy and Etiology

Signs and Symptoms

Diagnosis

Treatment

Surgical Techniques for Venous TOS

This chapter is a revision of: Sanders RJ, Haug CE: Subclavian vein obstruction and thoracic outlet syndrome: A review of etiology and management. Ann Vasc Surg 1990; 4:397–410. With permission.

Because subclavian vein compression in the costoclavicular space can cause venous obstruction, it is regarded as a form of TOS. Technically, since the subclavian vein is the inflow to the thorax, venous TOS might more accurately be called thoracic "inlet" syndrome. However, the label "thoracic outlet" has become an all-inclusive one, being used as an anatomic rather than a mechanistic term. It therefore seems reasonable and less confusing to use the term "thoracic outlet" to describe all forms of compression in this area.

Primary and Secondary Thrombosis

Axillosubclavian vein thrombosis is generally classified as primary or secondary. Secondary thrombosis involves an obvious etiology, such as central venous cannulation or malignancy. Primary thrombosis is spontaneous; it has no readily discernible etiology. Most authors have regarded TOS-associated venous thrombosis as primary rather than secondary, because the anatomy is grossly normal and the mechanism speculative.

Primary subclavian vein thrombosis has many pseudonyms—e.g., as idiopathic, spontaneous, traumatic, or effort thrombosis. In 1884, von Schroetter suggested that movements of the shoulder girdle could damage the axillary vein and cause venous thrombosis.[1] This theory introduced the term "traumatic or effort" thrombosis. However, when it was realized that neither trauma nor thrombosis was a constant feature in these cases, Hughes recommended that venous blockage be called a syndrome, to indicate that venous obstruction can be due to one of several causes.[2] He used the names of the first two men to describe this condition and coined the term Paget-Schroetter Syndrome.[3]

Nonthrombotic Venous Obstruction

Many cases initially diagnosed as axillosubclavian vein thrombosis prove to be cases of nonthrombotic venous obstruction. When Roelsen reviewed all of the operated cases of axillary vein thrombosis reported through 1938, he found that nine of the 21 patients (43%) explored for axillary vein thrombosis had no clot found at surgery.[4] In 1973, Mercier reported 21 cases of upper limb venous obstruction, seven with thrombosis, and 14 without thrombosis.[5] The symptomatic, nonthrombotic patients must be treated, not only to relieve symptoms, but also to avoid thrombosis, for which they are at greater risk.[6]

Incidence and Side

The incidence of venous obstruction in all TOS patients is small, from 1.5%[7] to 5%.[8] In a large review of 969 TOS patients, venous symptoms were present in 3.5%.[9] In most series, the right side is involved in at least two-thirds of the patients, and the left side in less than one-third.[10–13] The usual explanation is that the majority of these cases involved "effort" with the dominant arm; since most people are right handed, the right subclavian vein is more apt to be injured. However, another theory to explain right-sided predominance is the difference in anatomy between the right and left brachiocephalic vessels. The junction of subclavian and innominate veins is quite different on the two sides, with the right side having a much more acute angle than the left. Because the curve in the right subclavian-innominate junction is immediately beneath the costoclavicular ligament, the right subclavian vein may be more predisposed to extrinsic compression and trauma than the left subclavian vein (Fig. 15-1).

Anatomy and Etiology

Primary venous obstruction is probably the result of normal structures or their variants being placed in abnormal positions by extremes of activity.[14] This is supported by observations that some type of physical exertion is associated with most cases of venous obstruction.[15] The proposed mechanism is chronic, subclinical, intermittent compression that damages the vein wall and eventually leads to scarring, narrowing, and finally thrombosis. According to this theory, occlusion is not a matter of acute thrombosis of a previously normal subclavian vein precipitated by a single traumatic event; rather, it is the culmination of multiple small traumata over a prolonged period of time, similar to various overuse syndromes described in athletes. "The last straw" is the final exertional event associated with

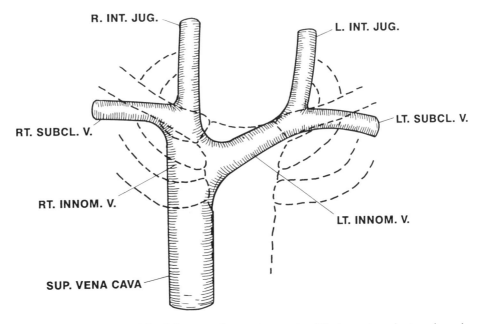

Fig. 15-1.   Anatomy of the right and left subclavian and innominate veins. The innominate begins where the internal jugular vein meets the subclavian vein. The costoclavicular ligament lies just distal to the subclavian-innominate junction. There is a sharper angulation of the right subclavian at this point than the left.

"effort thrombosis." In many cases, symptoms begin while extrinsic compression is developing and before complete occlusion or thrombosis occurs.

Historically, investigators have suggested different normal anatomical structures and sites as the primary instigator of venous compression. The normal structures bordering the costoclavicular space include the clavicle, first rib, subclavius muscle, the costoclavicular ligament, and the anterior scalene muscle (Fig. 15-2). The pectoralis minor space lies under that tendon near its attachment to the coracoid process a few cm lateral to the costoclavicular space. The axillary vein passes through the pectoralis minor space and arbitrarily changes its name to subclavian vein as it crosses the first rib to enter the costoclavicular space. The vein normally travels through this tunnel of musculoskeletal structures unimpeded. However, it is easy to appreciate how venous compression can develop with extensive movements of the shoulder girdle and slight variations in the size and positions of the surrounding muscles and ligaments.

Lowenstein performed the first thorough anatomical study and believed that the sharp edge of the costocoracoid ligament pinched the vein against the ribs as the arm was abducted.[16] Veal and McFetridge suggested that the head of the humerus, acting through the subscapularis muscle, constricted the vein when the arm was abducted.[17] Wright, like Lowenstein, thought that the vessel was damaged during hyperabduction by the pectoralis minor tendon or the coracoid process.[18] Direct compression between first rib and clavicle, or costoclavicular narrowing, was also suggested as the cause by several authors.[14, 19, 20]

In 1989, Kunkel and Machleder reported observations in 17 patients undergoing transaxillary first rib resection following axillosubclavian vein thrombosis. All patients exhibited mechanical abnormalities capable of compressing the sub-

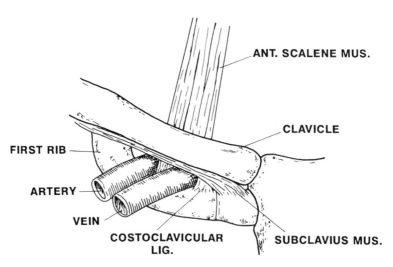

Fig. 15-2.   Anatomy of the costoclavicular space. The subclavian vein can easily contact the costoclavicular ligament, subclavius muscle, clavicle, first rib, or anterior scalene muscle.

clavian vein where it crossed the first rib. These included nine patients with prominent exostosis at the insertion of the subclavius or scalene anterior tendons and 12 patients with notable hypertrophy of these muscles and tendons.[13]

Prevenous Phrenic Nerve

The phrenic nerve normally passes posterior and medial to the subclavian vein. However, at least three anatomical studies have found a small, but significant, incidence of phrenic or accessory phrenic nerves lying anterior to the subclavian vein. Shroeder and Green were the first to note this, recording a 4% incidence of this variation and, in their cases, all of the prevenous phrenic nerves were on the right side.[21] In 1936, Havelaque found the phrenic nerve to lie anterior to the subclavian vein in 7% of 138 anatomical dissections[22] while Hughes, in 1948, noted a 5% incidence (one in 20 dissections).[2]

Clinically, there is only a single reported case of subclavian vein compression by a phrenic nerve.[23] However, the only way this anatomical variation can be clinically recognized is by surgically removing the medial half of the clavicle or opening the mediastinum, procedures that are seldom performed. We have observed this variation in one patient following claviculectomy and it is likely that this anomaly is more common than realized but often goes unrecognized because most cases of subclavian vein obstruction are treated nonsurgically. When surgery is performed, it is usually through infraclavicular or transaxillary approaches through which the subclavian-innominate junction is seldom seen (Fig. 15-3).

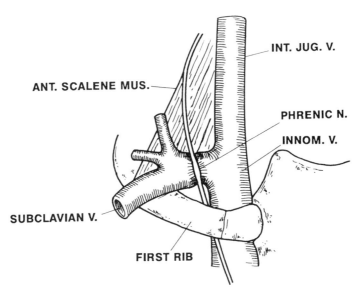

Fig. 15-3.   Prevenous (anterior lying) phrenic nerve compressing the subclavian vein. Normally, the phrenic nerve lies posterior to the subclavian vein.

Other Causes

Other possible causes of venous obstruction include congenital bands and ligaments that may encroach on the path of the axillosubclavian vein as well as the pectoralis minor tendons.[6]

Hypertrophy and malformation of the venous valves in the subclavian vein were first described in the early 1960s.[24, 25] They appear to be intrinsic venous abnormalities not related to extrinsic venous compression.

After reviewing this list of possible causes of subclavian vein obstruction, it is obvious that no single action or anatomical structure is the sole etiology. The causes are several and in any individual case it is difficult or impossible to ascertain a specific one. For this reason, the use of a generic term, such as primary venous obstruction or Paget-Schroetter Syndrome, permits the pathology to be acknowledged and treated even though the precise etiology remains obscure.

Venous Collaterals

The major collateral veins around the axillary-subclavian vein are the cephalic, transverse cervical, transverse scapular, and external jugular veins. When these collaterals are occluded as well, the lateral thoracic-intercostal-internal mammary veins are used. Venous collaterals are usually adequate for sedentary activities, but are often inadequate for performing strenuous tasks (Fig. 15-4).

Signs and Symptoms

Thrombotic Subclavian Vein Obstruction

The primary symptoms and signs of chronic venous obstruction are swelling, pain, cyanosis, and venous distention in the upper extremity. In the acute stage, the same findings are present, but can be severe and accompanied by a blue, cold, and tender arm, with distended collateral veins over the chest wall. Although rare, clot can propagate to the superior vena cava and produce massive swelling of the entire upper body (SVC Syndrome). Pulmonary emboli are uncommon[15] but have been noted in as many as 12% of patients and can be life threatening.[26]

Nonthrombotic Subclavian Vein Obstruction

Intermittent occlusion without thrombosis can present acutely, but more often it begins with the subtle onset of intermittent pain and swelling caused by partial or complete occlusion at the level of the costoclavicular ligament. The severity of symptoms depends upon the degree of collateralization. Symptoms are typically aggravated by exercise or work with the arm and are relieved by rest.

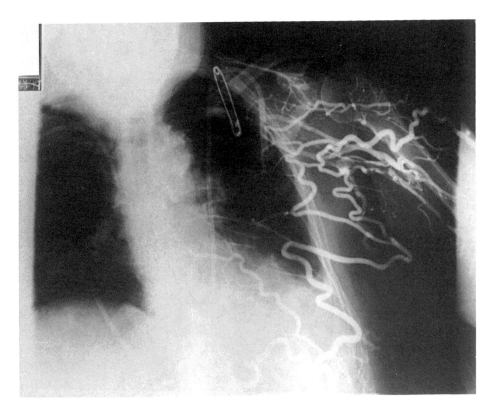

Fig. 15-4.   Venogram of massive brachial-axillary-subclavian vein thrombosis demonstrating the collateral veins over the upper arm and chest.

Diagnosis

Venography

The primary diagnostic tool is venography. It is diagnostic of thrombosis when a persistent filling defect is present, totally occluding the vein for several centimeters (Fig. 15-5). Nonthrombotic occlusion is more difficult to diagnose. It is suspected by delayed emptying of a patent subclavian vein or by the appearance of venous constriction at the subclavian-innominate junction (Fig. 15-6). Digital subtraction techniques, by "subtracting" out common elements such as bone, can improve venographic resolution in complicated cases (Fig. 15-7).

In patients with nonthrombotic venous obstruction, positional venography, with the arm abducted to 90 degrees or with the shoulders braced (hyperabducted, military position), is sometimes needed to demonstrate subclavian vein compression. Such venograms may be abnormal in asymptomatic individuals as well. In a study of normal people, Dunant noted a 70% incidence of venous compression: 20% in the costoclavicular space, 38% at the head of the humerus, and 12% in

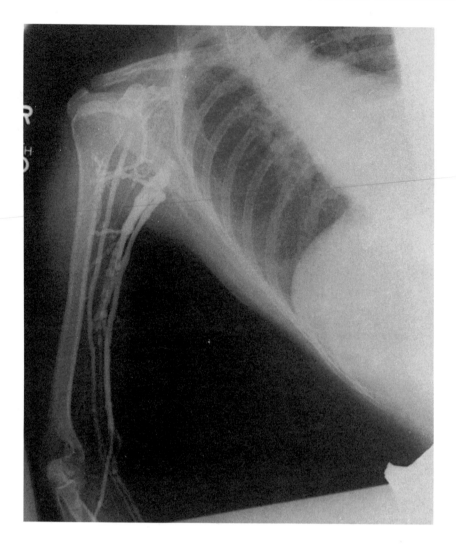

Fig. 15-5.   Venogram of typical subclavian vein thrombosis.

both areas.[26] Nevertheless, while abnormal venograms can be elicited with positioning in asymptomatic people, in a symptomatic patient an abnormal venogram is significant.

Duplex Scanning

In recent years, venous duplex scanning has been used to detect venous obstruction in the axillary-subclavian veins. This can be helpful with major venous occlusion, but misleading results have been obtained. Patent large collaterals can be mistaken for the occluded main channel; recanalized veins cannot always be distinguished from normal veins; and partial or intermittent obstructions are sometimes difficult to evaluate. For complete venous evaluation, venography is still

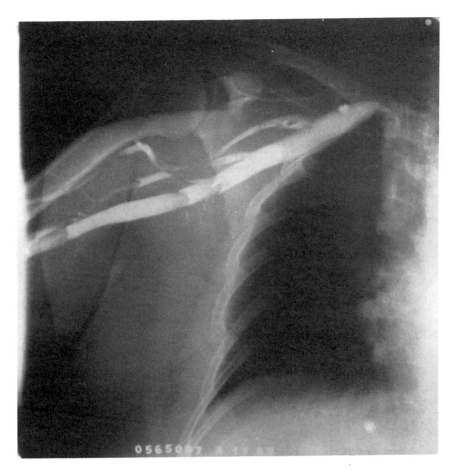

Fig. 15-6. Venogram of nonthrombotic venous obstruction, typically located at the subclavian-innominate vein junction. This proved to be an anterior lying phrenic nerve as diagrammed in Figure 3. The distal subclavian and axillary veins are normal.

needed. For screening and followup of therapy, duplex scanning can be used with a view toward its limitations.

Venous Pressure

Measurement of brachial venous pressure is another diagnostic modality for the nonthrombotic patient. Normal venous pressure in the upper extremity is 6–15 cm H_2O and is determined by inserting a needle into a peripheral vein in each arm. During shoulder bracing while sitting (military position), the pressure may double in normal people, while in patients with nonthrombotic occlusion, the pressure may increase 3 or 4 times[28] (Fig. 15-8). Daskalakis has found significant differences in resting venous pressures between normals and patients with venous obstruction. He recorded an average venous pressure in control subjects of 8.3 cm H_2O compared to pressures of 22.9 cm H_2O in patients with nonthrombotic

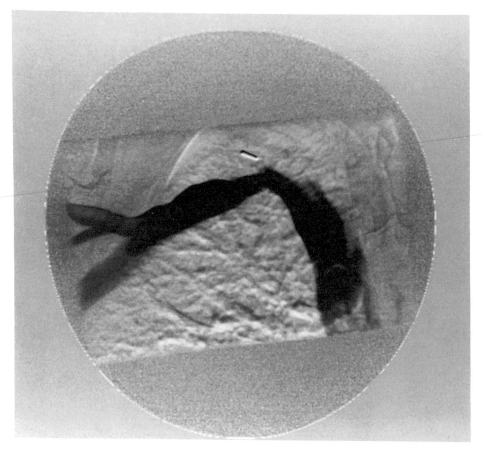

Fig. 15-7.   Venogram using digital subtraction angiography (DSA) in which bony structures are removed by subtraction techniques. This is the postoperative study of the patient in Figure 6 following repair of a prevenous phrenic nerve by reanastomosis of the subclavian to the innominate vein anterior to the nerve.

obstruction and 30.9 cm H_2O in patients with venous thrombosis. With exercise by repeated fist clenching, the pressures increased about 50% higher than the resting values. Following surgical decompression in the nonthrombotic patients, resting venous pressures fell to an average of 10.9 cm H_2O[6] with no increase on exercise.

Treatment

Options and Indications

The treatment of subclavian vein obstruction should be separated into the treatment of acute and chronic venous obstruction. The choice of therapy depends upon the intensity of the symptoms, the degree of disability, and the venographic findings.

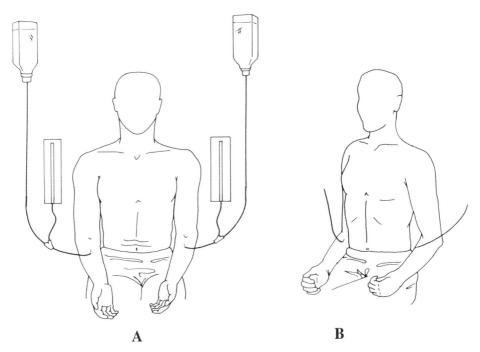

Fig. 15-8.   Technique of venous pressure measurements at rest (**A**) and with the shoulders braced in the military position (**B**).

Acute

Acute occlusion can be managed by anticoagulants, fibrinolytic therapy, or by surgical thrombectomy as outlined in the algorithm in Fig. 15-9. In general, all cases of thrombosis secondary to indwelling catheters or intravenous medication are treated nonsurgically; they rarely develop severe disabilities. Patients with primary venous thrombosis and mild to moderate symptoms should initially be managed conservatively. Those with severe symptoms may be handled conservatively or with surgical thrombectomy. When thrombectomy is performed, efforts should be made to determine whether the subclavian vein is narrowed or occluded by extrinsic compression or intrinsic disease. Extrinsic compression can be treated by first rib resection, claviculectomy, and/or division of the costoclavicular ligament and subclavius muscle at the time of thrombectomy. If appropriate, direct venous reconstruction can also be performed at this time, but in most cases reconstruction is deferred pending failure of thrombectomy and extrinsic decompression alone.

Chronic

The symptoms of chronic venous obstruction, either postthrombotic or nonthrombotic, usually do not improve with conservative measures. The options are either to modify lifestyle and live with the symptoms or to consider surgical

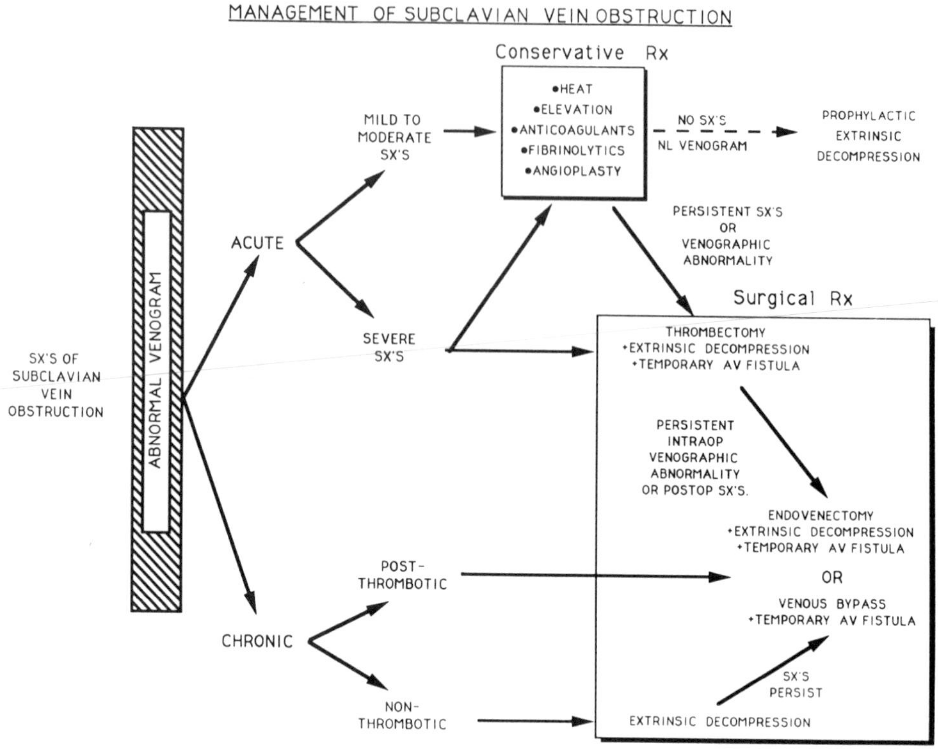

MANAGEMENT OF SUBCLAVIAN VEIN OBSTRUCTION

Fig. 15-9.   Algorithm of management of subclavian vein obstruction.

reconstruction. The choices for repair are extrinsic decompression, direct repair by endovenectomy and patch graft, or venous bypass. The choice of venous repair depends upon the findings at the time of operation. The surgeon should be equipped to apply an appropriate repair to a variety of situations. Currently there is not enough data to provide clear guidelines to recommend any single procedure over any other, perhaps with the exception of first rib resection. For intermittent, nonthrombotic subclavian vein obstruction, first rib resection is the simplest and least complicated procedure to perform. However, it is often inadequate, and more aggressive operations are necessary to relieve symptoms.

Acute Obstruction

Heat and elevation are adjuncts to conservative therapy. Their role is to alleviate symptoms during the acute phase, but they do not affect the thrombotic process. Elevation of the arm should be anterior, with the arm over the abdomen or chest, not over the head. Abducting the shoulder by raising the arm over the head may further narrow an already tight costoclavicular space.

Anticoagulants

The role of anticoagulants is to prevent clot propagation in the axillosubcla-vian-innominate venous system and its collaterals, as well as to prevent pulmonary emboli. Anticoagulants do not lyse clots. Recanalization of the vein is possible, but there is no evidence to confirm that it is promoted by anticoagulants. The reason for the effectiveness of anticoagulants is that they stabilize the clotting process. In time, the preserved venous collaterals enlarge and recanalization via the bodies' fibrinolytic system may occur. This results in improvement of symptoms even though the thrombus is still present.

Most cases of axillosubclavian vein thrombosis are treated with intravenous heparin for 8 to 10 days followed by warfarin therapy for 3 to 12 months. The general therapeutic guideline is to maintain a prothrombin time at one and one-half to two times the control level. This therapy is similar to the treatment of lower extremity deep venous thrombosis.

The results of anticoagulant treatment alone vary widely as the incidence of disabling arm swelling ranges from 4% to 100%, averaging 49% (Table 15–1). This wide variation in "successful results" stems from a lack of randomization, no uniformity in definition of success, and variable follow-up. Following initial anticoagulant therapy, if patients continue to have disabling symptoms, some form of surgical reconstruction can be considered. Only venography can determine the feasibility of such surgical correction.

Fibrinolytic Therapy

Lytic enzymes, streptokinase and urokinase, and more recently tissue plasminogen activator (tPA) have the potential, like heparin, to prevent clot propagation. However, unlike heparin, lytic enzymes can also dissolve clot and more quickly establish venous outflow. Lytic therapy is more effective if the catheter tip is buried in the clot, which is more difficult to achieve in venous than in arterial thrombosis. Systemic heparin should be given coincident with fibrinolysis to avoid thrombus formation around the indwelling catheter sitting in the brachial vein.

Table 15–1. **Results of Anticoagulant Therapy for Axillosubclavian Thrombosis**

Author	Year	No. Cases	Successful[a] No.	Successful[a] %
Adams et al.[29]	1965	10	3	30%
Drapanas, Curran[30]	1966	4	0	
Swinton et al.[10]	1968	23	2	9%
Tilney et al.[15]	1970	11	3	28%
Dalal Pitney[31]	1972	4	2	50%
Prescott, Tikaff[32]	1979	13	13	100%
Campbell et al.[33]	1977	25	1	4%
Glovickzki et al.[9]	1986	69	48	70%
Ameli et al.[26]	1987	20	15	75%
Brochneret al.[34]	1989	6	4	67%
TOTALS		185	91	49%

[a]Success indicates patient was "improved," which was usually a subjective evaluation of a postphlebitic arm and not clearly defined. Few cases had follow up venograms.

Fibrinolytic therapy is only recommended for acute venous thrombosis, usually less than 5 days old. If therapy successfully lysis the clot, venography is performed at the completion of therapy to be certain that the vein is patent, as improvement in clinical signs and even duplex scans can be misleading. If there is a compressing or obstructing lesion in or around the subclavian vein or even if the vein appears normal, surgical correction should be considered to prevent recurrent thrombosis, although there is no unanimity of opinion on this point. Long-term anticoagulants may prevent recurrence as long as the medication is taken, but committing a young person to the long-term risks of anticoagulants may be unwarranted. In addition, thrombosis can still occur in the presence of therapeutic levels of anticoagulants.

There are two options regarding the timing of first rib resection following successful lytic therapy. One is to perform rib resection shortly after the vein has been opened and a few days of heparin therapy have been given. The rationale for this is to decompress the vein before it reclots. The other option is to maintain the patient on warfarin therapy for 3 months and then perform rib resection for persistent and significant symptoms. At this time, there is not sufficient data to favor one option over the other. In the series by Kunkel and Machleder, although all patients received at least 3 months of nonoperative treatment prior to considering surgery, 72% of their 25 patients eventually underwent an operation.[13]

If the vein has not recanalized with lytic therapy, concurrent surgery should not be considered. The patient should be continued on anticoagulants for several months and symptoms reevaluated after this time. If the symptoms are significant, the patient should be managed as a case of chronic obstruction as described below.

The experiences with fibrinolytic therapy indicate that it is usually combined with additional types of invasive treatment. Of the 82 cases collected from the literature, there were 43 patients (52%) who had 45 definitive corrective procedures following the lytic therapy: 41 first rib resections; three angioplasties; and one venous repair. The success rate for combined therapy was 79% (Table 15–2).

Experience with angioplasty is new. While angioplasty can help intrinsic venous narrowing, it cannot relieve extrinsic venous compression. Following angioplasty, patients who continue to be symptomatic, or whose venograms indicate irregularities around the subclavian vein, should be considered candidates for surgical decompression.

Thrombectomy

Surgical thrombectomy has been performed since 1926. Its indications are acute thrombosis (no more than a few days old) and severe pain and swelling in the arm. The purpose is to prevent chronic disability.

Axillosubclavian vein thrombectomy can be accomplished by a balloon catheter through a peripheral vein or by direct removal via a transaxillary, infraclavicular, supraclavicular, and transclavicular route.[12] In large patients, removal of the medial portion of the clavicle provides the best exposure and will not

Table 15–2. Results of Fibrinolysis

Author	Year	No. Cases	Drug[a]	Successes[b] No.	Successes[b] %	Other Treatment[c] 1st Rib	Other Treatment[c] Angpl	Other Treatment[c] Recnst
Becker et al.[35]	1983	4	Local UK	4/4	100%		1	1
Dunant[27]	1984	25	Not stated	17/25	68%	25		
Taylor et al.[14]	1985	2	Syst SK	2/2	100%	2		
Dury et al.[36]	1985	5	Local SK,UK	3/5	60%	2		
Vogel, Jenen[37]	1985	1	SK	1/1	100%	1		
Gloviczki et al.[9]	1986	2	SK	2/2	100%			
Smith-Behn et al.[38]	1986	1	Syst SK	1/1	100%			
Steed et al.[39]	1986	7	Syst SK	7/7	100%[d]			
Huey et al.[40]	1987	9	Local SK	6/9	66%			
Landercasper et al.[41]	1987	4	Syst SK,UK	4/4	100%	2		
O'Leary et al.[42]	1987	2	Local SK	1/2	50%	2	2	
Shuttleworth et al.[43]	1987	3	Syst SK	3/3	100%	2		
Wiles et al.[44]	1987	4	Syst SK	2/4	50%			
Rauwerda et al.[45]	1988	5	Local SK	5/5	100%[e]	5		
Wilson et al.[46]	1990	8	Syst SK	7/8	87%[f]			
TOTALS		82		65/82	79%	41	3	1

[a]Local = infusion of lytic agent directly into thrombus; syst = systemic administration of lytic agent; SK = streptokinase; UK = urokinase.
[b]Success indicates patient was "improved," which was usually a subjective evaluation of a postphlebitic arm and not clearly defined. Few cases had follow up venograms.
[c]1st Rib = first rib resection; Angpl = transcutaneous balloon dilatation (angioplasty); Recnst = venous reconstruction.
[d]Venograms demonstrated recanalization of thrombus in only one of seven cases, in spite of clinical improvement in all seven. Five of seven were secondary to central catheters; only two cases were "effort" thromboses.
[e]All five cases were open on venography.
[f]Partial or complete recanalization in seven of eight cases on venography.

result in serious cosmetic deformity. Following thrombectomy, catheters, probes, and venography are used to evaluate the proximal subclavian and innominate veins. If there has been no venous narrowing, the first rib is removed and the costoclavicular ligament divided to eliminate extrinsic pressure. If there has been venous narrowing or occlusion, venous reconstruction may be needed to prevent postphlebitic symptoms. Following thrombectomy, a temporary arteriovenous fistula is created.

The reported results of surgical thrombectomy indicate that 94% of 33 patients had improvement in symptoms (Table 15–3). However, not all of this improvement is attributable to the thrombectomy because only a few cases had follow-up venograms. Among those who did have venograms, many were found to have venous reocclusion even though their symptoms had lessened. Obviously, some of the improvement was due to recanalization and increased collaterals. However, this criticism is not unique to thrombectomy; the same applies to all of the treatment modalities discussed here.

Table 15–3. Results of Subclavian Vein Thrombectomy

Author	Year	No. Cases	No. Successes[a]
Drapanas, Curran[30]	66	2	2/2
Dale[47]	48	1	1/1
DeWeese et al.[12]	70	6	5/6 includes 4 with claviculectomy
DeWeese et al.[b 12]	26–64	20[b]	20/20 (only short term)
Gaylis[48]	74	4	3/4
TOTALS		33	31/33 (94%)

[a]Success indicates clinical improvement. In some instances, the vein reoccluded and recanalization or collateral circulation accounted for the improvement.
[b]20 cases collected from the surgical literature.

Chronic Obstruction

Nonthrombotic and Postphlebitic Venous Obstruction

Axillosubclavian vein thrombosis generally has been regarded as a nonsurgical condition and most cases have been treated with anticoagulants. Surgical therapy for upper extremity venous obstruction is still evolving. Operations for subclavian vein obstruction began about 1960 and, by 1990, less than 200 cases of all types of subclavian venous surgery has been reported in the medical literature.

Most patients treated with anticoagulants develop some degree of postphlebitic obstruction; still they experience enough symptomatic improvement to live comfortable lives with an acceptable disability. However, what is regarded as "acceptable disability" includes various degrees of pain, swelling, and weakness of the arm in the majority of patients.[45] Many disabilities are in young, active individuals whose lifestyles are impaired by their symptoms. Today, this level of disability may *not* be "acceptable" in the face of new surgical techniques.

Extrinsic Decompression

First Rib Resection

Extrinsic pressure on the subclavian vein, near the point where the vein crosses the first rib, is thought to be responsible for initiating axillosubclavian vein obstruction, thrombotic as well as nonthrombotic. First rib resection is the simplest way to relieve this pressure and may be performed alone or with other reconstructive procedures. Theoretically, first rib resection should not help total venous occlusion without recanalization; it cannot reopen the vein. However, in some patients with total venous occlusion, the axillary vein is occluded while the subclavian vein reopens and receives the cephalic vein collateral (Fig. 15-10A & 10B). In such situations, compression at the subclavian-innominate vein junction is still present, as demonstrated by positional changes (Fig. 15-10B); first rib resection in these cases may be followed by symptomatic improvement.[50]

First rib resection for venous TOS must include the anterior portion of the rib, up to the costochondral junction. In some instances, removal of a portion of the

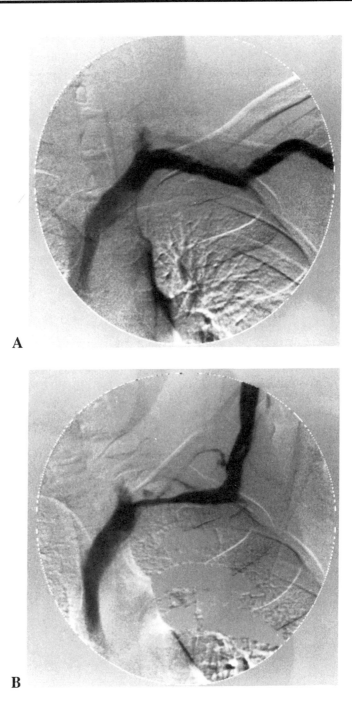

Fig. 15-10.   Venogram in 20-year-old man eight months following a left axillosubclavian vein thrombosis treated with lytic therapy and now experiencing minimal symptoms. **A.** With the arm at the patient's side, the axillary vein is occluded and does not visualize but the cephalic vein flows nicely into the patent subclavian vein. **B.** Repeat dye injection with the arm above his head reveals significant compression at the subclavian-innominate junction, presumably the underlying pathology.

costal cartilage is necessary to insure that all pressure against the vein has been relieved. Therefore, rib resection must be accomplished by the transaxillary or infraclavicular routes, as the supraclavicular approach cannot reach the costochondral junction.

First rib resection was successful in 92 of 114 cases (81%) reported in the medical literature (Table 15–4). In 43 cases, fibrinolytic therapy preceded rib resection and in six of these, angioplasty was also employed.

Contralateral First Rib Resection

Axillosubclavian vein compression is often bilateral. Kunkel and Machleder performed bilateral venograms in 15 of their patients with unilateral symptoms. Twelve (80%) demonstrated axillosubclavian vein compression on the contralateral side, three of whom already had thrombosis. Because of the high incidence of contralateral thrombosis, they performed prophylactic transaxillary rib resection on the contralateral side in four of these patients.[13]

Table 15–4. **Results of Extrinsic Decompression**

Author	Year	First Rib Resection			Other Treatment[a]	
		No. Cases	Successes[b] No.	%	Lysis	Angpl
Siegel, Steichen[51]	1967	1	1/1	100%		
Adams et al.[11]	1968	2	1/2	50%		
Mercier et al.[5]	1973	13	12/13	92%		
Charrette et al.[52]	1974	4	4/4	100%		
Glass[53]	1975	8	8/8	100%		
Etheredge et al.[50]	1979	6	6/6	100%		
Dunant[27]	1984	25	17/25	68%	25	
Dury et al.[36]	1985	2	1/2	50%	2	
Schubart et al.[7]	1985	1	1/1	100%		
Vogel, Jensen[37]	1985	1	1/1	100%	1	
Taylor et al.[14]	1985	2	2/2	100%	2	
Gloviczki et al.[9]	1986	12	7/12	58%		
Landercasper et al.[41]	1987	2	2/2	100%	2	
O'Leary et al.[42]	1987	2	1/2	50%	2	2
Shuttleworth et al.[43]	1987	2	2/2	100%	2	
Pittam, Drake[54]	1987	7	5/7	71%		
Salo et al.[55]	1988	5	2/5	60%		
Brochner et al.[34]	1989	2	2/2	100%		
Kunkel, Machlela[13]	1989	17	17/17	100%	7[c]	4
TOTALS		114	92/114	81%	43	6

[a]Lysis = therapy with lytic enzymes, urokinase or streptokinase; Angpl = transcutaneous balloon dilatation (angioplasty).
[b]Success indicates patient was "improved," which was usually a subjective evaluation of a postphlebitic arm and not clearly defined. Few cases had follow up venograms.
[c]Estimated number.

Claviculectomy

Another method of extrinsic decompression is claviculectomy. Only a few cases of claviculectomy alone have been reported with improvement in five of the six cases (83%) (Table 15–5). Since both the subclavius muscle and costoclavicular ligament, which can contribute to extrinsic compression of the vein, attach to the clavicle, claviculectomy also removes these structures.

Although most surgeons report no complications from removal of the clavicle,[57] Pairolero noted an unstable shoulder in two of five patients who underwent partial claviculectomy for arterial repairs.[58] In one patient, the lateral portion compressed the subclavian vein and required later removal. This experience suggests that claviculectomy should be performed only when absolutely necessary, and when done most or all of the clavicle should be removed along with its periosteum.

Soft Tissue Decompression

This includes division of the anterior scalene muscle, subclavius muscle, congenital bands, and/or the costoclavicular ligament. Nineteen of 23 cases (83%) experienced clinical improvement following soft tissue division, and in the patients of Daskalakis, there was objective reduction in venous pressure as well[6] (Table 15–6).

Intrinsic Repair or Bypass

Venous reconstruction may be performed immediately following thrombectomy if there is residual stenosis or occlusion. It may also be done electively for chronic swelling and aching in patients initially treated without surgery and in patients with nonthrombotic venous obstruction. Two options are available: venous bypass or direct excision of the stenosis by endovenectomy.

Table 15–5. **Results of Extrinsic Decompression**

Author	Year	Claviculectomy	
		No. Cases	No. Successes[a]
Adams et al.[11]	1968	2	2/2
Rabinowitz, Goldfarb[56]	1971	1	0/1
Charrette et al.[52]	1974	1	1/1
Etheredge et al.[50]	1979	1 (with Rib Res.)	1/1
Gloviczki et al.[9]	1986	1	1[b]/1
TOTALS		6	5/6 (83%)

[a]Success indicates patient was "improved," which was usually a subjective evaluation of a postphlebitic arm and not clearly defined. Few cases had follow up venograms.
[b]This patient had a "fair" result.

Endovenectomy

Excision of intimal webs and bands in the subclavian and innominate veins (Fig. 15-11) has been reported in only 10 patients (Table 15-7). In several, the operation included thrombectomy, excision of the medial clavicle, division of the costoclavicular ligament and extrinsic bands, complete excision of the strictures within the subclavian vein, and closure with a vein patch to avoid restenosis. In

Table 15–6. Results of Extrinsic Decompression

| | Soft Tissue Release | | |
| | Anterior Scalene, Subclavius, Costoclavicular Ligament | | |
Author	Year	No. Cases	No. Successes[a]
McLaughlin, Popma[59]	1939	1	1/1
McCleery et al.[60]	1951	5	5/5
Adams et al.[11]	1968	3	0/3
Rabinowitz, Goldfarb[56]	1971	1	0/1
Charrette et al.[52]	1974	1	1/1
Daskalakis, Bouhoutsos[6]	1980	11	11/11
Salo et al.[55]	1988	1	1/1
TOTALS		23	19/23 (83%)

[a]Success indicates patient was "improved," which was usually a subjective evaluation of a postphlebitic arm and not clearly defined. Few cases had follow up venograms.

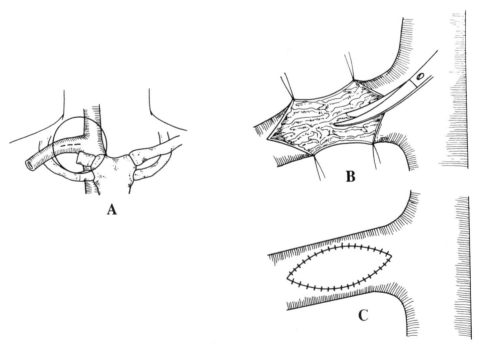

Fig. 15-11.   Technique of endovenectomy of the subclavian-innominate junction and patch graft with autogenous vein or prosthetic material.

two patients, temporary arteriovenous fistulae were added to improve patency. Good results were obtained in nine of the ten patients (90%) and a fair result in one patient (Table 15–7).

Venous Bypass

Rerouting venous flow around the subclavian-innominate junction has been performed in several ways. The internal jugular vein was used in seven of the 15 cases in Table 15–8 (Fig. 15-12). The anastomoses were either end-to-end or end-to-side and patency was confirmed in six of the seven patients by venography. Saphenous vein interposition between axillary and jugular veins was successful in two of four cases. A single case of a crossover cephalic vein graft and a spiral graft were each successful. A prevenous phrenic nerve compressing the right subclavian vein in one patient was treated by dividing the subclavian vein, placing the phrenic nerve behind the vein, and reanastomosing the subclavian to the innominate vein, end-to-side. Temporary arteriovenous fistulae were inserted in eight cases and seven had patent veins. The only failure occluded more than one year post-operatively (Table 15–8).

Experimental venous bypass with small and large diameter grafts have revealed that higher flow rates and less venous hypertension were seen when venous grafts were larger in diameter than the recipient vessels.[68] Applying this principle to subclavian vein bypass, the larger internal jugular vein or a spiral vein[67, 69] can be expected to achieve the highest success rates. Prostheses in the venous system have a high failure rate, particularly in smaller veins. If autogenous vein is not available, endovenectomy is probably preferable to a prosthesis.

Endovenectomy vs. Bypass

Patients who do not improve following rib resection, and patients who have partial or complete subclavian vein obstruction, are candidates for venous reconstruction by endovenectomy or bypass. Too few of either of these procedures have been reported to establish distinct indications for selecting one operation over the other. Endovenectomy requires better exposure, either a claviculectomy or mediastinotomy; once exposed, the vein may be too badly scarred to use. Internal jugular vein bypass can be done without claviculectomy and obviates dealing with

Table 15–7. **Endovenectomy**

Author	Year	No. Cases	No. Successes[a]
Campbell et al.[61]	1977	3	3/3
Jacobson, Haimov[62]	1977	1	1/1
Aziz et al.[63]	1986	4	4/4
Gloviczki et al.[9]	1986	2	1[b]/2
TOTALS		10	9/10 (90%)

[a]Success indicates patient was "improved," which was often a subjective evaluation of a postphlebitic arm and not clearly defined. Several of these patients did have follow up venograms.
[b]This patient had a "fair" result.

Table 15–8. Results of Venous Reconstruction with Venous Bypass

Author	Year	No. Cases	Type[a]	Clav[b]	AVF[c]	No. Successes[d]
Witte, Smith[64]	1966	1	IJ, EEA	Y	0	1/1
Inahara[65]	1968	1	Saph, ESA	Y	0	1/1
Rabinowitz, Goldfarb[56]	1971	1	Saph	?	1	1/1
Hashmonai et al.[66]	1976	1	Ceph X-over	N	1	1/1
Campbell et al.[61]	1977	2	IJ, teflon	1/2	0	0/2
Jacobson, Haimov[62]	1977	2	IJ, ESA	N	1	2/2
Pittam, Drake[54]	1987	2	Saph	?	0	0/2
Jain, Smejkal[67]	1988	1	Spiral	N	1	1/1
Sanders, Haug[e]	1990	4	IJ, ESA (3 patients)	1/4	4	3/4
TOTALS		15		4/15	8/15	10/15
PERCENTAGE				27%	53%	67%

[a]Type = IJ = internal jugular vein; EEA = end-to-end anastomosis; Saph = saphenous vein; ESA = end-to-side anastomosis; Ceph = cephalic vein; X-over = crossover vein graft from opposite side; teflon = teflon graft; spiral = spiral vein graft.
[b]Clav = Claviculectomy; Y = yes; N = no.
[c]AVF = Temporary arteriovenous fistula.
[d]In most cases, venography confirmed success.
[e]Four cases: One patient with phrenic nerve compression was treated by dividing the subclavian-innominate junction, letting the nerve fall behind the vein, and reanastomosing the veins. 3 patients were treated by end-to-side internal jugular vein bypass. In one of these three, a saphenous vein graft between the internal jugular and subclavian veins had failed within 24 hours in spite of an AV fistula.

a diseased vein. Its disadvantages are the sacrifice of one internal jugular vein, a scar high in the neck, and the potential for the clavicle to obstruct the bypass if the clavicle is not removed. If endovenectomy is tried first and is not successful, bypass can always be performed.

Temporary Arteriovenous Fistula (AVF)

Venous reconstructions are prone to early thrombosis because they are low pressure systems. In 1969, Johnson and Eiseman introduced the concept of a temporary arteriovenous fistula (AVF) in this setting to increase flow and improve patency.[70] In recent years, an AVF has also been added to axillosubclavian venous repairs with favorable results. A temporary AVF is created at the brachial or axillary level. While adjacent artery and vein can be sewn together to form the fistula, this is more difficult to ligate at a later date than a loop of teflon-reinforced PTFE. The fistula is defunctionalized 6 to 12 weeks later by dividing and ligating each half of the fistula[71] (Fig. 15-13).

Summary

Acute subclavian vein thrombosis has generally been treated with heparin and conservative measures. The data show that at least half of such patients develop some degree of chronic postphlebitic symptoms, swelling and aching.

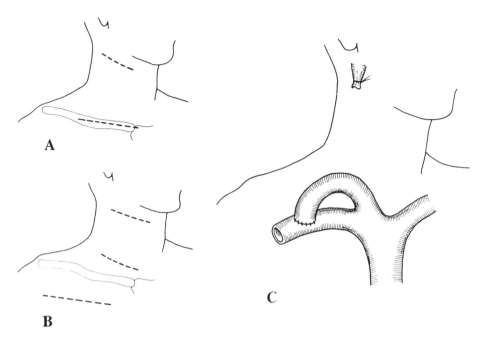

Fig. 15-12.   Diagram of end-to-side internal jugular vein to subclavian vein bypass.

Therefore, a more aggressive approach based on new nonoperative and operative techniques is recommended. Many treatment alternatives involve extrinsic decompression in recognition of the importance of TOS etiologically. Other treatment options, which may be used separately or in combination, include fibrinolysis, angioplasty, thrombectomy, endovenectomy, and bypass; the vein can be resurrected or replaced. The data does not allow a definitive choice among these treatment options and therefore an individualized approach, starting with the least invasive procedure, is justified.

Surgical Techniques for Venous TOS

Subclavian Vein Thrombectomy With Claviculectomy

The skin incision is made directly over the medial two thirds of the clavicle, beginning at the midline. The subcutaneous tissue is divided down to the clavicle, which is freed of all muscle attachments by cautery or knife dissections. A periosteal elevator may be used to detach some of the muscles from the clavicle, but the elevator is not used to peel back periosteum. The periosteum is removed along with bone to prevent regrowth.

A bone cutter or giggli saw is used to divide the clavicle moving from lateral to medial on a 45–60-degree angle. This avoids leaving a sharp bony corner at the skin level.

The divided medial end of the clavicle is mobilized bluntly. A knife or cautery divides remaining muscle and fascial attachments down to the costo-chondral-

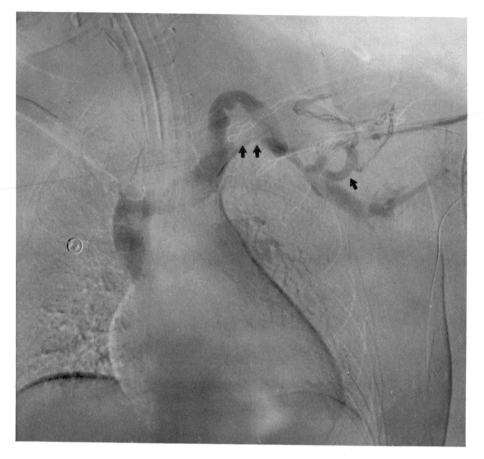

Fig. 15-13.   Arteriovenous fistula between the axillary artery and axillary vein (single arrow) in case of jugular-subclavian bypass (double arrow).

sternal junction. The clavicle is then disarticulated at the junction by cutting the remaining ligamentous attachments.

Once the medial portion of the clavicle is gone the sternal portion of the sternocleidomastoid muscle is divided to expose the subclavian vein. The vein lies in the center of the field. On the right side, the junction of the innominate and subclavian veins can be dissected free. On each side, a prevenous (located anteriorly) phrenic or accessory phrenic nerve can be identified, if one is present.

The subclavian/axillary vein is mobilized for at least 4 cm and surrounded with plastic vessel loops. At this time, it is also appropriate to dissect out the axillary artery, which lies deep to the vein. This will be used later for a temporary arteriovenous fistula (AVF).

The patient is heparinized and a 2-cm vertical venotomy is performed in the subclavian vein. Thrombectomy can be performed with a variety of instruments, such as endarterectomy forceps, endarterectomy elevators, common bile duct stone forceps, and balloon thrombectomy catheters. The distal vein is opened first by passing an endarterectomy elevator distally, freeing the thrombus from the venous intima. The thrombectomy forceps is then passed as far as possible into the vein with its jaws open. The thrombus is lightly engaged and withdrawn slowly. By squeezing the thrombus gently, not closing the forceps completely, it is sometimes possible to remove not only the clot in the forceps, but also a tail of more distal adherent thrombus with it. The arm, which was sterilely draped into the field, is now wrapped from fingers to axilla with an Esmarch elastic bandage to squeeze out more clot from the arm into the subclavian vein. Finally, a venous balloon catheter is passed down the arm, inflating the balloon at the valves in order to traverse them. Squeezing the arm with the elastic bandage and passing the balloon catheter are repeated until no more clot can be removed. The vein is then filled with heparinized saline and occluded with the distal plastic loop.

Proximal venous thrombectomy is performed primarily with the embolectomy forceps because the venotomy is within a few centimeters of the innominate vein and the proximal termination of the thrombus. It should be possible to pass instruments easily into the innominate vein. If the passage is small, it can be sounded gently with metal dilators (either common bile duct or arterial dilators). If the dilators will not pass, chronic intrinsic venous obstruction is probably present. It must be excised by endovenectomy or bypassed. If the proximal vein can be opened, thrombectomy is complete.

Arteriovenous Fistula (AVF)

The venotomy is closed by using it as the venous anastomosis of a temporary AVF. The arterial anastomosis lies deeper, and it will be easier to perform if it is done before the venous anastomosis. The axillary artery rather than the more proximal subclavian artery is used for the fistula to permit a little more distance between the arterial and venous anastomoses.

The axillary artery, which was dissected free earlier, has two plastic loops passed around it about 3 cm apart. Doubling the plastic vessel loops and pulling them up will both control arterial bleeding and bring the artery closer to the surface of the skin to facilitate exposure. A 6-mm externally supported PTFE graft is prepared by trimming the external support from around the graft no more than 1 cm back from the end of the graft. This will make sewing easier but will keep the external support near the anastomosis to prevent kinking. An 8-mm longitudinal arteriotomy is made and the end of the graft is sewn end-to-side to the axillary artery. The suture line is begun in the center of the posterior wall with a horizontal mattress suture of monofilament permanent suture (6–0 polypropylene) with double-ended needles. The suture is left loose, untied, as each of the two needles is run along the posterior wall and around each corner. The suture is then carefully pulled tight and the anterior suture line completed. The suture line can be tested for major leaks by injecting saline into the open end. When the leaks are repaired the vessel loops around the artery are released.

The PTFE graft is occluded with a vascular clamp just beyond the arterial anastomosis until the venous anastomosis is completed. No harm comes from clamping across the reinforced rings on the graft. Bleeding through the needle holes in the PTFE is controlled by packing the suture line with a sponge. Chemical hemostatic materials can be used but seldom are needed.

With the artery returned to its natural bed, the length of the PTFE graft is determined by making it long enough to lie in the subcutaneous tissue, within 1 cm of the skin. The graft then continues deep to the venotomy in the subclavian vein. The venous anastomosis is performed by bevelling the PTFE so it will cover the venotomy. The graft is sewn to the subclavian vein with a running monofilament permanent suture and the arterial clamp released.

If the wound is fairly dry, the heparin is not neutralized. If the wound is wet, protamine is given to neutralize the heparin. A closed suction drain is usually left in the wound for 18 to 24 hours.

AV Fistula Closure

Two to three months postoperatively, an arteriogram or duplex scan is used to determine patency of the AV fistula. If it is still open, it will be surgically closed under local anesthesia. The graft is identified in the subcutaneous tissue and divided in half. Each end is dissected free as deep as possible and the graft then suture ligated. The stumps of the PTFE will thrombose within a few hours. No attempt is made to dissect out the arteriotomy and venotomy site to remove all of the PTFE. If the fistula closed spontaneously, it is not removed.

If the patient's symptoms are greatly improved by the venous repair with the AVF functioning, current thought tends toward permitting the AVF to remain open permanently. The reason for this is to maintain the high flow through the repair to prevent late thrombosis. At the present time, there is no long term data on the results of such a permanent fistula.

Venous Bypass

The internal jugular vein is mobilized through two transverse incisions, one at the base, and the other at the apex of the neck; or through a vertical incision along the anterior border of the sternocleidomastoid muscle. The vein is ligated near the base of the skull, divided, and the caudal end mobilized down to the level of the clavicle. The vein is passed through a tunnel superficial or deep to the clavicle and sewn, end-to-side, to the axillary vein (Fig. 15-13). In our cases, we have found the plane deep to the clavicle to feel tight and have therefore, passed the graft superficial to the clavicle. If the medial half of the clavicle has been removed, the graft will sit more comfortably.

An axillary-axillary bypass can be performed by mobilizing the contralateral cephalic vein and tunnelling it across the sternum to the axillary vein distal to the occluded subclavian vein.[66] Prosthetic grafts can also be used in this position. Their diameter should be a little larger than the recipient vein.[68]

References

1. von Schrotter L. Handbuch der allgemeinen pathologie und therapie (Nothnagel). Berlin. A. Hirschwald, 1884:533. Cited by Sampson JJ. Am Heart J 1943; 25:313.

2. Hughes ESR. Venous obstruction in the upper extremity. Brit J Surg 1948; 36:155–163.

3. Paget J. Clinical lectures and essays. London, 1975.

4. Roelson E. So-called traumatic thrombosis of the axillary and subclavian veins. Acta Med Scand 1939; 98:589–622.

5. Mercier CP, Branchereau A, Dimarino V, Adhoute B, Tournigand P. Venous thrombosis of the upper limb: effort or compression. J Cardiovasc Surg (Torino) 1973; Spec. No:519–522.

6. Daskalakis E, Bouhoutsos J. Subclavian and axillary compression of musculoskeletal origin. Br J Surg 1980; 67:573–576.

7. Schubart PJ, Haeberlin JR, Porter JM. Intermittent subclavian venous obstruction: utility of venous pressure gradients. Surgery 1986; 99:365–368.

8. Perler BA, Mitchell SE. Percutaneous transluminal angioplasty and transaxillary first rib resection: a multidisciplinary approach to the thoracic outlet syndrome. Am Surgeon 1986; 52:485–488.

9. Gloviczki P, Kazmier FJ, Hollier LH. Axillary subclavian venous occlusion: the morbidity of a nonlethal disease. J Vasc Surg 1986; 4:333–337.

10. Swinton NW Jr, Edgett JW Jr, Hall RJ. Primary subclavian-axillary vein thrombosis. Circulation 1968; 38:737–745.

11. Adams JT, DeWeese JA, Mahoney EB, Rob CG. Intermittent subclavian vein obstruction without thrombosis. Surgery 1968; 63:147–165.

12. DeWeese JA, Adams JT, Gaiser DL. Subclavian venous thrombectomy. Circulation 1970; 41 and 42 (suppl II):158–164.

13. Kunkel JM, Machleder HI. Treatment of Paget-Schroetter syndrome: a staged multi-disciplinary approach. Arch Surg 1090; 124:1153–1158.

14. Taylor LM Jr, McAllister WR, Dennis DL, Porter JM. Thrombolytic therapy followed by first rib resection for spontaneous ("effort") subclavian vein thrombosis. Am J Surg 1985; 149:644–647.

15. Tilney NL, Griffiths HJG, Edwards EA. Natural history of major venous thrombosis of the upper extremity. Arch Surg 1970; 101:792–796.

16. Lowenstein PS. Thrombosis of the axillary vein: an anatomical study. JAMA 1924; 82:854–857.

17. Veal JR, McFetridge EM. Primary thrombosis of the axillary vein: an anatomic and roentgenologic study of certain etiologic factors and a consideration of venography as a diagnostic measure. Arch Surg 1935; 31:271–289.

18. Wright IS. The neurovascular syndrome produced by hyperabduction of the arms. Am Heart J 1945; 29:1–19.

19. Falconer MA, Weddell G. Costoclavicular compression of the subclavian artery and vein. Lancet 1943; 2:539–543.

20. Kobinia GS, Olbert OJ, Denck H. Chronic vascular disease of the upper extremity: radiologic and clinical features. Cardiovasc Intervent Radiol 1980; 3:25–41.

21. Schroeder WE, Green FR. Phrenic nerve injuries. report of a case. anatomical and experimental researches, and critical review of the literature. Am J Med Sci 1902; 123:196–220.

22. Hovelacque A, Monod O, Evrard H, Beuzart J. Etude anatomique du nerf phrenique pre-veineux. Ann D'Anatomie Path 1936; 13:518–522.

23. Jackson NJ, Nanson EM. Intermittent subclavian vein obstruction. Brit J Surg 1961; 49:303–306.

24. Cucci CE, Bottino CG, Ciampa V. Venous obstruction of the upper extremity caused by a malformed valve of the subclavian vein. Circulation 1963; 27:275–278.

25. Wilder JR, Haberman ET, Nach RL. Subclavian vein obstruction secondary to hypertrophy of the terminal valve. Surgery 1964; 55:214–219.

26. Ameli FM, Minas T, Weiss M, Provan JL. Consequences of "conservative" conventional management of axillary vein thrombosis. Can J Surg 1987; 30:167–169.

27. Dunant JH. Subclavian vein obstruction in thoracic outlet syndrome. Inter Angio 1984; 3:157–159.

28. DeWeese JA. Management of subclavian venous obstruction: In Bergen JJ, Yao JST (eds). Surgery of the veins; Orlando, FL: Grune & Stratton, 1985:365–382.

29. Adams JT, McEvoy RK, DeWeese JA. Primary deep venous thrombosis of upper extremity. Arch Surg 1965; 91:29–42.

30. Drapanas T, Curran WL. Thrombectomy in the treatment of "effort" thrombosis of the axillary and subclavian veins. J Trauma 1966; 6:107–119.

31. Dalal AR, Pitney WR. Primary thrombosis of the axillary-subclavian veins. Med J Aust 1972; 1:633–634.

32. Prescott SM, Tikaff G. Deep venous thrombosis of the upper extremity: a reappraisal. Circulation 1979; 59:350–355.

33. Campbell CB, Chandler JG, Tegtmeyer CJ, Bernstein EF. Axillary, subclavian, and brachiocephalic vein obstruction. Surgery 1977; 82:816–826.

34. Brochner G, Rojas M, Armas AJ, Silva Pereira JA, Mayall RC, Mayall ACDG, Mayall JC. Axillary-subclavian venous thrombosis. J Cardiovasc Surg 1989; 30:108–111.

35. Becker GJ, Holden RW, Rabe FE, Castaneda-Zuniga WR, Sears N, Dilley RS, Glover JL. Local thrombolytic therapy for subclavian and axillary vein thrombosis. Radiology 1983; 149:419–423.

36. Druy EM, Trout HH, Giordano JM, Hix WR. Lytic therapy in the treatment of axillary and subclavian vein thrombosis. J Vasc Surg 1985; 2:821–827.

37. Vogel CM, Jensen JE. "Effort" thrombosis of the subclavian vein in a competitive swimmer. Am J Sports Med 1985; 13:269–272.

38. Smith-Behn J, Althar R, Katz W. Primary thrombosis of the axillary/subclavian vein. South Med J 1986; 79:1176–1178.

39. Steed DL, Teodori MF, Peitzman AB, McAuley CE, Kapoor WN, Webster MW. Streptokinase in the treatment of subclavian vein thrombosis. J Vasc Surg 1986; 4:28–32.

40. Huey H, Morris DC, Nichols DM, Connell DG, Fry PD. Low-dose streptokinase thrombolysis of axillary-subclavian vein thrombosis. Cardiovasc Intervent Radiol 1987; 10:92–95.

41. Landercasper J, Gall W, Fischer M, Boyd WC, Dahlberg PJ, Kisken WA, Boland T. Thrombolytic therapy of axillary-subclavian venous thrombosis. Arch Surg 1987; 122:1072–1075.

42. O'Leary MR, Smith MS, Druy EM. Diagnostic and therapeutic approach to axillary-subclavian vein thrombosis. Ann Emer Med 1987; 16:889–893.

43. Shuttleworth RD, Van der Merve DM, Mitchell WL. Subclavian vein stenosis and axillary vein "effort thrombosis": age and the first rib bypass collateral, thrombolytic therapy and first rib resection. S Afr Med J 1987; 71:564–566.

44. Wiles PG, Birtwell JA, Davies JA, Chennells P. Subclavian vein notch: a phlebographic abnormality associated with subclavian-axillary vein thrombosis. Brit J Hosp Med 1987; 37:349–350.

45. Rauwerda JA, Bakker FC, van der Broek TAA, Dwars BJ. Spontaneous subclavian vein thrombosis: a successful combined approach of local thrombolytic therapy followed by first rib resection. Surgery 1988; 103:477–480.

46. Wilson JJ, Zahn CA, Newman H. Fibrinolytic therapy for idiopathic subclavian-axillary vein thrombosis. Am J Med 1990; 159:208–211.

47. Dale WA. Discussion of Adams JT, DeWeese JA, Mahoney EB, Rob CG: Intermittent subclavian vein obstruction without thrombosis. Surgery 1968; 63:163.

48. Gaylis H. A rational approach to venous thrombectomy. Surg Gynecol Obstet 1974; 138:864–868.

49. Horattas MC, Wright DJ, Fenton AH, Evans DM, Oddi MA, Kamienski RW, Shields EF. Changing concepts of deep venous thrombosis of the upper extremity—report of a series and review of the literature. Surgery 1988; 104:561–567.

50. Etheredge S, Wilbur B, Stoney RJ. Thoracic outlet syndrome. Am J Surg 1979; 138:175–182.

51. Siegel RS, Steichen FM. Cervicothoracic outlet syndrome: vascular compression caused by congenital abnormality of thoracic ribs. J Bone Joint Surg 1967; 49A:1187–1192.

52. Charrette EJP, Iyengar KSR, Lynn RB, Challis TW. Symptomatic non-thrombotic subclavian vein obstruction: surgical relief in six patients. Vasc Surg 1973; 7:220–231.

53. Glass BA. The relationship of axillary venous thrombosis to the thoracic outlet compression syndrome. Ann Thorac Surg 1975; 19:613–621.

54. Pittam MR, Drake SG. The place of first rib resection in the management of axillary-subclavian vein thrombosis. Eur J Vasc Surg 1987; 1:5–10.

55. Salo JA, Varstela E, Ketonen P, Ala-Kulja K, Luosto R. Management of vascular complications in thoracic outlet syndrome. Acta Chir Scand 1988; 154:349–352.

56. Rabinowitz R, Goldfarb D. Surgical treatment of axillosubclavian venous thrombosis: a case report. Surgery 1971; 70:703–706.

57. Lord JW Jr, Urschel HC Jr. Total claviculectomy. Surgical Rounds 1988; December:17–27.

58. Pairolero PC, Walls JT, Payne WS, Hollier LH, Fairbairn JF. Subclavian-axillary artery aneurysms. Surgery 1981; 90:757–763.

59. McLaughlin CW Jr, Popma AM. Intermittent obstruction of the subclavian vein. JAMA 1939; 113:1960–1963.

60. McCleery RS, Kesterson JE, Kirtley JA, Love RB. Subclavius and anterior scalene muscle compression as a cause of intermittent obstruction of the subclavian vein. Ann Surg 1951; 133:588–602.

61. Campbell CB, Chandler JG, Tegtmeyer CJ, Bernstein EF. Axillary, subclavian, and brachiocephalic vein obstruction. Surgery 1977; 82:816–826.

62. Jacobson JH, Haimov M. Venous revascularization of the arm: report of three cases. Surgery 1977; 81:599–604.

63. Aziz S, Straehley CJ, Whelan TJ Jr. Effort-related axillosubclavian vein thrombosis: a new theory of pathogenesis and a plea for direct surgical intervention. Am J Surg 1986; 152:57–61.

64. Witte CL, Smith CA. Single anastomosis vein bypass for subclavian vein obstruction. Arch Surg 1966; 93:664–666.

65. Inahara T. Surgical treatment of "effort" thrombosis of the axillary and subclavian veins. Amer Surgeon 1968; 34:479–483.

66. Hashmonai M, Schramek A, Farbstein J. Cephalic vein cross-over bypass for subclavian vein thrombosis: a case report. Surgery 1976; 80:563–564.

67. Jain KM, Smejkal R. Use of spiral vein graft to bypass occluded subclavian vein. J Cardiovasc Surg 1988; 29:572–573.

68. Lalka SG, Cosentino C, Malone JM, Reinert RL, Bernhard VM. Hemodynamics of revascularization for iliofemoral venous occlusion: a short-term canine model. J Vasc Surg 1988; 8:592–599.

69. Doty DB, Baker W. Bypass of superior vena cava with spiral vein graft. Ann Thorac Surg 1976; 22:490–493.

70. Johnson V, Eiseman B. Evaluation of arteriovenous shunt to maintain patency of venous autograft. Am J Surg 1969; 118:915–920.

71. Sanders RJ, Rosales C, Pearce WH. Creation and closure of temporary arteriovenous fistulas for venous reconstruction or thrombectomy: description of technique. J Vasc Surg 1987; 6:504–505.

72. Sanders RJ, Haug CE. Subclavian vein obstruction and thoracic outlet syndrome: a review of etiology and management. Ann Vasc Surg 1990; 4:397–410.

16
A Current Look at TOS—An Overview

Richard J. Sanders
Craig E. Haug

In the other chapters of this book, an attempt is made to present data on all aspects of thoracic outlet syndrome (TOS). In this chapter, the authors present their own views based upon this data and over 25 years of experience in managing patients with TOS. During this time, our results have periodically been reviewed and our approach, from initial history to surgical therapy, has been modified several times. The opinions being voiced today can likewise be expected to change as further studies and new data are added to our medical knowledge.

Vascular TOS

There is general agreement that patients with arterial or venous compression in the thoracic outlet area have an easily diagnosed condition requiring treatment. The options available for treating subclavian artery compression are relatively few, and sufficient cases have been reported to provide a reasonable and established protocol for the management of arterial complications in TOS patients. The repair or replacement of diseased arteries, accompanied by the removal of abnormal cervical and first ribs, has become the standard of care for these lesions.

On the other hand, there are several treatment modalities available for subclavian vein obstruction. As yet, none is clearly superior. Acute venous thrombosis can be treated with anticoagulants, thrombolytic agents, or thrombectomy; subacute, chronic, and partial venous obstruction can be managed by balloon dilation, extrinsic decompression (first rib resection, division of the subclavius muscle and costoclavicular ligament), or venous reconstruction by endovenectomy or venous bypass. The experiences with these various modalities are too sparse and the follow-ups too short to draw firm conclusions as to which of these procedures should be chosen in any given situation.

Neurogenic TOS

Neurogenic TOS With Objective Findings

When accompanied by objective neurologic findings, bony abnormalities, or typical neuroelectric diagnostic abnormalities, the diagnosis of neurogenic TOS is readily accepted. Unfortunately, once patients have reached this state, muscular atrophy and extremity weakness is seldom reversible.

Adson Maneuver

Obliteration of the radial pulse by certain positional maneuvers, as advocated in 1927 by Adson, was at one time thought to be the most reliable objective test for making a diagnosis of TOS. This test is the reason why TOS was thought to be a vascular compression disease and why it falls within the scope of the vascular surgeon. However, the Adson maneuver, and other positional maneuvers to demonstrate pulse obliteration, are positive in almost as many normal people as in those with TOS; they are no longer regarded as reliable tests for establishing a diagnosis of

TOS. Nevertheless, a positional pulse obliteration may be indicative of an anatomical predisposition to develop TOS symptoms following neck injuries.

Neurogenic TOS Without Objective Findings

The diagnosis of neurogenic thoracic outlet syndrome in the absence of positive objective tests is the controversial area of TOS and comprises more than 90% of the patients carrying this diagnosis today. While some physicians question the existence of this entity, more are learning how to recognize it.

A large number of physicians, from the United States as well as other countries, have published early success rates of 80–90% in large series of surgical TOS patients. The early success rate is a measure of diagnostic accuracy; the fact that this success rate deteriorates with time reflects the inadequacy of any surgical treatment for nerve compression conditions (see Table 1–1). Most TOS patients have no positive objective findings. The question to be asked is not "Does neurogenic TOS without objective findings exist?" but rather 1) "What are the criteria for establishing a diagnosis?" and 2) "What are the indications for surgery?"

Diagnostic Criteria

An overview of the management of TOS is presented in Figure 16-1. Suspicion of TOS is often raised when patients have paresthesia in their hand that cannot easily be explained. The diagnosis of neurogenic TOS is based primarily

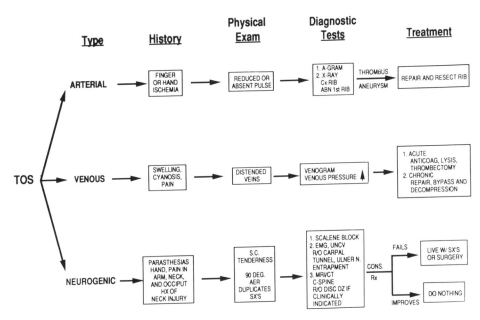

Fig. 16-1.   Algorithm of the management of TOS. The presenting history and symptoms, physical examination, and diagnostic tests are different for each of the three types. Treatment depends upon the nature and intensity of symptoms.

upon a clinical picture that usually includes a history of neck trauma; symptoms of numbness and tingling in the arm, hand, or fingers; pain in the arm, shoulder, and neck; occipital headaches; and aggravation of symptoms with the arms elevated. The most common physical findings are supraclavicular tenderness over the scalene muscles and duplication of symptoms with the arms abducted to 90 degrees in external rotation. Several other signs and symptoms are present in some patients, but the ones just mentioned are the most common. Relief of symptoms with a scalene muscle block is a helpful diagnostic tool. Although none of the symptoms and physical findings is specific for TOS, the combination of several of these criteria in one patient has proved fairly reliable for making a diagnosis of TOS.

Diagnoses that are important to rule out include cervical discs, cervical arthritis, carpal tunnel syndrome, ulnar nerve entrapment, biceps/rotator cuff tendinitis, and cervical radiculopathy. At times, these conditions are to be differentiated from TOS, but at other times, they coexist with TOS (the "double-crush syndrome"). This makes the establishment of a diagnosis with certainty almost impossible. Thus, the diagnosis of TOS is clinical and tenuous.

Indications for Surgery

Surgery is a last resort; conservative treatment should be tried first. Whether conservative therapy is treating TOS or some of the associated conditions is difficult to determine. If the symptoms improve, the diagnosis will never be known with certainty.

If symptoms do not improve with several months of conservative management, the patient regards the symptoms as disabling, and all other treatable conditions have been adequately excluded, the patient must either live with the symptoms or undergo surgery. While surgery is not an ideal solution, if there is persistent nerve compression, surgery is the only alternative. Although the failure rate of surgery is significant, when failure occurs patients are seldom made worse; the incidence of permanent nerve injuries is under 1%.

Choice of Operation

Scalenectomy vs. First Rib Resection

There is no evidence to support the view that first rib resection is needed in all cases of TOS. Data available indicate that in the absence of an osseous abnormality, anterior and middle scalenectomy has the same success rate as first rib resection. This is true for both upper and lower plexus symptoms.

Middle Scalenectomy

Whenever anterior scalenectomy is performed, middle scalenectomy should accompany it. While there is no data to support this, anatomical studies of the scalene triangle reveal that many ligaments and bands lie in the belly of the middle scalene and that the middle scalene muscle encircles and may easily press against C-7 and C-8. For these reasons, routine middle scalenectomy seems reasonable.

Complications

First rib resection, regardless of the route, carries a risk of plexus injury. Although low—in the 1% range for permanent injury—it is a risk that cannot be overlooked and cannot always be averted because of the need sometimes to retract the plexus to avoid injuring it. Most plexus injuries have been temporary, but occasionally they have been permanent. In comparison, plexus injuries are rare with scalenectomy.

First Rib Resection

When first rib resection is indicated, there are several effective routes. An experienced surgeon should have in his armamentarium several choices in order to select the most appropriate one for each situation. Reoperations are often best performed through an approach different from the one that was used the first time. We started our experience with the transaxillary approach but now prefer the supraclavicular route because it permits complete scalenectomy with or without rib resection, as the situation requires. An infraclavicular incision is added if better exposure of the anterior part of the rib is needed.

Pathophysiology

Traumatic TOS

In the large majority of patients, the onset of TOS symptoms follows a neck injury and is accompanied by head and neck complaints as well as extremity symptoms. It is easy to explain the symptoms of TOS as the result of scalene muscle injury followed by scarring, tightening or spasm of the scalenes, and subsequent compression of the plexus. This is the basis for scalenectomy as appropriate treatment. It is more difficult to understand how a hyperextension neck injury, in the absence of a fracture of the first rib or clavicle, could cause narrowing of the costoclavicular space, which would be the rationale for first rib resection. In most cases, rib resection is successful not because the rib is out, but because the anterior and middle scalene muscles were cut in order to remove the rib.

Supporting the hypothesis that scalene muscle injury is the cause of TOS are histologic studies showing increased connective tissue in the scalenes of most TOS patients. Although type I and type II fiber changes have also been observed in these patients, the significance of these findings awaits further studies to determine the histology of normal scalene muscle. An additional supporting fact is that in our experience the success rate following scalenectomy alone has not been improved by adding first rib resection at the same operation.

Nontraumatic TOS

In a minority of TOS patients there is no history of neck trauma immediately preceding the onset of their symptoms. In these cases, there may be a variety of different causes of neurovascular compression. Cervical ribs, abnormal first ribs, and healed fractures of the clavicle or first rib are each capable of narrowing the anatomical tunnel through which the nerves and vessels pass to the arm; these can easily be diagnosed by x-ray.

The congenital bands and ligaments described by Roos cannot be detected without surgery, and even in the operating room they are difficult to identify. These structures often lie within the belly of the anterior and middle scalene muscles and are hard to differentiate from the normal tendinous transformation that frequently occurs within a muscle. In almost all of the scalenectomies we have performed, we have observed thick bands within the anterior and middle scalene muscles that look like thin strips of tendon. We have been reticent to label these "congenital bands or ligaments" since they are present in almost every patient. Congenital bands and ligaments may be the etiology of some cases of TOS although it is difficult to determine how often.

Anatomical Predisposition To Develop TOS

The reason some patients develop TOS following neck injuries and others do not is unknown. However, anatomical predisposition could be a factor. Observations of the scalene triangle in cadavers and in TOS patients reveal wide variations in the normal relationships of the brachial plexus and the scalene muscles. For example, the nerves of the brachial plexus emerged high in the apex of the scalene triangle in 83% of TOS patients compared with only 40% of cadaver controls. This suggests that patients who develop TOS are those in whom the nerves exit from the narrow portion of the scalene triangle; this, in turn, permits the muscle fibrosis that accompanies neck injuries to increase the pressure against the nerves and produce symptoms. The narrow triangle can be regarded as a predisposing factor for TOS, and structures such as cervical ribs or congenital ligaments and bands may contribute to this predisposition.

Results of Surgery

In general, during the first few weeks following TOS surgery about 90% of patients notice significant improvement. This improvement rate falls in the first two years to about 75%. Beyond this time, recurrences are still seen, but they are infrequent. After two years, almost half of the recurrences are the result of another neck injury.

The definition of improvement is relief of symptoms. Most patients experience disappearance of paresthesia and significant reductions in intensity of head, neck, and arm pain. However, there are often minor symptoms remaining with which the patient can easily live. Only a minority of patients are truly asymptomatic.

Included in the success rate are 5–10% who have "fair" improvement. In these cases, the operation relieved enough symptoms to have made surgery worthwhile, but the patient continues to have several complaints. Often, they are the result of associated injuries in areas outside of the thoracic outlet such as the shoulder girdle or cervical spine.

Variables

General observations suggest that patients whose symptoms follow neck injuries from automobile accidents have a higher success rate following TOS surgery than patients whose symptoms develop following work-related injuries. Some people have a predisposition to develop neck, shoulder, arm, and hand symptoms from certain types of occupations requiring extensive use of their upper extremities. While the nature of this problem has yet to be defined, it has been observed in the workplace in cities around the world. Future investigative work will hopefully clarify this condition and how it relates to TOS. The presence of pending litigation has little influence on the results of treatment in most patients with TOS.

Staging the Operative Treatment

The results of performing both scalenectomy and first rib resection at the time of the primary operation have not been better than the results of each of these procedures alone. By performing these operations in two stages, the secondary success of either rib resection followed by scalenectomy or scalenectomy followed by rib resection yielded about 15% higher success rates than combining the two procedures in one operation (statistically significant, $P < 0.01$).

Therefore, a reasonable plan of treatment when surgery is indicated for neurogenic TOS (as differentiated from arterial or venous TOS) is to perform only one of these procedures at a time. The second procedure is reserved for recurrence. Our preference is to perform anterior and middle scalenectomy as the first procedure because its complications are fewer and the postoperative recovery is smoother and faster as compared to rib resection (through any route). If there is recurrence or persistence of hand symptoms, either transaxillary or supraclavicular rib resection is offered.

The primary advantage of performing the combined operation is that if there is no immediate improvement from surgery, the diagnosis is incorrect and no further surgery need be considered. It is our practice to discuss the advantages and disadvantages of these surgical options with the patients and permit them to share in choosing the procedure.

17
Medico-Legal Matters

Richard J. Sanders
Roger F. Johnson

Influence of Pending Litigation on Results of Treatment

The Doctor Who Treats Patients With Pending Litigation

The Doctor in Court

Influence of Pending Litigation on Results of Treatment

Should a patient be operated upon while a law suit is pending? This is a question frequently raised when patients with TOS do not improve on conservative therapy. Three studies have been found that address this point.

Woods, in 1965, followed 116 patients who were operated upon for traumatic TOS and had unsettled lawsuits at the time of surgery.[1] Eighty percent had improvement in headaches and 73% had relief of neck pains, which were the same rates as in his TOS patients without lawsuits. Woods points out that malingerers would be unlikely to have such a high success rate much less submit to surgery. In addition, patients whose primary goal was to collect a large monetary award would be unlikely to admit symptomatic improvement before the settlement.

Parisien, in 1975, studied 105 patients with neck injuries who were treated conservatively and were followed for a minimum of three months.[2] Forty-four of the patients in this study had litigation pending and a small number had industrial accidents. He found that the improvement rate in those with pending litigation was similar to that of those with no ongoing litigation, but the failure rate was higher among the eight patients with industrial accidents than in those with auto accidents.

A third study, performed by Youmans in 1980, included over 100 patients who received transaxillary first rib resection for traumatic TOS.[3] Two-thirds of those TOS cases followed auto accidents and the other one-third were job-related traumatic TOS, all with attorneys. The good-to-excellent results in the automobile accident groups were similar—82% among 35 patients with attorneys and 79% among 34 patients without attorneys. However, fair improvement was noted by 18% and failure by only 3% of those with no pending litigation compared to no partial improvement and 18% failures among those with attorneys. Industrial-related TOS in 34 patients had poorer results—only 48% with good to excellent relief, 37% with fair improvement, and 14% failures.

It can be concluded from these three studies that when TOS develops following an automobile accident, the results of treatment are not significantly affected by the status of pending litigation. However, although the numbers are small, the findings of Parisien and Youmans, as well as our data as noted in Chapter 12, suggest that patients whose symptoms develop at work do not have as much improvement as patients who develop symptoms following automobile accidents. The differences in our data were not statistically significant, but that could be a function of our small number of cases.

Settling a Claim Before Surgery

Patients sometimes ask if they should settle their claim before having surgery. In cases where surgery is a possibility, it is best to delay settlement. If there is pressure to settle the case before a decision is made regarding surgery, the patient should ask the insurance carrier to cover all future medical costs as a part of the settlement package. In this way, the insurance carrier will not have to be concerned about granting an award to be used for an operation the patient decides not to undergo after the settlement is complete. The patient will not have to be concerned about receiving enough money to cover the full costs of surgery and the potential complications.

The Doctor Who Treats Patients With Pending Litigation

Because the majority of patients with TOS today had the onset of their symptoms following an accident or injury, most commonly an auto accident or work-related injury, the physician will be requested by insurance carriers or attorneys to provide medical reports and sometimes to testify at hearings, depositions, or in court. A number of patients will already have retained an attorney to assist them in recovering damages for their injuries. Many of those who do not have an attorney when first seen will be finding one in the future. While this should not affect the way medicine is practiced, physicians should be aware of some of the ways these cases differ from other medical cases that have no medico-legal involvement.

Causation

Perhaps the most important question the physician is asked is the cause of the patient's present symptoms. The insurance carrier that is paying the patient's medical expenses will ask the doctor if the accident in question was the etiology. Frequently, a letter from the physician stating that the accident was the cause will result in settling the patient's claim, and the matter is concluded.

However, if the insurance carrier for any reason has questions regarding a case, it may hire attorneys and investigators to look further into the patient's claim. The doctor may be asked for more information by letter or may be subpoenaed to testify. Although giving testimony under oath regarding a patient should not be difficult for a physician, it helps to know what type of questions to expect and to have good office notes from which to refresh one's memory.

Low Impact Accidents

An insurance carrier may question the relationship of the severity of an injury to a low speed, minimal damage, motor vehicle accident. It is hard for lay people to see how minor accidents can produce injuries that eventually lead to major surgery. In such cases, it is the role of the physician to explain that TOS can be caused by a whiplash type injury that is produced by a quick hyperextension action of the neck and that these events frequently occur at low speeds. Medically, this statement is true. However, its acceptance by an insurance company, an attorney, or a jury may depend upon the credibility established by the physician.

Thorough History To Assess Cause

It is certainly standard practice to take a complete history from all patients. In TOS patients, it is particularly important to find out about all previous accidents and injuries the patient has experienced. When there have been previous accidents, notes should be made as to whether or not symptoms developed in the head, neck, or upper extremities; how long they persisted; whether or not the patient saw a doctor; the type of treatment that was administered; and over how long a period of time the treatment was given.

While obtaining this information may or may not be helpful in treating the patient for this illness, documenting previous injuries can become very important in a legal case when the physician is asked if the current accident was the cause of the patient's present problems. If the patient has been involved in previous accidents that had resulted in symptoms similar to the ones now being treated, the question will arise as to which accident the present symptoms should be attributed. There are three possible scenarios:

1. The patient had symptoms from a previous accident and those symptoms persist, *unchanged,* since the current accident. In this situation, the most recent accident is probably not the cause of the patient's present condition and the party responsible for the recent accident will most likely be relieved of liability.

2. The patient did have symptoms from a previous accident, but those symptoms were completely gone when the recent accident occurred. In this case, a question that helps to document the absence of symptoms prior to the recent accident is to ask if the patient was under medical care for the previous symptoms at the time of the recent accident. If there were no symptoms prior to the present accident, the patient's present symptoms can be attributed to the most recent accident.

3. The patient did have symptoms from a previous accident that had partially improved until the recent accident occurred. Since then, the patient's symptoms have gotten worse. In this scenario, the recent accident will be regarded as having aggravated a preexisting condition. The law may regard an accident that aggravates a preexisting condition and produces disability in the same way as if it had caused all the disability. Depending upon how symptomatic the patient was before and after the most recent accident, this accident could be regarded as the sole cause of the present symptoms, or it could be regarded as a partial cause and the liability apportioned between the two accidents.

Apportionment for More Than one Accident

Patients who have been involved in more than one accident frequently have more than one insurance carrier involved in paying for their medical care. In these cases, the physician is often asked to apportion the patient's present condition between the accidents so that each insurance carrier can pay its share. Objectively, there is no test that will assist in making this type of determination. We have handled this situation by asking the patient to estimate the percentage of his current discomfort that was present after the first accident. The remaining percentage is attributed to the second accident. When giving this apportionment to the insurance carrier, it may be helpful to state that the apportionment is based upon the patient's assessment of the intensity of symptoms after each incident.

Attorneys will ask the treating physician for his opinion as to the cause of the patient's symptoms. If the physician does not know about previous accidents the patient has sustained, a very embarrassing moment can occur during cross-examination when an attorney asks if the physician knew about a previous accident the patient had encountered. Although the patient may have been asymptomatic prior to the recent accident and a previous accident is of no significance to the matter at hand, an attorney can take advantage of failure to obtain all the facts in a history to discredit a doctor in the eyes of a jury.

Questionnaire

One way of being sure the patient is asked about previous accidents is to have the patient fill in a questionnaire in the doctors waiting room that contains all of the questions that should be asked (see Chapter 6, Fig. 6-2). Among the questions is a request to list all previous accidents and dates. When the doctor interviews the patient, this form is reviewed by the doctor with the patient and it is quite simple for the doctor to fill in the details of any injuries in the patient's chart. Should the patient forget to tell the doctor about previous injuries, the doctor can pull out the patient's questionnaire from the chart, while on the witness stand, so the jury can see that the patient was asked that question. This preserves the doctor's credibility before the jury—an important concern. The doctor can then continue to give opinions that will be respected based upon the new information regarding previous injuries. The doctor will also have an opportunity to tell the jury that it is a human error for patients to sometimes forget remote events that occurred some time ago, particularly when symptoms have long since disappeared.

The Doctor in Court

Many books and articles have been written to help doctors prepare to be witnesses. This information will not be duplicated here except to comment on a few personal observations about simple things that the authors have found particularly helpful.

Preparation for Testimony at Trial or Deposition

A well prepared attorney will review with the doctor the questions that will be asked so that the doctor can read the patient's records and have the details fresh in mind. If the attorney does not schedule a pretestimony conference, the doctor should feel free to request such a meeting in order to be better prepared for his appearance. By doing so, there should be no surprises or embarrassments and the doctor will be a better witness.

Type of Witness

In court, the doctor may be either a fact witness, an expert witness, or both. In giving evidence, the doctor may be asked to relate what the patient told the doctor, what the physical examination revealed, and what the results were of the x-rays and laboratory tests. When giving the facts that were observed and recorded the doctor is giving factual evidence.

When asked the significance of the examination and what the findings indicate, the doctor is being asked for an opinion. This requires a level of expertise in the field of medicine, and it is necessary for the doctor to be qualified as an expert witness before he can give the opinion. This is a legal matter which the attorney calling the doctor to court should discuss with the doctor prior to the court appearance. The doctor's qualifications to be an expert witness should be reviewed.

Address the Jury

In court it is the jury that will make the decision and the doctor should talk to the jury, try to establish eye contact with each juror at least once, and use as few medical terms as possible. *Lay terminology is a MUST.*

Video Deposition

When giving a video deposition that will be used in court in place of the doctor's live appearance, there is no live jury to address. However, the doctor should talk to and face the lens of the camera most of the time. When the video is shown in court, the doctor looks better if he or she is talking directly to the audience rather than looking to the side.

Correcting Records

When adding information or correcting information in medical records or office notes, the date the changes are made should be written on the record at the time. There is nothing wrong with correcting records, but failing to note that the changes are later corrections made to original records could cause someone to think that the doctor tried to alter the records after the fact. This can prove embarrassing if copies of the medical records happen to have been made prior to the time the corrections were made. However, if the corrections are dated, that dating should permit the physician to give the reason for the correction when testifying.

Repeat or Restate the Question

Attorneys can ask long, complicated, and at times unintelligible questions. When a question is unclear, is compound, or could not be followed, ask the questioner to restate or repeat it. If the doctor is distracted or for some other reason has lost part of a question, or if the doctor wants more time to consider the question, asking to have the question read back or restated can help.

Think Before Answering

Even when ready with an answer, it is a good idea to pause a moment before speaking. Pausing provides an opportunity to be sure the response is appropriate and gives the impression to the jury that the doctor has thoughtfully considered his testimony.

"I Don't Know"

There can be many reasons for answering "I don't know," the most frequent being that the doctor really does not know the answer. Doctors are not expected to be able to answer every question and should not be embarrassed to admit it.

Probability vs. Possibility

A common term heard in medical questions is "to a reasonable degree of medical certainty" or "medical probability." Since few things are 100% certain in the field of medicine, doctors are asked to state their opinions in terms of "degrees of medical probability." This means that the opinion is more likely true than not true, or that there is a greater than 50% probability that the opinion is true. When the doctor is asked by an attorney the cause of a patient's condition, it is realized that the doctor cannot be absolutely certain. The court recognizes this and asks the doctor to give the most likely cause or the most probable cause.

A possibility in this context is something that is less than 50% likely. While there may be many possibilities in each case, there can be only one probability. If in the doctor's opinion there are several possibilities but no probabilities, the doctor should so state. A possibility may be considered to be speculation and excluded from testimony by the court (the judge).

Ask for Continuance

Some court appearances can last for hours and the doctor becomes fatigued and may stop thinking clearly. Under those circumstances, requesting a recess or rescheduling the remainder of the testimony is appropriate.

References

1. Woods WW. Personal experiences with surgical treatment of 250 cases of cervico-brachial neurovascular compression syndrome. J Int Coll Surg 1965; 44:273–283.
2. Paresien VM. The "cervical syndrome." J Maine Med Assoc 1976; 67:66–68.
3. Youmans CR Jr, Smiley RH. Thoracic outlet syndrome with negative Adson's and hyperabduction maneuvers. Vasc Surg 1980; 14:318–329.

Annotated Bibliography

This bibliography represents an extensive search of the medical literature for all articles related to thoracic outlet syndrome (TOS). Only a few articles on this subject have been omitted, primarily because they were reviews of small numbers of cases that did not add significantly to our knowledge. Information within the earlier individual references is as complete as practicable.

The articles are listed chronologically so that readers can easily find the more recent references. Articles on a particular aspect of TOS may be easier to find at the end of the chapter in this book on that subject; a synopsis of those articles can then be found in this bibliography because all chapter references are included here. Within each year, the articles are listed alphabetically.

Bibliography—Thoracic Outlet Syndrome

1740   Hunauld. Sur le nombre des cotes, moindre ou plus grand qu a l'ordinaire. Histoire Acadamie Royale de Sciences de Paris, 1740.

1821   Cooper A. On exostosis. In Cooper, Cooper, and Travers. Surgical Essays, 3rd Ed. London: 1821; 128.

       First recorded description of the symptoms of vascular compression from a cervical rib.

1831   Mayo. Exostosis of the first rib, with strong pulsation of the subclavian artery. London Med Phys J 1831; 11:40.

       Case report of a man with a pulsating neck tumor and a bony prominence thought to be an exostosis of the first rib. The artery was occluded below the mass. No treatment was offered. Just of historical interest.

1860   Willshire. Lancet 1860; 2:633.

       Case report of a woman with a supraclavicular pulsation thought to be due to a cervical rib. The woman was not treated.

1861   Coote H. Exostosis of the left transverse process of the seventh cervical vertebra, surrounded by blood vessels and nerves; successful removal. Lancet 1861; 1:360–361.

       First case report of cervical rib resection in a case of arterial TOS performed under chloroform anesthesia. Postoperatively, the patient's absent wrist pulse returned.

1869   Gruber W. Ueber die halsrippen des menschen mit vergleichend-anatomischen. Bemerkungen, St. Petersburg, 1869.

       Anatomical classification of cervical ribs into four types. In German.

1875   Paget J. Clinical lectures and essays. London, 1875.

       First description of axillary vein thrombosis.

1884   von Schrotter L. Handbuch der allgemeinen pathologie und therapie (Nothnagel). Berlin. A. Hirschwald, 1884: 533. Cited by Sampson JJ. Am Heart J 1943; 25:313.

Second description of axillary vein thrombosis.

1901   Kammerer F. Cervical ribs. Ann Surg 1901; 34:637–648.

Good review of cervical ribs and one case report involving arterial TOS.

1902   Schroeder WE, Green FR. Phrenic nerve injuries; report of a case. Anatomical and experimental researches, and critical review of the literature. Am J Med Sci 1902; 123:196–220.

In 100 anatomical studies of the origin of the phrenic nerve, C-4 was a source of origin in 100%. The phrenic arose in 25% from C-4 alone; in 37% from C-4 and C-5; in 23% from C-3, C-4, and C-5; and in 15% from C-3 and C-4. In 51 dissections, a pre-venous, or anterior-lying phrenic nerve was noted on the right side three times: twice anterior to the vein and once running through the vein.

1903   Bramwell E. Lesion of the first dorsal nerve root. Rev Neurol Psychiat 1903; 1:236–239.

1905   Murphy JB. A case of cervical rib with symptoms resembling subclavian aneurysm. Ann Surg 1905; 41:399–406.

Case report of cervical rib resection followed by reduction in diameter of dilated subclavian artery. The significance of cervical ribs and the anterior scalene muscle is discussed.

1906   Murphy JB. The clinical significance of cervical ribs: Surg Gynecol Obstet 1906; 3:515–520.

Embryology, anatomy, classification, and diagnosis of cervical ribs are reviewed. The symptoms may be vascular or nervous. Technique of surgical excision of the rib is described.

1907   Howell CMH, Oxon MB. A consideration of some symptoms which may be produced by seventh ribs. Lancet 1907; 1702–1707.

Report of 16 cases of cervical ribs, 14 in women; 70% bilateral. Symptoms and management of each case is detailed.

1907   Keen WW. The symptomatology, diagnosis, and surgical treatment of cervical ribs. Am J Med Sci 1907; 133:173–218.

Review of 42 operated cases of cervical ribs from literature. Neurological symptoms were present in two-thirds; vascular symptoms in less than one-half. Ten patients had subclavian artery aneurysms; Trauma brought on symptoms in some cases. Surgical incisions and technique are described.

1907   Russel CK. Supernumerary cervical ribs and their effects on the brachial plexus and subclavian artery. Med Rec 1907; 71:253–258.

Three case reports of patients with cervical ribs; one underwent rib excision with improvement. Extensive discussion of state of knowledge of neurologic and vascular symptoms and complications of cervical ribs.

1908   Thorburn W. The symptoms due to cervical ribs. Dreschfeld Memorial 1908; 85–111.

Report of nine cases of cervical rib; six were operated upon, five improved. Complications included nerve damage at surgery. Rudimentary first rib was questioned in one case. Extensive discussion of all aspects of cervical ribs.

1910   Murphy T. Brachial neuritis caused by pressure of first rib. Aust Med J 1910; 15:582–585.

First case report of excision of normal first rib for TOS symptoms with excellent result at three months.

1912   Todd TW. Costal anomalies of the thoracic inlet, their interpretation and significance. Anat Anz 1912; 41:257–271.

1912   Todd TW. The descent of the shoulder after birth: its significance in the production of pressure-symptoms on the lowest brachial trunk. Anat Anz 1912; 41:385–397.

Theory to explain cervical rib symptoms in the absence of a cervical rib: Brachial plexus is stretched over a normal first rib due to the descent of the clavicle in infancy.

1913   Jones FW. Discussion on cervical ribs: the anatomy of cervical ribs. Proc R Soc Med 1913; 6:95–112.

A theory is presented explaining cervical ribs. In fetal life, ribs from cervical vertebrae are normally blocked early in their development by larger developing nerves. The nerves are positioned by descent of the upper limb bud. If a nerve fails to block the rib, a cervical rib results, most often at C-7.

1913   Morley J. Brachial pressure neuritis due to a normal first thoracic rib: its diagnosis and treatment by excision of rib. Clin J 1913; 42:461–464.

Case report of normal first rib resection resulting in relief of symptoms of brachial plexus compression.

1913   Sargent P. Some points in the surgery of cervical ribs. Proc R Soc Med 1913; 6: Pt 1, 117–126.

Report of 34 operations for cervical ribs. With short ribs, just dividing the band relieved symptoms.

1916   Halsted WH. An experimental study of circumscribed dilation of an artery immediately distal to a partially occluded band, and its bearing on the dilation of the subclavian artery observed in certain cases of cervical rib. J Exp Med 1916; 24:271–286.

Review of 716 cases of cervical rib from the medical literature revealed at least 27 subclavian aneurysms. In dogs, by constricting the aorta with a band, aneurysms were produced distal to the band. Halsted carefully recorded his observations of poststenotic dilatation and presented his theory of increased turbulence and distal diastolic pressure as the cause. Dr. Montgomery Reid worked with Dr. Halsted on this study.

1916   Murphy JB. Cervical rib excision: collective review on surgery of cervical rib. Clin John B Murphy 1916; 5:227–240.

Summary of a collective review of 112 articles on cervical ribs.

1919   Stopford JS, Telford ED. Compression of the lower trunk of the brachial plexus by a first dorsal rib: with a note on the surgical treatment. Br J Surg 1919; 7:168–177.

Report of 10 cases with TOS symptoms due to normal first ribs; Two cases were due to trauma. Treatment is first rib resection and scalenotomy.

1920   Law AA. Adventitious ligaments simulating cervical ribs. Ann Surg 1920; 72:497–499.

Four cases of congenital bands from transverse process of C-7 to first rib causing symptoms of cervical rib syndrome without a cervical rib. The patients were treated by surgically dividing the bands and all four improved.

1923   Stiles H. In: Jones R and Lovett R, Orthopedic surgery. 2d ed. New York: William Wood & Co., 1923.

Discussion of diagnosis and treatment of torticollis, cervical ribs, and first ribs.

1924   Lowenstein PS. Thrombosis of the axillary vein: an anatomical study. JAMA 1924; 82:854–857.

On the basis of anatomical dissections it is suggested that marked abduction or extension of the arm produces pressure by the costoclavicular ligament and/or the subclavius muscle on the distended axillosubclavian vein. This results in injury to the vascular endothelium and subsequent venous thrombosis.

1924   Southam AH, Bythell WJ. Cervical ribs in children. Br Med J 1924; 2:844–855.

Nine cervical ribs were found in 2,000 children, an incidence of 0.45%. Girls were twice as common as boys and bilaterality was noted in 77%.

1925   Brickner WM, Milch H. First dorsal, simulating cervical rib—by maldevelopment or by pressure symptoms. Surg Gynecol Obstet 1925; 40:38–44.

One of the first discussions of abnormal first ribs.

1925   Agassiz CDS, Sykes AH. Cervical ribs in children. Br Med J 1925; 1:71–72.

Two short case reports of asymptomatic cervical ribs found on x-ray.

1927   Adson AW, Coffey JR. Cervical rib: a method of anterior approach for relief of symptoms by division of the scalenus anticus. Ann Surg 1927; 85:839–857.

Classic article on cervical rib syndrome. Thirty-six cases, 31 with rib resection, 5 with just anterior scalenotomy done to avoid the frequent nerve complications of rib resection. Good results in 83%.

1927   Brickner WM. Brachial plexus pressure by the normal first rib. Ann Surg 1927; 85:858–872.

Six case reports of symptoms due to normal first rib.

1927   Symonds CP. Two cases of thrombosis of subclavian artery with contralateral hemiplegia of sudden onset, probably embolic. Brain 1927; 50:259–260.

Two case reports of right sided cervical ribs as probable cause of emboli causing left hemiplegia.

1928   Gould EP, Patey DH. Primary thrombosis of the axillary vein: a study of eight cases. Brit J Surg 1928; 16:208–213.

All eight patients were male; seven were on the right side. Trauma was the usual etiology. Recommended treatment was elevation of the arm for 2–3 weeks, followed by massage.

1930   Telford ED, Stopford JSB. The vascular complications of cervical rib. Br J Surg 1930; 18:557–564.

Three cases of cervical ribs causing arterial occlusion, white, cold, numb fingers, with gangrenous digital changes in two cases. All three were treated by cervical rib excision with excellent improvement. Symptoms can also occur from normal first rib and are thought to be due to sympathetic nerve stimulation by the rib.

1934   Lewis T, Pickering GW. Observations upon maladies in which the blood supply to the digits ceases intermittently or permanently and upon bilateral gangrene of the digits: observations relevant to so called "Raynaud's disease." Clin Sci 1934; 1:327–366.

Elaborate discussion and report of several cases of Raynaud's phenomenon, bilateral digital gangrene, and those conditions associated with arterial disease: thromboangeitis and cervical ribs. Two possible causes for vascular symptoms in patients with cervical ribs are reviewed: irritation of sympathetic nerve fibers running in lower nerves of the brachial plexus and distal emboli from the subclavian artery.

1934   Matas R. Primary thrombosis of the axillary vein caused by strain: report of a case with comments on diagnosis, pathogeny and treatment of this lesion in its medico-legal relations. Am J Surg 1934; 24:642–666.

Discussion of primary (spontaneous) and secondary (usually traumatic) causes. Failure of patient to respond to conservative measures is indication for surgical exploration, thrombectomy, or excision of vein segment.

1935   Blair DM, Davies F, McKissock W. The etiology of the vascular symptoms of cervical rib. Br J Surg 1935; 22:406–414.

Suggests that the vascular symptoms seen in cervical rib patients are due to sympathetic nerve irritation by the rib. This is based upon a case report and detailed microscopic anatomical studies of the brachial plexus.

1935   Ochsner A, Gage M, Debakey M. Scalenus anticus (Naffziger) syndrome. Am J Surg 1935; 28:669–695.

Report of six cases of scalenus anticus syndrome treated by anterior scalenectomy; none had cervical ribs. Describes hypertrophy, degeneration, and fibrosis of muscle and suggests elevation of first rib by tight muscle as etiology. Three patients had history of trauma. First article to discuss muscle pathology.

1935   Telford ED. The technique of sympathectomy. Br J Surg 1935; 23:448–450.

Author became dissatisfied with results after 35 cases using posterior technique. He switched to anterior approach (supraclavicular?) leaving the stellate ganglion and removing the second and third ganglia. This avoids Horner's syndrome and early results are good.

1935   Veal JR, McFetridge EM. Primary thrombosis of the axillary vein: an anatomic and roentgenologic study of certain etiologic factors and a consideration of venography as a diagnostic measure. Arch Surg 1935; 31:271–289.

Report of two cases and extensive discussion of etiology and treatment. This is first introduction of venography, using stabilized thorium dioxide solution (thorotrast). On venography, compression of the axillary vein was noted with the arm abducted and externally rotated, suggesting that trauma with the arm in this position might be an etiologic factor.

1936   Hovelacque A, Monod O, Evrard H, Beuzart J. Etude anatomique du nerf phrenique preveineux. Ann D'Anatomie Path 1936; 13:518–522.

Anatomical dissections of 138 phrenic nerves demonstrated the phrenic running anterior to the subclavian vein in ten cases, 7.2%. In eight cases it was the main phrenic, in two cases, an accessory branch. In French.

1937   Craig W McK, Knepper PA: Cervical rib and the scalenus anticus syndrome. Ann Surg 1937; 105:556–563.

Six cases, three with and three without cervical ribs. Five were treated with scalenotomy only; only one with cervical rib excision. All six had excellent improvement.

1938   Adson AW. Vascular Clinics. VI.2 Thrombosis of arteries of the right upper extremity resulting from anomalous first rib. Proc Staff Meet Mayo Clin 1938; 13:637–640.

Single case report of rudimentary first rib, thrombosed subclavian artery aneurysm, and digital gangrene. Treatment was anterior scalenectomy and cervicothoracic sympathectomy. There was partial symptomatic improvement, but fifth finger amputation was necessary.

1938   Baumgartner A, Clerc A, Macrez C. Sur L'anevrysme arteriel de voisinage et la gangrene ischemique des doigts. Press Med 1938; 46:1665–1667.

1938   Freiberg JA. The scalenus anterior muscle in relation to shoulder and arm pain. J Bone Joint Surg 1938; 20:860–861.

In 20 patients with scalenus anticus syndrome, most had associated trauma or inflammation of the shoulder or cervical spine. Most patients improved by treating the associated injury. Scalenotomy was performed in the few who did not improve on three months of conservative therapy with good improvement in all.

1938   Naffziger HC, Grant WT. Neuritis of the brachial plexus mechanical in origin: the scalenus origin. Surg Gynecol Obstet 1938; 67:722.

Coined the term "scalenus anticus syndrome." Reports 18 cases, six with cervical ribs. Five of the 12 without cervical ribs had traumatic histories. Notes importance of supraclavicular tenderness as a diagnostic sign. Scalenotomy must be accompanied by cervical rib excision in some patients.

1938   Spurling RG, Bradford FK. Scalenus neurocirculatory compression. Ann Surg 1938; 107:708–715.

Reports 20 cases of cervical rib with neurologic symptoms. Good late results followed rib excision in 18 of the 20. All had temporary phrenic nerve palsy postoperatively. Trauma precipitated symptoms in five patients, and perhaps two more.

1939–40   Eden KC. Complications of cervical rib: vascular complications of cervical ribs and first thoracic rib abnormalities. Br J Surg 1939–40; 27:111–139.

Review of literature from 1818 to 1937 and report of 48 cases of vascular complications. All were due to cervical ribs except two, which were due to abnormal first ribs.

1939   Gage M. Scalenus anticus syndrome: a diagnostic and confirmatory test. Surgery 1939; 5:599–601.

Description of the scalene muscle block as a diagnostic test. One percent Novocaine was injected into the belly of the anterior scalene muscle. Improvement in symptoms was a positive response compatible with a diagnosis of scalenus anticus syndrome.

1939   Haven H. Neurocirculatory scalenus anticus syndrome in the presence of developmental defects of the first rib. Yale J Bio 1939; 11:443–448.

A review of 5,000 chest x-rays revealed 38 anomalous first ribs (0.76%) and 37 cervical ribs (0.74%). Anomalous first ribs were seldom bilateral and were equally distributed between men and women. Two-thirds of cervical ribs were bilateral and two-thirds were in women.

1939   McLaughlin CW Jr, Popma AM. Intermittent obstruction of the subclavian vein. JAMA 1939; 113:1960–1963.

Single case report of intermittent right subclavian vein obstruction relieved by anterior scalenotomy.

1939   Roelson E. So-called traumatic thrombosis of the axillary and subclavian veins. Acta Med Scand 1939; 98:589–622.

Report of seven cases of axillosubclavian vein obstruction. Three patients underwent operation and no clot was found in the axillary vein; the other four patients were not operated upon. A review of 21 reported cases in the medical literature disclosed similar findings: Thrombus was found in 12 and no thrombus was found in 9. Etiology is discussed with the conclusion that thrombosis is a complication of venous obstruction and stasis but the primary cause of thrombosis is still obscure.

1939   Theis FV. Scalenus anticus syndrome and cervical ribs. Surgery 1939; 6:112–125.

Three of 20 patients with scalenus anticus syndrome underwent scalenotomy. One patient had no improvement from a previously resected cervical rib but improved following scalenotomy. The other two patients failed to benefit from surgery. A thorough workup and long trials of conservative therapy are advocated before offering operation in neurological cases. Oscillometry is unreliable in diagnosis because abnormalities are found in normals.

1940   Aynesworth KH. The cervicobrachial syndrome: a discussion of the etiology with report of twenty cases. Ann Surg 1940; 111:724–742.

The term "cervicobrachial syndrome" is presented as a comprehensive term, like "thoracic outlet syndrome," to include all causes of neurovascular compression in the supraclavicular area. Of 20 reported cases, 80% had histories of trauma as the precipitating cause. Most patients also had cervical ribs. Nine of 10 operated cases obtained relief.

1940   Donald JM, Morton BF. The scalenus anticus syndrome with and without cervical rib. Ann Surg 1940; 111:709–723.

Cervical ribs were present in two and an abnormal first rib in one of 16 patients undergoing scalenotomy. Excellent results were seen in 14 patients. Microscopic examination revealed scattered areas of fibrosis in three of nine cases. The other cases had normal findings.

1940   Smithwick RH. The problem of producing complete and lasting sympathetic denervation of the upper extremity by preganglionic section. Ann Surg 1940; 112:1085–1100.

Description of technique of posterior dorsal sympathectomy, removing the second and third dorsal ganglia. Postoperatively, nerve regeneration is the cause for recurrent symptoms. Discussion is presented of the physiology of pre- and post-ganglionic nerve division.

1941   Kaplan L. Relation of the scalenus anticus muscle to pain in the shoulder: diagnostic and therapeutic value of procaine infiltration. Arch Surg 1941; 42:739–757.

Procaine injections in 40 patients were used for both diagnosis and therapy for scalenus anticus syndrome with mixed results. Scalene muscle spasm is often associated with supraspinatus tendinitis and other shoulder pathology. Scalene injection gave prolonged relief of shoulder symptoms in some patients.

1942   Judovich B, Bates W. The scalenus anticus syndrome: faulty diagnosis in the presence of Horner's syndrome—a modified technic of infiltration. Am J Surg 1942; 57:523–524.

Reports that Horner's syndrome should be avoided in performing scalene muscle blocks for diagnosis: misleading information is obtained. However, if a successful block is achieved, there is good correlation with results of scalenotomy.

1943   Falconer MA, Weddell G. Costoclavicular compression of the subclavian artery and vein. Lancet 1943; 2:539–543.

Classical description of costoclavicular compression. Report of four cases, three with arterial compression and one with neurological compression. Military position easily occludes pulses in those patients, although it occludes pulses in 54% of normals also. Treatment was excision of a portion of first rib under local anesthesia after demonstrating a tight space between clavicle and rib with a forefinger "pinch" at surgery.

1944   Etter LE. Osseous abnormalities of the thoracic cage seen in forty thousand consecutive chest photoroentgenograms. Am J Roentg 1944; 51:359–363.

Review of 40,000 male chest x-rays revealed only 68 cervical ribs (.17%) and 114 first rib abnormalities (0.29%). First rib abnormalities were an anomalous rib, 31 cases; rudimentary rib, 67 cases; and bifid rib 16 cases.

1944   Swank RL, Simeone FA. Scalenus anticus syndrome: types; their characterization, diagnosis, and treatment. Arch Neurol Psych 1944; 51:432–445.

First description of upper and lower plexus types of scalenus anticus syndrome. Of 15 patients, seven responded to conservative treatment and eight (two bilateral) improved following scalenotomy. Several scalene muscle abnormalities were observed at operation. Muscle hypertrophy was noted in all patients.

1944   Sycamore LK. Common congenital anomalies of the bony thorax. Am J Roentg 1944; 51:593–599.

Review of 2,000 male chest x-rays at Dartmouth college revealed cervical ribs in 10 (0.5%) and rudimentary first ribs in 10 (0.5%). Anomalies of the other ribs were also noted in another 1.8%.

1944   Walshe FMR, Jackson H, Wyburn-Mason R. On some pressure effects associated with cervical and with rudimentary and "normal" first ribs, and the factors entering into their causation. Brain 1944; 67:141–177.

Extensive discussions of cervical, rudimentary, and normal first ribs and symptoms related to them.

1945   Love JG. The scalenus anticus syndrome with and without cervical rib. Proc Mayo Clin 1945; 20:65–70.

Review of 303 patients with cervical ribs at the Mayo clinic in which 36, 11%, were symptomatic enough to require surgery. The paper reviews the clinical features.

1945   White JC, Poppel MH, Adams R. Congenital malformations of the first thoracic rib: a cause of brachial neuralgia which simulates the cervical rib syndrome. Surg Gynecol Obstet 1945; 81:643–659.

Report of 10 cases of abnormal first ribs, five requiring surgery and five asymptomatic. The embryology, anatomy, and clinical features are extensively discussed.

1945   Wright IS. The neurovascular syndrome produced by hyperabduction of the arms. Am Heart J 1945; 29:1–19.

First description of the pectoralis minor or hyperabduction syndrome. Treatment is learning to sleep with the arms down; surgery is seldom indicated. In 150 normals, 82% cut off their radial pulses when abducting their arms above their heads. In performing Adson's maneuver, some individuals occluded their radial pulses by turning their head towards the symptomatic side, others by turning their head away from the symptomatic side.

1946   Eaton LM. Neurologic causes of pain in the upper extremities: with particular reference to syndromes of protruded intervertebral disk in the cervical region and mechanical compression of the brachial plexus. Surg Clin North Am 1946; 26:810–833.

General review of compression syndromes and description of their clinical features.

1946   Shumacker HB. A case of costoclavicular compression of the subclavian artery simulating arterial aneurysm. Surgery 1946; 20:478–481.

Case report of costoclavicular compression of the subclavian artery in a young man with no symptoms and no aneurysm. The mechanics and hemodynamics are discussed.

1947   Adson AW. Surgical treatment for symptoms produced by cervical ribs and the scalenus anticus muscle. Surg Gynecol Obstet 1947; 85:687–700.

This is Adson's last article on this subject. Clinical features and Adson's "pathognomonic" maneuver are described. Results of surgery in three groups of patients were: 90% improvement in 63 patients with cervical ribs in whom anterior scalenectomy only was done; 81% improvement in 26 patients following both scalenectomy and cervical rib resection; and 81% improvement following scalenectomy alone in 53 patients with scalenus anticus syndrome and no cervical rib. Adson recommended rib resection only if the cervical rib was a complete one.

1947   Annersten S. Studies on the scalenus anticus syndrome. Acta Surg Scand 1947; 95:419–439.

Among 27 patients with scalenus anticus syndrome, scalenotomy was performed in 21 and first rib resection in six. The results were good to excellent in 70%.

1947   Gage M, Parnell H. Scalenus anticus syndrome. Am J Surg 1947; 73:252–268.

In 100 cadavers, the space between anterior and middle scalene muscle insertions on the first rib ranged from 0.3 to 2.3 cm; C-5 and C-6 went through anterior scalene muscle fibers in 30%; scalene minimus was seen in 60%. Microscopic studies of the anterior scalene muscles of TOS patients demonstrated muscle hypertrophy, inflammation, and degeneration. Physical findings of scalene muscle tenderness were present in 100% of patients; positive Adson's maneuver was present in 50% of normals. Good discussion of these points.

1947   Telford ED, Mottershead S. The costoclavicular syndrome. Br Med J 1947; 1:325–328.

Review of observations on the anatomy of the supraclavicular area based upon 120 operations, 30 cadaver dissections, and 120 normal students. The study concluded that loss of the radial pulse with positional changes was due to causes distal to the clavicle and has nothing to do with costoclavicular compression.

1948   Hughes ESR. Venous obstruction in the upper extremity. Br J Surg 1948; 36:155–163.

Thorough discussion of the many etiologies of upper extremity venous obstruction. When neither trauma nor thrombosis are present, a phrenic nerve lying anterior to the subclavian vein may be the cause. In such cases, the author suggests that a venous bypass may be the treatment, although he presents no data. In 20 autopsies, one instance of a prevenous phrenic nerve was found (5%).

1948   Kirgis HD, Reed AF. Significant anatomic relations in the syndrome of the scalene muscles. Ann Surg 1948; 127:1182–1201.

Classical article discussing anatomical variations of the scalene muscles and triangle. Many anterior scalene muscle variations occur too often to call them anomalies. Anterior scalene fibers frequently pass below C-6; scalene minimus occurs in 55%; middle scalene has several variations of insertion on the first rib. It is recommended that middle scalenectomy accompany anterior scalenectomy when surgical decompression is indicated.

1948   Telford ED, Mottershead S. Pressure at the cervico-brachial junction: an operative and anatomical study. J Bone Joint Surg 1948; 30:249–265.

Review of anatomical findings in 122 operated cases of TOS. There were 70 cervical ribs; 12 more had fibrous bands running in the middle scalene muscle from a short cervical rib to the first rib; and a variety of other abnormalities were observed. Causative factors include scalene muscle trauma, fibrosis, and spasm. Costoclavicular compression occurs only when there is a cervical or anomalous first rib. Most vascular symptoms are due to irritation of sympathetic nerve fibers accompanying T-1 or C-8; only a few are due to emboli arising from subclavian artery aneurysms.

1949   Kleinsasser LJ. "Effort" thrombosis of the axillary and subclavian veins: an analysis of 16 personal cases and 56 cases collected from the literature. Arch Surg 1949; 59:258–274.

Review of the etiology, symptoms, diagnosis, and treatment of effort thrombosis. All 16 of the author's cases were treated with rest, heat, elevation, and stellate ganglion block. Anticoagulants were not regarded as useful. The results were poor: all 16 patients had residual swelling; 14 had symptoms on activity.

1949   McGowan JM, Velinsky M. Costoclavicular compression: relation to the scalenus anticus and cervical rib syndrome. Arch Surg 1949; 59:62–73.

Diagnosis of costoclavicular compression is based upon symptoms and a reduced radial pulse when assuming a shoulder braced (military) position. In normals, Falconer (1943) found 54% had reduced radial pulses in the military position, but current study noted an incidence of only 16%. Improvement occurred in all 14 patients undergoing first rib resection for this condition.

1949   Rogers L. Upper limb pain due to lesions of the thoracic outlet. Br Med J 1949; 2:956–958.

Neurovascular compression of the lower extremity does not occur as it does in the upper extremity. This is because acute angulation of the nerve trunks leaving the thorax is not replicated in the lower extremity. Relief of symptoms requires dividing the structure over which the nerves angulate, which means the anterior scalene muscle is not enough. Underlying ribs, bands, middle scalene muscle, or other abnormal scalene muscle must be sectioned to eliminate the point over which the plexus is stretched.

1950   Harvey EN. Bubble formation in liquids. In Glasser O, ed. Medical physics, Vol 2; Chicago: Yearbook Publishers, 1950; 137–150.

A chapter from a textbook on medical physics discusses the possibilities and conditions under which bubbles might be found in animal or human blood. The conclusion was that if bubbles do exist, they must come from gas nuclei that stick to or are formed on or within the endothelial linings of the vascular system or extravascular spaces; and only when they have enlarged to the point of instability do they pass into the blood stream.

1950   Stammers FAR. Pain in the upper limb from mechanisms in the costoclavicular space. Lancet 1950; 1:603–607.

Review of the several factors in the costoclavicular space that can cause neurovascular compression. These include cervical rib, scalenus medius muscle, abnormal first rib, enlarged C-7 transverse process, scalenus anticus muscle, and costoclavicular space. Surgical treatment, through the supraclavicular approach, requires removing the anterior scalene muscle first, observing the anatomy of the area which is now exposed, and excising any and all structures that appear to be compressing the neurovascular structures.

1951   Holden WD, Murphy JA, Portmann AF. Scalene anticus syndrome: unusual diagnostic and therapeutic aspects. Am J Surg 1951; 81:411–416.

Scalene muscle tenderness and improvement following scalene muscle block were very helpful in establishing a diagnosis. Trauma precipitated symptoms in 28%. In 28 patients, 79% had complete symptomatic relief following scalenotomy.

1951   Imler RL Jr, Hayne RA, Stowell A. Aneurysm of the subclavian artery associated with cervical rib: report of two cases. Am Surg 1951; 17:478–485.

Two case reports of subclavian aneurysms, one with a cervical rib, the other an anomalous first rib. Both were treated with anterior scalenectomy only. In one case, the aneurysm shrunk 50% in size following scalenectomy. Follow-up was only a few months.

1951   Lawson FL, McKenzie KG. The scalenus minimus muscle. Can Med Assoc J 1951; 65:358–361.

Description of the anatomy of the scalenus minimus muscle, which had been observed in about one-half of normal dissections. A case is reported in which division of a scalenus minimus muscle relieved symptoms of the scalene syndrome.

1951   McCleery RS, Kesterson JE, Kirtley JA, Love RB. Subclavius and anterior scalene muscle compression as a cause of intermittent obstruction of the subclavian vein. Ann Surg 1951; 133:588–602.

Report of five cases of intermittent subclavian vein obstruction without thrombosis. Treatment was excision of the subclavius muscle through an infraclavicular incision combined with anterior scalenectomy through a supraclavicular incision. All five patients improved with 3–9 month follow-up.

1952   Edwards H. Thoracic inlet syndrome with recurrence of symptoms after operation. Proc R Soc Med 1952; 45:439–441.

Case report of a man with swelling, cyanosis, and paresthesia in his hand. This was relieved for 10 months by division of a tight scalenus minimus muscle band, then symptoms recurred. The question of first rib resection is discussed as the more appropriate operation for someone with these symptoms.

1952   Luke JC. The costobrachial syndrome. Can Med Assoc J 1952; 66:127–131.

Good review of the clinical presentation of cervical rib, scalenus anticus, costoclavicular, venous obstruction, and hyperabduction syndromes. Forty cases of cervical ribs were observed; 72% were women; 63% were bilateral; 50% had symptoms. Treatment is not presented.

1953   Lord JW Jr. Surgical management of shoulder girdle syndromes: new operative procedure for hyperabduction, costoclavicular, cervical rib, and scalenus syndromes. Arch Surg 1953; 60:69–83.

Claviculectomy is introduced as a new and better approach for the treatment of symptomatic patients with vascular compression in the thoracic outlet area. Good results were achieved in eight of nine patients.

1953   Ziss RC. Paget-Schroetter's syndrome. US Armed Forces Med J 1953; 4:127–129.

Single case report of acute axillary vein thrombosis treated conservatively with warfarin. Pain and function of the arm improved, although the swelling was unaltered after six months.

1954   Holman E. The obscure physiology of poststenotic dilatation: its relationship to the development of aneurysms. J Thor Surg 1954; 28:109–133.

Presentation of the theory that poststenotic dilatation is caused by an increase in lateral wall pressure resulting from widening of the vessel and reduced blood flow. This theory was later disproved by Robicsek, 1958, who measured no increase in lateral wall pressure.

1955   Raaf J. Surgery for cervical rib and scalenus anticus syndrome. J Am Med Assoc 1955; 157:219–223.

Less than 50% of 17 patients with scalenus anticus syndrome improved following anterior scalenotomy alone; better results were obtained when another structure, such as a cervical rib or middle scalene muscle, was excised. Emphasis is placed on doing more than dividing the anterior scalene muscle in patients with symptoms of thoracic outlet compression.

1955   Phillips AM, Yurko AA. Primary thrombosis of the axillary vein caused by strain (effort thrombosis). W Virg Med J 1955; 198–199.

Single case report of axillary vein thrombosis diagnosed by clinical criteria and treated with a stellate ganglion block only. Symptoms improved, venous collaterals became less dilated, and function was restored.

1956   Lord JW Jr, Stone PW. Pectoralis minor tenotomy and anterior scalenotomy with special reference to the hyperabduction syndrome and "effort thrombosis" of the subclavian vein. Circulation 1956; 13:537–542.

Report of five cases with hyperabduction syndrome, three with axillosubclavian thrombosis. Treatment was pectoralis minor tenotomy and anterior scalenotomy followed by good clinical results in four of the five patients.

1956   Palumbo LT. Anterior transthoracic approach for upper thoracic sympathectomy. Arch Surg 1956; 72:659–666.

Technical description of the transthoracic technique of dorsal sympathectomy via an anterior approach through the third interspace. The sympathetic chain is removed from the fifth thoracic ganglion to the lower third of the stellate ganglion. This gave good results in 20 patients and avoided a Horner's syndrome according to the author. [Editorial comment: In our experience, Horner's syndrome has been common when removing only one quarter of the stellate ganglion.]

1956   Peet RM, Hendriksen JD, Anderson TP, Martin GM. Thoracic outlet syndrome: evaluation of a therapeutic exercise program: Proc Mayo Clin 1956; 31:281–287.

Introduction of the term "thoracic outlet syndrome" to include all of the compression syndromes in this area, such as scalenus anticus and costoclavicular. Of 55 patients treated conservatively with an exercise program at the Mayo clinic, 71% improved.

1956   Schein CJ, Haimovici H, Young H. Recent advances in surgery: arterial thrombosis associated with cervical ribs: surgical considerations. Report of a case and review of the literature. Surgery 1956; 40:428–443.

The first extensive review of arterial TOS due to cervical ribs from 1815 to 1955. A total of 29 reported cases were found; their symptoms and treatments were tabulated. This is also the first report of utilizing an homologous subclavian arterial graft for managing this condition.

1956   Stowell A. The scalenus anticus syndrome. J Int Coll Surg 1956; 26:711–717.

Eighty-four percent of 130 patients with scalenus anticus syndrome improved following anterior scalenectomy. Whiplash neck injuries were a common etiology; supraclavicular tenderness was the most reliable physical finding; responses to scalene muscle blocks with procaine correlated poorly with results; and occipital headaches were frequently cured by scalenectomy.

1957   Shenkin HA. Cervical rib and thrombosis of the subclavian artery. JAMA 1957; 165:335–338.

Report of three cases of subclavian artery thrombosis due to cervical rib. Treatment was scalenotomy, thrombectomy, and dorsal sympathectomy. All three patients improved.

1958   Palumbo LT. New surgical approach for upper thoracic sympathectomy: a method to avoid Horner's syndrome. Arch Surg 1958; 76:807–810.

Description of technique of anterior thoracotomy approach for dorsal sympathectomy. This is similar to the 1956 article by the same author. Limiting stellate ganglionectomy to the lower third is emphasized again as the method to avoid a Horner's syndrome.

1958   Rob CG, Standeven A. Arterial occlusion complicating thoracic outlet compression syndrome. Br Med J 1958; 2:709–712.

Introduction of the term "thoracic outlet compression syndrome." Report of eleven cases: nine cervical ribs; one abnormal first rib; and one fractured first rib. Treatment included: eight cervical rib and one abnormal first rib resections with dorsal sympathectomy; two patients were not treated. Results were good in seven, poor in three, and there was one amputation.

1958   Robicsek F, Sanger PW, Taylor FH, Magistro R, Fori E. Pathogenesis and significance of post-stenotic dilatation in great vessels. Ann Surg 1958; 147:835–844.

Pressure measurements in the poststenotic segment of an artery revealed no increase in lateral pressure. The theory is proposed that cavitation is the cause of poststenotic dilatation. This was later disproved.

1958   Upmalis IH. The scalenus anticus and related syndromes. Surg Gynecol Obstet 1958; 107:521–529.

A good historical review of the state of TOS in 1958.

1959   Cobb LA, Thomas GI, Dillard DH, Merendino KA, Bruce RA. An evaluation of internal mammary artery ligation by a double-blind technic. N Engl J Med 1959; 260:1115–1118.

Eight patients with angina had internal mammary artery ligations while nine similar patients had a sham operation. The improvement in chest pain was similar in both groups, illustrating the placebo effect of a sham operation.

1959   Daseler EH, Anson BJ. Surgical anatomy of the subclavian artery and its branches. Surg Gynecol Obstet 1959; 108:149–174.

Good review of anatomical variations of the subclavian artery, its branches, and the variations in length of the base of the scalene triangle.

1960   Dimond EG, Kittle CF, Crockett JE. Comparison of internal mammary artery ligation and sham operation for angina pectoris. Am J Cardiol 1960; 5:483–486.

Sham operations in five patients with angina resulted in the same degree of improvement in pain as in 13 patients receiving internal mammary artery ligation. This stresses the placebo effect of an operation in relieving subjective symptoms.

1960   Crowell DL. Effort thrombosis of the subclavian and axillary veins: review of the literature and case report with two-year follow-up with venography. Ann Int Med 1960; 52:1337–1343.

Single case report of axillary vein thrombosis. Initial venogram and follow-up venogram two years later showed no change in the venous occlusion, but the later films demonstrated increased size of collateral veins. Since few axillary veins recanalize, it is proposed that the thrombosed vein be ligated to prevent pulmonary emboli, although no data is presented to support this.

1960   Javid H. Compression vascular syndrome of the neck and shoulder. Surg Clin N A 1960; 40:231–240.

Review of osseous and soft tissue causes of subclavian artery compression. Diagnosis is by arteriography and treatment is directed at removing the offending structure.

1960   Lord JW Jr. Thrombosis of the subclavian artery. West J Surg Obstet Gyn 1960; 68:11–12.

Eleven patients with 13 instances of subclavian artery thrombosis are reported. Treatment included eight claviculectomies, five scalenotomies, and three dorsal sympathectomies. Some patients received more than one procedure. Results were good in 12 and poor in one.

1961   Jackson NJ, Nanson EM. Intermittent subclavian vein obstruction. Brit J Surg 1961; 303–306.

First case report of intermittent subclavian vein obstruction caused by an anterior lying accessory phrenic nerve. This was treated by division of the accessory phrenic nerve. Through 1989, no additional reports of this condition have appeared in the English-speaking literature.

1961   Rosati LM, Lord JW Jr. Neurovascular compression of the shoulder. Modern Surg Monographs. NY: Grune and Stratton, 1961.

Monograph on shoulder compression syndromes including scalenus anticus, costoclavicular, and hyperabduction; arterial and venous thrombosis; differential diagnosis; and treatment.

1962   Clagett OT. Presidential address: research and prosearch. J Thorac Cardiovasc Surg 1962; 44:153–166.

Classical article by president of the American Association for Thoracic Surgery introducing first rib resection as a better operation than scalenotomy for scalenus anticus syndrome. The article claimed about 60% of scalenectomies done at the Mayo clinic failed, but actual data were not presented. Of 12 patients undergoing first rib resection through a posterior thoracotomy approach, eight had good improvement, two fair improvement, and two failed. This article stimulated surgeons around the country to consider rib resection for TOS.

1962   Eastcott HH, Lond MS. Reconstruction of the subclavian artery for complications of cervical rib and thoracic outlet syndrome. Lancet 1962; 2:1243–1246.

Report of five cases with arterial complications from cervical ribs. Treatment included resection of the cervical rib, resection of the subclavian aneurysm with end-to-end anastomosis if possible, and dorsal sympathectomy if necessary. Claviculectomy can be done for exposure if needed; arterial bypass can be done if direct anastomosis is not feasible.

1962   Falconer MA, Li WP. Resection of the first rib in costoclavicular compression of the brachial plexus. Lancet 1962; 1:59–63.

Twelve of 13 cases of costoclavicular syndrome were relieved by supraclavicular first rib resection. The two useful physical findings were reproducing symptoms by shoulder bracing (military position) and eliciting arm pain by pressure over the brachial plexus in the supraclavicular area.

1962   Lang EK. Roentgenographic diagnosis of the neurovascular compression syndromes. Radiology 1962; 79:58–63.

Introduces arteriography by the Seldinger technique in the diagnosis of TOS. [Editorial comment: Its claim of being able to pinpoint the exact cause of arterial obstruction, i.e., bone, muscle, or ligament, is overly optimistic. Few patients have arteriography today except when arterial obstruction is suspected, usually with osseous abnormalities.]

1963   Brannon EW. Cervical rib syndrome: an analysis of nineteen cases and twenty-four operations. J Bone Joint Surg 1963; 45:977–998.

Twenty-four cervical rib resections were performed in 19 patients, most for neurologic symptoms. Only a few had vascular symptoms and these were probably due to sympathetic nerve irritation. Results were 18 excellent, 4 improved, and 1 failure.

1963   Cucci CE, Bottino CG, Ciampa V. Venous obstruction of the upper extremity caused by a malformed valve of the subclavian vein. Circulation 1963; 27:275–278.

First case report of subclavian vein obstruction by a thickened valve with a 2 mm opening. Diagnosis was by antegrade and retrograde venography. This was treated by claviculectomy and open excision of the valve with a good clinical result.

1963   Gilroy J, Meyer JS. Compression of the subclavian artery as a cause of ischemic brachial neuropathy. Brain 1963; 86:733–745.

The authors suggest that neurologic symptoms of TOS are due to ischemia of the nerves produced by mechanical compression of the subclavian artery. [Editorial comment: This theory is not generally accepted.]

1963   Roach MR. Changes in arterial distensibility as a cause of poststenotic dilatation. Am J Cardiol 1963; 12:802–815.

Poststenotic dilatation in canine arteries occurred only if the stenosis created enough turbulence to produce vibrations and a thrill in the arterial wall. The vibrations weaken the elastin fibers so that the wall becomes more distensible. Even though poststenotic dilatation seems to be a hemodynamic paradox, it can be explained by simple physical principles, i.e., a structural weakness of the wall due to turbulence.

1963   Shenkin HA, Somach FM. Scalenotomy in patients with and without cervical ribs. Arch Surg 1963; 87:30–34.

Scalenotomy was performed in 64 patients. Only one-third of those with cervical ribs had the rib removed, yet all improved postoperatively. Eleven of 14 patients with associated cervical spine disease improved following scalenotomy. About 50% of patients with no cervical rib or spine disease improved postoperatively.

1963   Shucksmith HS. Cerebral and peripheral emboli caused by cervical ribs. Br Med J 1963; 2:835–837.

Case reports of six patients, five with cervical ribs and one with abnormal first rib, treated by a variety of methods: cervical rib excision and scalenotomy; repair and patch graft; ligation of subclavian artery (three cases); and thrombectomy. Dorsal sympathectomy was added in two cases.

1963   Smith CA, Schisgall RM. The effect of a distal arteriovenous fistula upon an autogenous vein graft in the venous system. J Surg Res 1963; 3:412–415.

A side-to-side arteriovenous fistula in dogs did not improve the patency rate of autogenous vein grafts in the venous system.

1963   Wickham JEA, Martin P. Aneurysm of the subclavian artery in association with cervical abnormality. Br J Surg 1963; 50:205–209.

Two case reports, one with a cervical rib and one an anomalous first rib, both treated successfully with vein grafts.

1963   Williams CL, Takaro T. Subclavian arterial occlusion. Ann Surg 1963; 157:48–55.

Report of seven cases, five due to arteriosclerosis and two to cervical ribs, plus a review of the literature on arterial repair.

1964   Gunning AJ, Pickering GW, Robb-Smith AHT, and Russell RR. Mural thrombosis of the subclavian artery and subsequent embolism in cervical rib. Q J Med 1964; 33:133–159.

Report of three cases of cervical rib and one of abnormal first rib with arterial thrombosis and distal emboli treated by thrombectomy (two cases), Dacron graft (one case), and scalenotomy (one case). Results were good in three of the four cases.

1964   Harris JD, Jepson RP. Vascular complications of cervical ribs: Aust NZ J Surg 1964; 269–274.

Report of four cases of cervical ribs in four women, two treated by rib resection alone and two with rib resection and cervico-thoracic sympathectomy. All four patients improved.

1964   Wilder JR, Haberman ET, Nach RL. Subclavian vein obstruction secondary to hypertrophy of the terminal valve. Surgery 1964; 55:214–219.

Report of three cases of nonthrombotic subclavian vein obstruction, two due to intrinsic venous valve thickening and one due to an extrinsic tumor. The three were treated by excising the abnormality with good results in all.

1965   Adams JT, McEvoy RK, DeWeese JA. Primary deep venous thrombosis of upper extremity. Arch Surg 1965; 91:29–42.

In 25 cases of primary upper extremity deep vein thrombosis, the process usually started in the subclavian vein at the first rib level. Conservative therapy in 23 patients was followed by residual or recurrent symptoms in 68%; three patients, 12%, had pulmonary emboli. The 10 patients who received anticoagulants did no better than those receiving none. Two patients treated with thrombectomy were asymptomatic at follow-up, two and five years later, respectively.

1965   Bonney G. The scalenus medius band: a contribution to the study of the thoracic outlet syndrome. J Bone Joint Surg 1965; 47B:268–272.

Report of 13 cases of TOS due to a tight band in the middle scalene muscle. All were relieved by surgical division of the band. The band arose from the tip of the C-7 transverse process and inserted on the first rib, running on the anterior edge of the middle scalene muscle. X-rays demonstrated a long transverse process of C-7 in six instances, a short cervical rib in four cases, and no bony abnormalities in three cases.

1965   Kleinert HE, Cook FW, Kutz JE. Neurovascular disorders of the upper extremity: treated by transaxillary sympathectomy. Arch Surg 1965; 90:612–616.

Dorsal sympathectomy, removing the lower third of the stellate ganglion and the ganglia of C-2, C-3, and C-4, was performed 51 times through the second interspace via a transaxillary, transpleural approach. Follow-up in 31 cases at 3 months to 5 years revealed 77% asymptomatic and 23% improved. This approach permits a more complete and safe sympathectomy than the supraclavicular approach. Its primary disadvantage is that the chest is entered exposing the patient to the potential complications of any thoracotomy.

1965   Lang EK. Arteriographic diagnosis of the thoracic outlet syndrome. Radiology 1965; 84:296–303.

Good review of the role of arteriography in TOS. This is applicable for cases of arterial involvement and osseous abnormalities but is not appropriate for neurogenic TOS.

1965   Woods WW. Personal experiences with surgical treatment of 250 cases of cervicobrachial neurovascular compression syndrome. J Int Coll Surg 1965; 44:273–283.

Report of 250 cases of TOS treated with scalenotomy; 80% had improvement of headaches and 73% improvement in neck pain. All patients failed conservative therapy; 66% had neck trauma; all had supraclavicular tenderness on physical exam; 96% had paresthesia, 94% arm pain, 73% neck pain, and 66% headache. EMG studies were usually normal. Pending litigation did not affect results.

1966   Coon WW, Willis PW. Thrombosis of axillary and subclavian veins. Arch Surg 1967; 94:657–663.

Twenty-seven patients receiving no specific treatment for upper extremity venous thrombosis were compared to 31 patients treated with anticoagulants. Only three of the 27 patients not receiving anticoagulants were edema-free; the others were lost, died, or had postphlebitic symptoms. Almost all of 31 patients anticoagulated were edema-free at various follow-up periods to 11 years.

1966   deBruin TR. Costoclavicular space enlargement: eight methods for relief of neurovascular compression. Int Surg 1966; 46:340–360.

Description of method for enlarging the costoclavicular space by cutting the first rib and pulling it toward the second rib. Anterior and middle scalenotomy are also performed. There was only one failure in 22 cases. [Editorial comment: It is hard to determine how important the osteotomy was in these cases.]

1966   De Villiers JC. A brachiocephalic vascular syndrome associated with cervical rib. Br Med J 1966; 2:140–143.

Case report of 15-year-old girl with a left hemiparesis due to an embolus from the right subclavian artery. This was treated by arterial repair, cervical rib resection, and cervical sympathectomy with some improvement. All eight cases from the medical literature reported to this date are reviewed and summarized.

1966   Drapanas T, Curran WL. Thrombectomy in the treatment of "effort" thrombosis of the axillary and subclavian veins. J Trauma 1966; 6:107–119.

Two patients with axillosubclavian vein thrombosis were asymptomatic with normal venograms following thrombectomy in the acute phase. They are compared to four other patients with the same condition treated conservatively, all of whom had postphlebitic symptoms.

1966   McBurney RP, Howard H. Resection of the first rib for thoracic outlet compression: report of nine cases. Am Surgeon 1966; 32:165–169.

Report of nine cases of TOS, several with cervical ribs, treated by posterior first rib resection with good results in seven patients and fair results in two. Follow-up was short, a few months.

1966   Roos DB. Transaxillary approach for first rib resection to relieve thoracic outlet syndrome. Ann Surg 1966; 163:354–358.

The first description of the transaxillary technique of first rib resection. Twelve patients received a total of 15 operations, all of whom had initial good results. This is the classical article on this approach.

1966   Roos DB, Owens JC. Thoracic outlet syndrome. Arch Surg 1966; 93:71–74.

In 87 patients, 106 first rib resections were performed, 92 through the axilla. There were 5% failures and two temporary plexus injuries.

1966   Winsor T, Brow R. Costoclavicular syndrome: its diagnosis and treatment. J Am Med Assoc 1966; 196:109–111.

In 100 patients with symptomatic costoclavicular compression, postural maneuvers obliterated radial pulses in 94% compared to only 14% in 50 controls. [Editorial comment: Later studies by other investigators have shown a higher incidence of cutoff in controls.]

1966   Witte CL, Smith CA. Single anastomosis vein bypass for subclavian vein obstruction. Arch Surg 1966; 93:664–666.

First report of internal jugular-subclavian vein bypass for subclavian vein obstruction with good long-term result.

1967   Brannon EW Jr, Wickstrom J. Surgical approaches to neurovascular compression syndromes of the neck. Clin Ortho Rel Res 1967; 51:65–70.

Review of the technique of several surgical approaches: supraclavicular, transaxillary, and transclavicular scalenectomy and rib resection.

1967   Jebsen RH. Motor conduction velocities in the median and ulnar nerves. Arch Phys Med 1967; 48:185–194.

First description of technique for measuring motor conduction velocity over proximal segments of the median and ulnar nerves, using Erb's point as the proximal point of stimulation and calipers for measuring distance. Values from 50 normal subjects are presented.

1967   Kirtley JA, Riddell DH, Stoney WS, Wright JK. Cervicothoracic sympathectomy in neurovascular abnormalities of the upper extremities: experiences in 76 patients with 104 sympathectomies. Ann Surg 1967; 165:869–879.

Good presentation of 104 dorsal sympathectomies in 76 patients by four different approaches. The authors prefer the transthoracic transaxillary approach because of the good exposure, the extensive sympathectomy it permits, and minimal complications. Severe postoperative neuralgia occurred in some of their posteriorly approached patients and severe neuralgia of the breast occurred in three patients approached anteriorly.

1967   Roos DB. Thoracic outlet syndrome. Rocky Mtn Med J 1967; 49–55.

Early experiences with transaxillary first rib resection in 130 patients noting 93% good results with short follow up. There were a significant number of patients with histories of neck trauma and headache as well as other patients with spontaneous onset of symptoms. Only seven patients had cervical ribs.

1967   Siegel RS, Steichen FM. Cervicothoracic outlet syndrome: vascular compression caused by congenital abnormality of thoracic ribs; a case report. J Bone Joint Surg 1967; 49A:1187–1192.

First reported case of subclavian vein compression by an anomalous first rib inserting on a second rib. Treatment was resection of both first and second ribs and reconstruction of the defect with Dacron mesh. Symptoms were relieved; postop venogram at five months showed absence of venous compression with the arm abducted.

1967   Whelan TJ, Baugh JH. Non-atherosclerotic arterial lesions and their management. Curr Probl Surg 1967; March:3–15.

General review of arterial entrapment syndromes, including cervical and first rib abnormalities and popliteal artery entrapment.

1968   Adams JT, DeWeese JA, Mahoney EB, Rob CG. Intermittent subclavian vein obstruction without thrombosis. Surgery 1968; 63:147–165.

Classical article calling attention to the entity of nonthrombotic venous obstruction and its management. Diagnostic tests are dynamic venography and venous pressure. Report of eight cases; three were followed without surgery and no thrombosis developed. Five were operated upon: three scalenectomies were unsuccessful but later rib resection or claviculectomy was successful.

1968   Bertelsen S, Mathiesen FR, Ohlenschlaeger HH. Vascular complications of cervical rib. Scand J Thor Cardiovasc Surg 1968; 2:133–139.

Report of six cases, five treated, one not treated. Several forms of treatment were used, including rib resection, thrombectomy, endarterectomy, and arterial resection with end-to-end anastomosis.

1968   Dale WA. Discussion of Adams JT, DeWeese JA, Mahoney EB, Rob CG: Intermittent subclavian vein obstruction without thrombosis. Surgery 1968; 63:163.

Case report of lady with massive axillosubclavian vein thrombosis relieved by thrombectomy and division of a large anterior scalene muscle.

1968   Eriksson I, Hiertonn T. The brachiocephalic vascular syndrome. Acta Chir Scand 1968; 134:93–97.

Report of the 12th case of left hemiparesis from an embolus associated with subclavian artery thrombosis and cervical rib. The other 11 cases are reviewed. In this case, arterial compression was thought to be due to the anterior scalene muscle and not the rib; treatment was thrombectomy and scalenotomy.

1968   Gol A, Patrick DW, McNeel DP. Relief of costoclavicular syndrome by infraclavicular removal of first rib. J Neurosurg 1968; 28:81–84.

First description of the infraclavicular approach for first rib resection. Report of one case.

1968   Inahara T. Surgical treatment of "effort" thrombosis of the axillary and subclavian veins. Amer Surgeon 1968; 34:479–483.

Report of successful treatment of two cases, one with venous thrombectomy, the other with an axillosubclavian vein bypass using reversed saphenous vein and medial claviculectomy.

1968   Sanders RJ, Monsour JW, Baer SB. Transaxillary first rib resection for the thoracic outlet syndrome. Arch Surg 1968; 97:1014–1023.

Report of 69 cases of transaxillary first rib resection with 90% improvement. Follow-up was short. Plethysmography and arteriography are discussed as diagnostic tools, but these are no longer used in this way.

1968   Swinton NW Jr, Edgett JW Jr, Hall RJ. Primary subclavian-axillary vein thrombosis. Circulation 1968; 38:737–745.

Long-term follow-up of 23 patients with axillosubclavian vein thrombosis who were treated conservatively was disappointing. While initial results were good, after an average follow-up period of eight years, nine patients had major and 12 had minor postphlebitic symptoms. Venous collaterals were present in all patients.

1968   Urschel HC, Paulson DL, McNamara JJ. Thoracic outlet syndrome. Ann Thorac Surg 1968; 6:1–10.

Report of 70 cases of TOS treated as follows: scalenotomy, 26 cases; posterior first rib resection, 33 cases; and transaxillary rib resection, 10 cases. Results were better with rib resection, but follow-up was also much shorter.

1969   Johnson V, Eiseman B. Evaluation of arteriovenous shunt to maintain patency of venous autograft. Am J Surg 1969; 118:915–920.

First clinical case, along with animal studies, demonstrating improved patency rates in venous reconstruction by utilizing a temporary arteriovenous fistula. The principle is to maintain a high flow rate across suture lines and rough areas until they are covered by an endothelial layer.

1969   Lang EK. Arteriographic diagnosis of thoracic outlet syndromes: improved surgical results of corrective procedures selected on basis of arteriographic studies. Medical Times 1969; 97:195–203.

Describes the use of arteriographic findings to select appropriate decompressive operations for TOS. [Editorial comment: This has not been accepted by most surgeons.]

1969   Nelson RM, Davis RW. Thoracic outlet compression syndrome. Ann Thorac Surg 1969; 8:437–451.

Review article on the history and status of TOS in 1969.

1969   Payan J. Electrophysiological localization of ulnar nerve lesions. J Neurol Neurosurg Psychiat 1969; 32:208–220.

A study of measurements of sensory and motor conduction in 46 patients with ulnar neuropathies. The paper describes how electrophysiological tests are employed in localizing these lesions.

1969   Semple JC, Cargill AO. Carpal-tunnel syndrome: results of surgical decompression. Lancet 1969; 1:918–919.

Results of 150 carpal tunnel operations revealed 97% good results for 37 patients operated upon within six months of the onset of symptoms. After six months, the success rate in 113 patients fell to 71% . The overall success rate was 75%. The authors theorize that if fibrosis of the endoneurial and perineurial connective tissue is present for a long enough time, intractable neuropathy can occur.

1969   Woods WW, Compere WE Jr. Electronystagmography in cervical injuries. Int Surg 1969; 51:251–258.

Proposal of a theory that positional dizziness and nystagmus following neck injuries may be due to compression of the vertebral artery at its origin. Nine patients had symptomatic improvement following scalenectomy with removal of all connective tissue from around the subclavian and vertebral arteries. [Editorial comment: This observation has not been confirmed in the medical literature.]

1970   Brodsky AE, Gol A. Costoclavicular syndrome: relief by infraclavicular removal of first rib. South Med J 1970; 63:50–58.

A review of the different syndromes causing TOS symptoms with the conclusion that most cases are due to costoclavicular compression. The infraclavicular approach to first rib resection is described with a report of 22 cases, 20 of whom improved.

1970　　Brooke M, Kaiser K. Muscle fiber types: how many and what kind? Arch Neurol 1970; 23:369–379.

Discussion of the problems in classification of striated muscle. The article stresses the use of ATPase to differentiate type I and type II muscle fibers. Incubation at acid pH can further differentiate type II fibers into three subtypes.

1970　　DeWeese JA, Adams JT, Gaiser DL. Subclavian venous thrombectomy. Circulation 1970; 41 and 42 (suppl. II):158–164.

Report of six new cases of axillosubclavian vein thrombectomy, five with claviculectomy, and one with scalenectomy. Follow-up of 1–12 years showed good results in all patients. The literature, to date, of 23 cases is reviewed and summarized. Claviculectomy is stressed as the best means of exposure for this procedure.

1970　　Gilliatt RW, Le Quesne PM, Logue V, Sumner AJ. Wasting of the hand associated with a cervical rib or band. J Neurol Neurosurg Psychiat 1970; 33:615–624.

Nine cases of brachial plexus palsy due to either a cervical rib or a band running from C-7 to the first rib. Surgical division of the band or removal of the cervical rib resulted in improved sensory symptoms but no recovery of motor function.

1970　　Heymann RL, Whelan TJ. Vascular complications of the thoracic outlet syndrome: a case report. Military Med 1970; 135:793–796.

Single case report of anomalous first rib causing mural thrombus in the subclavian artery, distal emboli, and ischemia. This was treated by resection of the medial clavicle and first rib, resection of the subclavian artery, end-to-end anastomosis, and dorsal sympathectomy. The result was excellent with healing of the gangrene.

1970　　Nelson RM, Jenson CB. Anterior approach for excision of the first rib: surgical technique. Ann Thorac Surg 1970; 9:30–35.

Description of the infraclavicular approach for first rib resection with good results in 20 of 22 patients.

1970　　Roach MR. Reversibility of poststenotic dilatation in the femoral arteries of dogs. Circ Res 1970; 27:985–993.

Poststenotic dilatation in the femoral artery of dogs was produced by banding the artery. After nine days to five months, the band was removed and the poststenotic dilatation disappeared within a few hours in most animals. Disappearance of the dilatation was associated with loss of the murmur over the vessel, suggesting that turbulence causes the dilatation: when the turbulence disappears, so does the dilatation.

1970　　Tilney NL, Griffiths HJG, Edwards EA. Natural history of major venous thrombosis of the upper extremity. Arch Surg 1970; 101:792–796.

Long-term follow-up in 48 cases of upper extremity thrombosis, 17 cases of "effort" or primary thrombosis, and 31 cases of thrombosis secondary to a systemic disease, revealed 74% with residual disability. Late venography in 11 cases demonstrated continuing occlusion in 10. Venous pressure was significantly elevated in symptomatic patients but normal in asymptomatic ones. The right arm was involved in 76% of cases.

1971   Adams JT, DeWeese JA. "Effort" thrombosis of the axillary and subclavian veins. J Trauma 1971; 11:923–930.

Comparison of treatment in 34 cases of upper extremity venous thromboses revealed a 70% incidence of residual symptoms in 14 patients treated with rest and elevation and the same incidence in another 14 patients anticoagulated. In contrast, residual symptoms were present in only one of six patients, 16%, treated with thrombectomy.

1971   Andrews ET, Gentchos EJ, Beller ML. Results of anterior cervical spine fusions done at the hospital of the University of Pennsylvania: a nine year follow up. Clin Orthop 1971; 81:15–20.

Of 41 patients undergoing cervical spine fusion, 70% for degenerative disc disease and 30% for herniated discs, 56% had good improvement; 21% fair; and 23% failed.

1971   Caldwell JW, Crane CR, Krusen EM. Nerve conduction studies: an aid in the diagnosis of the thoracic outlet syndrome. South Med J 1971; 64:210–212.

Description of the technique and normal values of ulnar nerve motor conduction velocities in the diagnosis of thoracic outlet syndrome.

1971   Frankel SA, Hirata I Jr. The scalenus anticus syndrome and competitive swimming: report of two cases. JAMA 1971; 215:1796–1798.

Two case reports of swimmers who developed symptoms of TOS only while swimming. Following anterior scalenotomy, they were both able to return to competitive swimming symptom-free.

1971   Longo MF, Clagett OT, Fairbairn JF. Surgical treatment of thoracic outlet syndrome. Ann Surg 1971; 171:538–542.

Report of 44 cases of first rib resection for TOS symptoms using a posterior approach. Results were good to excellent in 73%, with a 5-month to 18-year follow-up. The pleura was opened in 59%.

1971   Petersen RE, Staab FD, Brintall ES. An evaluation of transaxillary removal of cervical and first rib. J Iowa Med Soc 1971; 61:554–556.

Temporary winging of the scapula occurred in four of six cases of transaxillary first rib resection. Recovery in all four was followed by good clinical results.

1971   Rabinowitz R, Goldfarb D. Surgical treatment of axillosubclavian venous thrombosis: a case report. Surgery 1971; 70:703–706.

Single successful case report of axillary-internal jugular vein bypass using reversed saphenous vein in a patient with postphlebitic symptoms who had previously undergone two unsuccessful repairs. A temporary arteriovenous fistula at the wrist was used for three weeks. The patient was asymptomatic at one-year follow-up.

1971   Roach MR, Melech E. The effect of sonic vibration on isolated human iliac arteries. Can J Physiol Pharmacol 1971; 49:288–291.

Human iliac arteries were exposed to sonic vibrations which made the arteries more distensible. The alteration appeared to be in the elastin rather than the collagen of the arterial wall.

1971   Roos DB. Experience with rib resection for thoracic outlet syndrome. Ann Surg 1971; 173:429–442.

Early results in 276 cases of transaxillary first rib resection demonstrated 88% improvement. Recurrence in 3.6% was treated by second rib resection in seven patients. The technique of rib resection, dorsal sympathectomy, and venous thrombectomy through the axillary incision is described.

1971   Schein CJ. A technic for cervical rib resection. Am J Surg 1971; 121:623–627.

Description of technique of supraclavicular cervical rib resection. Phrenic nerve injury is discussed. When injury is temporary, phrenic recovery occurs in 6 to 12 months. [Editorial comment: In our experience, some cases recover in a few days, others require up to a year or longer.]

1971   Urschel HC Jr, Razzuk MA, Wood RE, Parekh M, Paulson DL. Objective diagnosis (ulnar nerve conduction velocity) and current therapy of the thoracic outlet syndrome. Ann Thorac Surg 1971; 12:608–620.

Analysis of 155 first rib resections for TOS in which ulnar nerve conduction velocities (UNCV) were used as an important diagnostic test. There were 82 cases of transaxillary and 46 cases of posterior rib resection; improvement occurred in 84% with six-month to eight-year follow-up.

1972   Dalal AR, Pitney WR. Primary thrombosis of the axillary-subclavian veins. Med J Aust 1972; 1:633–634.

Four patients with primary upper extremity venous thrombosis were treated with heparin. Initial improvement was good in all four, but residual, postphlebitic symptoms were present in two.

1972   Lang EK. Arteriography and venography in the assessment of thoracic outlet syndromes. South Med J 1972; 65:129–136.

Description of the use of arteriography and venography to diagnose TOS and select the appropriate operation.

1972   Judy KL, Heymann RL. Vascular complications of thoracic outlet syndrome. Am J Surg 1972; 123:521–531.

Report of seven cases of subclavian artery thrombosis and/or aneurysm: five with cervical ribs (four bilateral); one with an abnormal first rib; and one with no osseous abnormality. Treatment included four medial claviculectomies for exposure; five direct arterial repairs, including three grafts; and several dorsal sympathectomies and rib resections. Also reviewed and summarized are 53 additional reported cases between 1956 and 1968.

1972   Ross CA, Uyas US. Thoracic outlet syndrome due to congenital anomalous joint of the first thoracic rib. Can J Surg 1972; 15:186–190.

Single case report of an extra joint in the middle of the first rib, treated by posterior resection of the first rib.

1972   Urschel HC, Razzuk MA. Management of the thoracic outlet syndrome. N Engl J Med 1972; 286:1140–1143.

Description of ulnar nerve conduction velocities (UNCV) and their use in diagnosing TOS. Following first rib resection, there is a high correlation between symptomatic improvement and a return of UNCV to normal range. [Editorial comment: These data have been disputed—see Wilbourn and Urschel, 1984.]

1973   Charrette EJP, Iyengar KSR, Lynn RB, Challis TW. Symptomatic nonthrombotic subclavian vein obstruction: surgical relief in six patients. Vasc Surg 1973; 7:220–231.

Cine-venography was used to diagnose intermittent subclavian vein obstruction, manifested by intermittent swelling, aching, and cyanosis. Report of six cases treated successfully by operation: four first rib resections, one claviculectomy, and one division of a congenital band.

1973   Cox CL, Cocks GR. Headaches treated by anterior scalenotomy. J Med Assoc State Ala 1973; 43:385–387.

Anterior scalenotomy gave good-to-excellent relief of occipital headaches in 82% of 258 patients with severe occipital headaches. The indications for surgery included an appropriate clinical picture and relief of scalene muscle tenderness and headaches with an occipital nerve block.

1973   Dubowitz V, Brooke M. Muscle biopsy: A modern approach, Philadelphia: W.B. Saunders, 1973.

Basic textbook on muscle physiology.

1973   Graham GG, Lincoln BM. Anterior resection of first rib for thoracic outlet syndrome. Am J Surg 1973; 126:803–806.

Technique of supraclavicular first rib resection is described with 90% improvement in 70 patients. Follow-up was beyond 2 years in 65%. Postop complications included two cases of temporary brachial plexus palsy, which cleared up within one month.

1973   Hoofer WD, Burnett AD. Thoracic outlet relief. J Kansas Med Soc 1973; 74:329–331, 352.

Report of 135 cases of transaxillary first rib resection with 100% good results. [Editorial comment: This is only article claiming 100% relief, which makes us question the follow-up.]

1973   Hobson RW, Croom RD, Swan KG. Hemodynamics of the distal arteriovenous fistula in venous reconstruction. J Surg Res 1973; 14:483–489.

In 10 dogs, arteriovenous fistulae maintained the patency of all venous reconstructions with venous grafts. Complications included a "steal" of blood from the distal limb, coldness, and edema. In this study, size of the fistula did not affect the results or complications.

1973   Krogness K. Ulnar trunk conduction studies in the diagnosis of the thoracic outlet syndrome. Acta Chir Scand 1973; 139:597–603.

Five TOS patients had delayed ulnar nerve conduction velocities (UNCV) preoperatively with return to normal in four of the five postoperatively. The fifth patient, whose UNCV did not return to normal, did not experience symptomatic relief either.

1973   Maxwell L, Faulkner J, Lieberman D. Histochemical manifestations of age and endurance training in skeletal muscle fibers. Am J Physiol 1973; 224:356–361.

Different muscle fibers were studied in guinea pigs 1–14 weeks of age, with and without muscle training. Training caused soleus muscle fibers to hypertrophy while plantaris muscle shifted composition to a higher proportion of high oxidative fibers without hypertrophy.

1973   Mercier CP, Branchereau A, Dimarino V, Adhoute B, Tournigand P. Venous thrombosis of the upper limb: effort or compression. J Cardiovasc Surg (Torino) 1973; Spec. No.: 519–522.

In 21 cases of upper limb venous compression, thrombosis was present in seven and intermittent, nonthrombotic obstruction in 14. Diagnosis was by dynamic venography. Transaxillary resection of not only the first rib, but also the subclavius muscle and tendon were performed in 13 patients with early symptomatic relief in all but one. The authors stress the importance of dividing the subclavius muscle.

1973   Mulder DS, Greenwood FAH, Brooks CE. Posttraumatic thoracic outlet syndrome. J Trauma 1973; 13:706–715.

Report of seven cases of TOS due to fractures of clavicle or first rib. These were treated by resection of clavicle or first rib, along with the bony callus, which is responsible for neurovascular compression and the symptoms.

1973   Roeder DK, Mills M, McHale JJ, Shepard BM, Ashworth HE. First rib resection in the treatment of thoracic outlet syndrome: transaxillary and posterior thoracoplasty approaches. Ann Surg 1973; 178:49–52.

The results of 26 transaxillary and 11 posterior first rib resections were identical—92% improvement. The advantages and disadvantages of each approach are compared.

1973   Somerdike JM, Ostermiller WE Jr, Salyer JM, Camarata SJ. Surgical management of thoracic outlet syndrome by first rib resection. Am Surg 1973; 39:250–253.

Report of 20 cases of transaxillary first rib resection with relief of symptoms in 19. Many patients had pain along the dorsal spine and edge of the scapula that was not relieved by surgery.

1973   Stayman JW. Thoracic outlet syndrome. Surg Clin North Am 1973; 667–671.

There were good results in 90% of 40 cases of first rib resection. Three different routes for surgery are discussed.

1973   Upton ARM, McComas AJ. The double crush in nerve-entrapment syndromes. Lancet 1973; 2:359–362.

In 115 patients with carpal tunnel syndrome or ulnar nerve lesions at the elbow, 81 cases (70%) also had electrophysiological evidence of a compressive neck lesion. This is the first description of the "double-crush syndrome."

1973   Urschel HC, Hyland JW, Solis RM, Paulson DL. Thoracic outlet syndrome masquerading as coronary artery disease (pseudoangina). Ann Thorac Surg 1973; 16:239–248.

Chest pain suggesting angina was the presenting complaint in 44 patients who proved to have TOS, although 13 patients also had coronary artery disease. Ulnar nerve conduction velocities (UNCV) were used to diagnose TOS. Treatment was conservative for UNCV above 55 m/sec, or transaxillary first rib resection for UNCV below 55 m/sec. Anatomic pain pathways of angina and irritation of the brachial plexus are similar.

1973   Van Echo DA, Sickles EA, Wiernik PH. Thoracic outlet syndrome, supraclavicular adenopathy, Hodgkin's Disease. Ann Int Med 1973; 78:608–609.

This is the only case report of TOS caused by neurovascular compression from enlarged lymph nodes in Hodkin's Disease. Shrinkage of the supraclavicular mass with irradiation relieved all symptoms.

1974   Buchthal F, Rosenfalck A, Trojaborg W. Electrophysiological findings in entrapment of the median nerve at wrist and elbow. J Neurol Neurosurg Psychiat 1974; 37:340–360.

Motor and sensory conduction velocities were measured in 117 patients with carpal tunnel syndrome and 11 with median nerve compression at the elbow. These were compared to 190 normals. Fifteen percent of carpal tunnel patients had clinical and electrophysiological signs of ulnar involvement. Electromyelography (EMG) was more useful than conduction velocities for nerve compression at the elbow.

1974   Gaylis H. A rational approach to venous thrombectomy. Surg Gynecol Obstet 1974; 138:864–868.

Report of four cases of upper extremity and three cases of lower extremity venous thrombectomy. In three of the arm cases claviculectomy was used for exposure; in two instances, vein patch closures were employed. Postoperatively, three of the four upper extremity cases were asymptomatic as were two of the three lower extremity cases. No disability resulted from removal of the medial two-thirds of the clavicle.

1974   Johnson CR. Treatment of TOS by removal of first rib and related entrapments through posterolateral approach: a 22 year approach. J Thorac Cardiovasc Surg 1974; 68: 536–545.

Using a posterior thoracotomy approach in 110 cases of TOS, good results were obtained in 92%.

1974   Mathes SJ, Salam AA. Subclavian artery aneurysm; sequela of thoracic outlet syndrome. Surgery 1974; 76:506–510.

Case report of subclavian artery aneurysm, thrombosis, distal emboli, and gangrene. This was treated by supraclavicular cervical rib excision, aneurysm resection, and arterial reconstruction with end-to-end anastomosis. Ischemia persisted, requiring later hand amputation. Reasons for preferring the supraclavicular approach are discussed.

1975   Colton T. Statistics in medicine. Boston: Little Brown, 1975; 237–250.

Description of the life-table method of statistically recording results.

1975   Dale WA. Management of thoracic outlet syndrome. Ann Surg 1975; 181:575–585.

Review of 153 cases of TOS. EMG and arteriography were of no help in making a diagnosis; history was most important. Conservative treatment should always be tried first. Results in 56 operations were excellent in 56%, partial improvement in 36%, and failure in 7%.

1975   Daube JR. Nerve conduction studies in thoracic outlet syndrome. Neurology (Minneap) 1975; 25:347.

Mean sensory and motor conduction velocities across the thoracic outlet were not statistically different between 27 TOS patients and 27 controls. There were significant differences in evoked potential amplitudes.

1975   Glass BA. The relationship of axillary venous thrombosis to the thoracic outlet compression syndrome. Ann Thorac Surg 1975; 19:613–621.

In a seies of 41 transaxillary first rib resections for TOS, there were eight patients with venous obstruction. Four had venous thrombosis, the other four nonthrombotic obstruction. The right arm was involved in seven of the eight cases. Management of four cases is described in detail.

1975   Kremer RM, Ahlquist RE Jr. Thoracic outlet compression syndrome. Am J Surg 1975; 130:612–616.

Report of 64 operations for TOS, including 48 transaxillary first rib resections, with 85% good to excellent results. There were six operations for rib regeneration. Most symptoms were neurologic; ulnar nerve conduction velocities (UNCV) were normal and of no help.

1975   London GW. Normal ulnar nerve conduction velocity across the thoracic outlet: comparison of two measuring techniques. J Neurol Neurosurg Psychiatry 1975; 38:756–760.

Compares caliper and tape measurement of nerve length in performing ulnar nerve conduction velocities (UNCV). The significance in the diagnosis of thoracic outlet syndrome is discussed.

1975   Paresien VM. The "cervical syndrome." J Maine Med Assoc 1976; 67:66–68.

A review of conservative treatment of 130 patients with pain and stiffness of the neck, shoulders, and dorsal spine area and often headache, dizziness, and eye and ear symptoms. Whiplash injury was a common cause. Electrical stimulation with needles gave better results than "standard" forms of therapy. Pending litigation did not affect the results of treatment.

1975   Porter JM, Seaman AJ, Common HH, Posch J, Eidemiller LR, Calhoun AD. A comparison of heparin and streptokinase in the treatment of venous thrombosis. Am Surgeon 1975; 41:511–519.

Complete lysis and restoration of valve function occurred in only one of 26 patients receiving heparin compared to 6 of 23 patients receiving streptokinase. Among patients with symptoms for three days or less, streptokinase achieved complete lysis in 50%. The incidence of complications was similar in the two groups but they were more severe in the patients treated with streptokinase.

1975   Sadler TR Jr, Rainer WG, Twombley G. Thoracic outlet compression: application of positional arteriographic and nerve conduction studies. Am J Surg 1975; 130:704–706.

Positional ulnar nerve conduction velocities (UNCV) are described as an aide in the diagnosis of TOS. They were positive in 88% of patients operated upon for thoracic outlet syndrome.

1975   Sanders RJ. Subcuticular skin closure: description of technique. J Dermatol Surg 1975; 1:61–64.

Technique of subcuticular skin closure showing how to bury all knots.

1975   Timmis H. Discussion in Dale WA: Management of thoracic outlet syndrome. Ann Surg 1975; 181:585.

In 175 cases of TOS, a history of hyperextension neck injury, headache, neck pain, and chest pain were common. Dizziness and tinnitus were seen less often. Scalene muscle injury is the probable cause.

1975   Tyson RR, Kaplan GF. Modern concepts of diagnosis and treatment of the thoracic outlet syndrome. Orthop Clin North Am 1975; 6:507–519.

Good general review of TOS. No data.

1976   Cherington M. Ulnar conduction velocity in thoracic outlet syndrome. N Engl J Med 1976; 294:1185.

Measurement of ulnar nerve conduction velocities (UNCV) in over 200 normal subjects yielded a value that was the same as the "abnormal" values in TOS patients as reported by Urschel in 1971. This questions the reliability of UNCV in the diagnosis of TOS.

1976   Clein LJ. The droopy shoulder syndrome. Can Med Assoc J 1976; 114:343–344.

Report of three cases of neck and shoulder pain, one with finger paresthesia, relieved by shoulder-strengthening exercises. Suggested theory is that droopy shoulders cause traction on the brachial plexus and subsequent neurologic symptoms.

1976   Doty DB, Baker W. Bypass of superior vena cava with spiral vein graft. Ann Thorac Surg 1976; 22:490–493.

Technique for creating a large-diameter vein graft is described in which a saphenous vein segment is opened longitudinally and sutured in spiral fashion over a mandrill of the desired caliber. The technique was used successfully in a 49-year-old man to bypass the superior vena cava. He was asymptomatic at 18-month follow-up.

1976   Gilliatt RW, Ebbetts JH, Jones BV. Thoracic outlet compression syndrome. Br Med J 1976; 1:1274–1275.

Editorial comment questioning the large number of rib resections being performed on patients with neurogenic TOS who lack objective diagnostic criteria. The authors claim the incidence of TOS is rare.

1976   Gjores JE, Svendler CA, Todoreskov R. Thrombosis of the subclavian vein—a feature of the thoracic outlet syndrome. Acta Chir 1976; 465:78–79.

Report of two patients who presented with upper extremity venous thrombosis and were initially treated conservatively, and whose subsequent history revealed symptoms of neurogenic TOS. First rib resection relieved symptoms in one patient and the other is considering surgery.

1976   Hashmonai M, Schramek A, Farbstein J. Cephalic vein cross-over bypass for subclavian vein thrombosis: a case report. Surgery 1976; 80:563–564.

Single case report of subclavian vein bypass using the cephalic vein of the normal side. A temporary arteriovenous fistula in the antecubital space of the diseased arm complimented the procedure. Venography six weeks postop at the time of fistula closure revealed good functioning of the graft and the patient noticed symptomatic relief.

1976   Hongladhrom T. "F"-Wave conduction velocity in thoracic outlet syndrome. N Engl J Med 1976; 295:1382–1383.

Editorial comment on F-wave conduction velocities as a way to avoid stimulating the nerve at Erb's point. This holds promise of providing an objective criterion with which to diagnose TOS. [Editorial comment: It is now felt that these changes are nonspecific.]

1976   Martin J, Gaspard DJ, Johnston PW, Kohl RD, Dietrick W. Vascular manifestations of the thoracic outlet syndrome: a surgical urgency. Arch Surg 1976; 111:779–782.

Two case reports of patients with cervical ribs, subclavian artery compression, poststenotic dilatation, and mural thrombosis. Treatment was surgical resection of the cervical and first ribs, thrombectomy, and arterial reconstruction using a combined supra- and infraclavicular approach.

1976   Peto R, Pike MC, Armitage P, Breslow NE, Cox DR, Howard SV, Mantel N, McPherson K, Peto J, Smith PG. Design and analysis of randomized trials required prolonged observations of each patient. I. introduction and design. Br J Cancer 1976; 34:585.

Description of statistical log-rank test used to evaluate differences between life-table results of different operations.

1976   Roos DB. Congenital anomalies associated with thoracic outlet syndrome: anatomy, symptoms, diagnosis and treatment. Am J Surg 1976; 132:771–778.

Nine-hundred-eighty transaxillary first rib resections in 776 patients plus 58 cadaver dissections led to the description of seven types of anomalous bands in the thoracic outlet area. There is a very high incidence of these bands in TOS patients, which probably predispose these patients to develop symptoms of neurovascular compression. Clinical features and diagnostic tests are discussed.

1976   Sadler TR Jr. Discussion in Urschel, et al.: Reoperation for recurrent thoracic outlet syndrome. Ann Thorac Surg 1976; 21:24–25.

In two patients with recurrent TOS, reoperation through a supraclavicular incision demonstrated the middle scalene muscle binding down the brachial plexus. It is not necessary to use the posterior approach, exclusively, for recurrent TOS.

1976   Urschel HD Jr, Razzuk MA, Albers JE, Wood RE, Paulson DL. Reoperation for recurrent thoracic outlet syndrome. Ann Thorac Surg 1976; 21:19–25.

Recurrent TOS following transaxillary or supraclavicular first rib resection was treated by a posterior thoracotomy approach in 30 patients. Most recurrences developed within three months of the original operation. Some improvement occurred in 90%.

1977   Banis JC, Rich N, Whelan TJ. Ischemia of the upper extremity due to noncardiac emboli. Am J Surg 1977; 134:131–139.

Mural thrombosis in the subclavian artery due to cervical or abnormal first ribs was the commonest etiology of microemboli in nine patients with upper extremity ischemia. An atheroma as the embolic source was found in only one patient. Treatment of the subclavian thrombus includes not only excision of the offending osseous structure, but also resection and reconstruction of the subclavian artery by either end-to-end anastomosis or a graft. In two of their five cases, the clavicle was removed for exposure.

1977   Campbell CB, Chandler JG, Tegtmeyer CJ, Bernstein EF. Axillary, subclavian, and brachiocephalic vein obstruction. Surgery 1977; 82:816–826.

Review of 25 patients with upper extremity venous obstruction, eight with primary or effort thrombosis; ten with secondary thrombosis; six with nonthrombotic obstruction; and one with a hypercoagulable state. Venography in 22 patients usually made the diagnosis but often failed to define the proximal extent of the disease. Twelve patients were anticoagulated; six had surgery to remove or bypass the obstruction. Chronic morbidity depended more on etiology than on treatment. Secondary thrombosis resulted in no persistent symptoms whether the patient was treated or not; nonthrombotic obstruction was most difficult to relieve. While operative treatment often improved venous outflow, it frequently did not relieve all symptoms.

1977   Capistrant TD. Thoracic outlet syndrome in whiplash injury. Ann Surg 1977; 185: 175–178.

TOS developed in 35 patients following whiplash or cervical strain injuries. Most improved on conservative therapy. Only two were operated upon. Physical exam revealed tenderness over the scalene and trapezius muscles and reduced range of motion of the neck.

1977   Crane C, Johnson R. Nerve conduction velocity and doppler evaluations of thoracic outlet syndrome. S Med J 1977; 67:269–270.

There was a high correlation between the results of ulnar nerve conduction velocities (UNCV) and Doppler flow studies in patients with paresthesia or pain in the involved arm.

1977   Eisen A, Schomer D, Melmed C. The application of F-wave measurements in the differentiation of proximal and distal upper limb entrapments. Neurology 1977; 27:662–668.

Conduction velocities of the proximal segments of median and ulnar nerves can be measured by evoking F-wave responses. This technique can be useful in differentiating between proximal and distal nerve entrapment.

1977   Gainer JB, Nugent GR. Carpal tunnel syndrome: report of 430 operations. South Med J 1977; 70:325–328.

Follow up in 71% of 430 patients who responded to a questionnaire revealed that 78% had occupations involving use of their hands and the dominant hand was involved in two-thirds. Relief was excellent in 51%, good in 31%, and fair in 10%.

1977   Jacobson JH, Haimov M. Venous revascularization of the arm: report of three cases. Surgery 1977; 81:599–604.

Postphlebitic arm symptoms were relieved in two patients with internal jugular-subclavian vein bypass and in one patient with direct subclavian endovenectomy. The latter procedure was performed through a median sternotomy with division of the clavicle and first rib. All three patients had permanent symptomatic relief.

1977   Lascelles RG, Mohr PD, Neary D, Bloor K. The thoracic outlet syndrome. Brain 1977; 100:601–612.

Supraclavicular cervical rib resection in 18 patients and scalenotomy in 11 patients resulted in improvement in all but two cases.

1977   Sargent A, Davies C, Edwards R, Maunder C, Young A. Functional and structural changes after disuse of human muscle. Clin Sci Mol Med 1977; 52:337–342.

Bilateral muscle biopsies from seven patients with unilateral casts revealed a 42% reduction in cross-sectional area form the vastus lateralis of the injured compared to the uninjured leg. Both type I and type II fibers were affected equally. Total leg volume was reduced 12% in the injured leg; net maximum oxygen consumption was also reduced.

1977   Stallworth JM, Quinn GJ, Aiken AF. Is rib resection necessary for relief of thoracic outlet syndrome? Ann Surg 1977; 185:581–592.

Operations were performed in 146 patients with upper extremity symptoms and a diagnosis of TOS. Muscle operations were the commonest: pectoralis minor tenotomy in 129 and scalenotomy in 38; bone resection was done in only 10 cases. Successful results were achieved in 92%.

1977   Tomonaga M. Histochemical and ultrastructural changes in senile human skeletal muscle. J Am Geriatr Soc 1977; 25:125–131.

Eight muscle biopsies from 79 patients aged 60–90 were examined by histochemical and electron microscopic methods. Various grades of type II fiber atrophy and neuropathic change were prominent features. There were several electron microscopic features that were similar to those reported for various neuromuscular diseases. Factors associated with aging apparently act on the motor neurons causing the neuropathic and myopathic changes seen in muscles of the elderly.

1978   Gilliatt RW, Willison RG, Dietz V, Williams IR. Peripheral nerve conduction in patients with a cervical rib and band. Ann Neurol 1978; 4:124–129.

Fourteen patients, 13 women, with hand wasting and cervical ribs and bands, underwent supraclavicular cervical rib excision and division of bands. Preoperatively, ulnar sensory action potentials (SAP) demonstrated a reduction in amplitude without a comparable change in velocity. Postoperatively, this did not improve, nor was muscle wasting corrected. The asymptomatic arms of the same patients, also with cervical ribs but no muscle wasting, had normal SAP amplitudes.

1978   Keens T, Chen V, Pravin P, O'Brien P, Levison H, Ianuzzo C. Cellular adaptations of the ventilatory muscles to a chronic increased respiratory load. J Appl Physiol 1979; 44: 905–908.

Increased respiratory loads were produced in rats by banding the trachea. Five weeks later, diaphragm muscle demonstrated an increase in the proportion of type I, slow twitch, fibers while intercostal muscles showed no change. This suggests that slow twitch fibers are better than fast twitch for sustained, prolonged fiber contraction and represents adaptation by the muscle to new loads.

1978   Keens T, Bryan C, Levison H, Ianuzzo C. Developmental pattern of muscle fiber types in human ventilatory muscles. J Appl Physiol 1978; 44:909–913.

High oxidative type I fibers have greater endurance and greater resistance to fatigue than type II fibers. Postmortem specimens from the diaphragms of premature, newborn, and older infants revealed only 19% type I fibers in premature infants compared to 54% in newborns and 65% in older infants. The lack of enough type I fibers in premature infants might explain their high rate of ventilatory failure.

1978   Stanton PE Jr, McClusky DA, Richardson HD, Lamis PA: Thoracic outlet syndrome: a comprehensive evaluation. South Med J 1978; 71:1070–1073.

There was 80% good and 10% fair improvement following transaxillary first rib resection in 50 patients. Ulnar nerve conduction velocities and directional doppler studies were useful in making a diagnosis.

1978   Thomas GI, Jones TW, Stavney LS, Manhas DR. Thoracic outlet syndrome. Am Surg 1978; 44:483–495.

Supraclavicular first rib resection was followed by 92% good to excellent results in 38 patients with TOS. Trauma was present in the history of 42%. Loss of the radial pulse with the arms at 90 degrees in AER was present in 92%. The operative technique is described. Temporary brachial plexus neuritis was a postop complication in 13%.

1978   Williams HT, Carpenter NH. Surgical treatment of the thoracic outlet syndrome. Arch Surg 1978; 113:850–852.

Following transaxillary first rib resection, 79% of 34 patients with neurologic symptoms had good improvement while only 50% of eight patients with arterial symptoms were better. Results of nerve conduction studies were disappointing.

1978   Woods WW. Thoracic outlet syndrome. West J Med 1978; 128:9–12.

Of 1,958 patients with cervical injuries, 459 (23%) were diagnosed as having TOS. Of these, 185 failed to respond to conservative treatment and underwent anterior scalenotomy and brachial plexus neuroplasty with 75% good and 11% fair improvement; average follow-up was a few years. Eight patients had undergone scalenotomy previously without improvement; reoperation in these patients consisted of complete neurolysis and resulted in improvement in all eight.

1979   Cox CJ, Cocks GR. Occipital neuralgia. J Med Assoc (Alabama) 1979; 23–32.

Occipital neuralgia and headaches were relieved in 86% of 395 patients who were treated with anterior scalenotomy. This suggests that the headaches were due to muscle spasm secondary to scalene anticus syndrome.

1979   Dorazio RA, Ezzet F. Arterial complications of the thoracic outlet syndrome. Am J Surg 1979; 138:246–250.

Report of five cases of distal emboli from subclavian artery thrombus secondary to arterial compression in the thoracic outlet. The cause was a cervical rib in three instances, one abnormal first rib, and one case of compression by an anomalous band with no osseous abnormality. Treatment was excision of the causative structure through a supraclavicular incision with removal of the medial half of the clavicle; arterial resection and repair by a variety of methods; and thrombectomy, if possible. Postoperatively, symptoms improved in all patients, but radial pulses were often not restored because the patients were operated upon too late in the course of their disease.

1979   Etheredge S, Wilbur B, Stoney RJ. Thoracic outlet syndrome. Am J Surg 1979; 138:175–182.

Vascular complications of TOS are reported in 11 patients, five arterial and six venous. All arterial cases were due to osseous abnormalities and treated through a supraclavicular approach. One claviculectomy and one infraclavicular incision were added for better exposure. All patients had direct arterial reconstruction and all received accompanying dorsal sympathectomies. There were four good results and one amputation. All six patients with venous obstruction, four due to thrombosis, improved following transaxillary first rib resection (five patients) or claviculectomy with rib resection (one patient).

1979   Kelly TR. Thoracic outlet syndrome: current concepts of treatment. Ann Surg 1979; 190:657–662.

Transaxillary first rib resection in 304 patients resulted in complete relief in 85% and partial relief in 7%. Diagnosis is by clinical criteria; angiography and EMG studies are of limited value. Symptoms were neurological in 96%.

1979   Lemmens HAJ. Thoracodorsal sympathectomy en bloc. Vasc Surg 1979; 13:331–335.

Technique of posterior, extended dorsal sympathectomy is described in which the dorsal roots and spinal ganglia of T-2 and T-3, the ventral roots of T-2 and T-3, and the sympathetic ganglia of T-2 and T-3 are excised, en bloc. Results of 78 operations in 63 patients depended upon the nature and progression of the primary disease. While the majority of patients improved initially, 24% had deterioration of the result due to disease progression.

1979   McGough EC, Pearce MB, Byrne JP. Management of thoracic outlet syndrome. J Ther Card Med 1979; 77:169–174.

Conservative therapy was used to treat 1,200 patients with TOS over a five-year period. Only 9% went on to transaxillary first rib resection, 80% of whom had complete relief and 13% partial relief. There was a history of trauma in 69% of men and 27% of women. Results of ulnar nerve conduction velocities (UNCV) did not correlate with results of surgery.

1979   Prescott SM, Tikaff G. Deep venous thrombosis of the upper extremity: a reappraisal. Circulation 1979; 59:350–355.

Twelve patients with upper extremity venous thrombosis were all treated with heparin and conservative measures. Of ten available for follow-up, six were asymptomatic and four had minimal symptoms.

1979   Prior AL, Wilson LA, Gosling RG, Yates AK, Russell RWR. Retrograde cerebral embolism. Lancet 1979; 2:1044–1047.

Report of four cases of cerebral emboli from the right subclavian artery: three had cervical ribs, the fourth arteriosclerosis. Retrograde propagation of thrombus was thought to be the cause in each case. Treatment is directed towards eliminating the source of the emboli, as little can be done for the cerebral damage already present.

1979   Roos DB. New concepts of thoracic outlet syndrome that explain etiology, symptoms, diagnosis, and treatment. Vasc Surg 1979; 13:313–321.

Nine different types of congenital bands in the thoracic outlet area, most accompanying the anterior or middle scalene muscles, are described as the cause or underlying predisposition for TOS symptoms. Diagnosis and treatment are discussed.

1979   Sanders RJ, Monsour JW, Gerber FG, Adams WRA, Thompson N. Scalenectomy versus first rib resection for treatment of the thoracic outlet syndrome. Surgery 1979; 85:109–121.

Using life-table methods, the improvement rate of transaxillary first rib resection (214 cases) and anterior and middle scalenectomy (239 cases) were virtually identical to five years. Good to excellent results were initially 85–86% and fell to 63–64% at five years.

1979   Sanders RJ, Monsour JW, Gerber WJ. Recurrent thoracic outlet syndrome following first rib resection. Vasc Surg 1979; 13:325–330.

Supraclavicular exploration was performed in 33 cases of recurrence following transaxillary first rib resection. In every case, the anterior scalene muscle had reattached to the subclavian artery and brachial plexus. Anterior scalenectomy gave good relief in 87% of patients with recurrent symptoms. In the three patients with persistent symptoms, there was no improvement.

1979   Taylor MF. Twelve years experience with thoracic outlet syndrome. J Fla Med Assoc 1979; 66:1022–1024.

Series of 351 transaxillary first rib resections in 256 patients. Bilateral operations at different times were done in 36%, suggesting that this number had derived enough improvement from the first side to undergo surgery again. Trauma was the cause in 60% indicating fibroses and contracture of the scalene muscles as the possible mechanism. In addition to paresthesia and pain, other common complaints were dropping objects, inability to comb the hair, and severe occipital headaches. Diagnosis was primarily by history and confirmed by supraclavicular tenderness and positional maneuvers. Angiography was helpful only in vascular cases. Postoperative improvement was seen in 90%.

1979   Thompson JB, Hernandez IA. The thoracic outlet syndrome: a second look. Am J Surg 1979; 138:251–253.

Supraclavicular first rib resection in 15 patients resulted in good improvement in 87% with an average follow-up of over two years. EMG studies were normal in five cases, abnormal in only three.

1979   Wulff CH, Gilliatt RW. F-waves in patients with hand wasting caused by a cervical rib and band. Muscle Nerve 1979; 2:452–457.

F-wave latencies were consistently prolonged following ulnar nerve stimulation at the wrist in patients with unilateral hand wasting. This change did not reverse following surgical decompression of the nerve.

1980   Chan RC, Paine KWE, Varughese G. Ulnar neuropathy at the elbow: comparison of simple decompression and anterior transposition. Neurosurgery 1980; 7:545–550.

Review of 235 cases of ulnar nerve compression at the elbow, 115 treated with simple decompression and 120 with anterior transposition. Eighty-two percent improved with a higher success rate in those treated with simple decompression.

1980   Craven PR Jr, Green DP. Cubital tunnel syndrome: treatment by medial epicondylectomy. J Bone Joint Surg 1980; 62A:986–989.

Thirty patients with ulnar nerve entrapment at the elbow underwent medial epicondylectomy with anterior transposition of the ulnar nerve. With an average followup of 22 months there was 81% improvement.

1980   Crawford FA. Thoracic outlet syndrome. Surg Clin North Am 1980; 60:947–956.

Good general review of subject. A summary of first rib resection from seven studies in the literature comprising a total of 1131 cases revealed 84% good-excellent, 10% fair, and 6% poor results.

1980   Daskalakis E, Bouhoutsos J. Subclavian and axillary compression of musculoskeletal origin. Br J Surg 1980; 67:573–576.

Twenty instances of upper extremity venous compression were found in 14 patients. Venography and venous pressures were the primary diagnostic tools. Large increases in venous pressure by fist clenching exercise was regarded as indicative of significant intermittent nonthrombotic venous obstruction. Nine patients had thromboses, five of whom had intermittent compression on the contralateral side. There were 11 cases of nonthrombotic venous obstruction, 10 of whom were operated upon. All operations were division of soft tissues, usually anterior scalene and subclavius muscles.

1980   Gergoudis R, Barnes RW. Thoracic outlet arterial compression: prevalence in normal persons. Angiology 1980; 31:538–541.

In 130 normal individuals, 53% had positive Adson's tests; 19% had positive hyperabduction maneuvers; and 14% had positive costoclavicular maneuvers. At least one thoracic outlet compression maneuver was abnormal in 60% of the subjects—47% of the women, and 80% of the men. Caution must be used in diagnosing TOS solely on the basis of an abnormal compression test.

1980   Kobinia GS, Olbert OJ, Denck H. Chronic vascular disease of upper extremity: radiologic and clinical features. Cardiovasc Intervent Radiol 1980; 3:25–41.

Upper extremity arterial disease occurs from arteriosclerotic changes, thoracic outlet compression, and angiospastic disease of the hand. The role of angiography in diagnosing these conditions is beautifully demonstrated by excellent x-ray examples of these various lesions.

1980   Murphy TO, Clinton AP, Kanar EA, McAlexander RA. Subclavicular approach to first rib resection. Am J Surg 1980; 139:634–636.

Infraclavicular first rib resection in 22 cases resulted in 73% excellent, 18% fair, and 9% poor results. The same incision is used for a transpleural dorsal sympathectomy.

1980   Pollack EW. Surgical anatomy of the TOS. Surg Gynecol Obstet 1980; 150:97–103.

Detailed description of the anatomical spaces in the thoracic outlet area, their borders, contents, and variations.

1980   Roos DB. Recurrent thoracic outlet syndrome after first rib resection. Acta Chir Belg 1980; 79:363–372.

Two symptom complexes, upper and lower plexus, are described for recurrent TOS. Reoperation removed the anterior scalene muscle from scarred attachments to the plexus in upper plexus recurrence; for lower plexus recurrence, the lower nerves of the plexus were freed from the chest wall by neurolysis. Good results were obtained in 95% of 76 patients.

1980   Wood VE, Frykman GK. Winging of the scapula as a complication of first rib resection. Clin Orthop 1980; 149:160–163.

Winging of the scapula occurred in six of 48 transaxillary first rib resections; four were temporary and two were permanent. Possible causes are cutting the nerve near the posterior corner of the rib by not staying close to rib or removal of the first interdigitation of the serratus anterior muscle.

1980   Youmans CR Jr, Smiley RH. Thoracic outlet syndrome with negative Adson's and hyperabduction maneuvers. Vasc Surg 1980; 14:318–329.

Review of 258 cases of transaxillary first rib resection with 75% excellent, 16% fair, and 9% poor results. Average follow-up was 34 months. Patients with pending litigation had slightly poorer results while those with job-related symptoms had a much lower incidence of good results.

1981   Glover JL, Worth RM, Bendick PJ, Hall PV, Markand OM. Evoked responses in the diagnosis of thoracic outlet syndrome. Surgery 1981; 89:86–93.

Introduction of somatosensory evoked potentials (SSEP) as a diagnostic test for TOS. In 22 operated cases, there were 15 abnormal results to testing. Postoperatively, there were good responses to surgery in patients with positive as well as in those with negative responses to SSEP; results of the test did not correlate well with results of surgery.

1981   Haggmark T, Jansson E, Eriksson E. Fiber type area and metabolic potential of the thigh muscle in man after knee surgery and immobilization. Int J Sports Med 1981; 2:12–17.

The immobilized quadriceps muscle underwent selective type I fiber atrophy and reduction in cross-sectional area of type I fibers.

1981   Hare WCS, Rogers WJ. The scalenus medius band and the seventh cervical transverse process. Diag Imaging 1981; 50:263–268.

Single case report of woman with TOS symptoms who was significantly relieved by transection of a short taut band between the tip of C-7 and the first rib. This was compressing the lowest nerve of the brachial plexus. X-rays in this patient and several others in the literature reveal the tip of the C-7 transverse process to be pointed and turned down. This appearance is probably more important than the length of the C-7 transverse process.

1981   Hempel GK, Rucher AH Jr, Wheeler CG, Hunt DG, Bukhari HI. Supraclavicular resection of the first rib for thoracic outlet syndrome. Am J Surg 1981; 141:213–215.

Following supraclavicular first rib resection in 433 cases, 84% had good, 13% fair, and 3% poor results. The surgical technique is described. Cervical ribs were present in 4%, abnormal first ribs in 1%, and venous compression in 3%. Adson's test was positive in 39%, but was also positive on the contralateral, asymptomatic side in 34%. Radial pulse decrease in the 90 degree AER position was noted in 66% and scalene tenderness in 28%.

1981   Iraci G, Negrin P, Zampieri P, Fardin P, Pardatscher K, Fiore D. Cervical rib syndrome: a neurosurgical experience with a series of 38 cases. Int Surg 1981; 66:325–330.

Following cervical and sometimes first rib resection, 15 of 27 patients (56%) were improved. Reasons for failure are discussed.

1981   Lord JW Jr. Thoracic outlet syndromes: real or imaginary? N Y State J Med 1981; 81:1488–1489.

Editorial questioning the use of clinical criteria alone to diagnose TOS. It is pointed out that in 1978, only seven patients were operated upon for TOS in four major hospitals in New York City. It is suggested that surgeons doing large numbers of these operations are doing so on inadequate indications (by the author's criteria).

1981   Pairolero PC, Walls JT, Payne WS, Hollier LH, Fairbairn JF. Subclavian-axillary artery aneurysms. Surgery 1981; 90:757–763.

Of 31 subclavian-axillary aneurysms operated upon at the Mayo Clinic between 1960 and 1980, six were due to poststenotic dilatation with TOS, 12 to atherosclerosis, and 10 to trauma. Treatment was TOS decompression in four; interposition graft in 11; lateral repair in eight; and ligation in four. In two of the five patients in whom the clavicle was removed for exposure, an unstable shoulder was present three and five years, respectively, postoperatively. Because of this, it is suggested that if claviculectomy is necessary, the clavicle should be reconstructed at the end of the operation.

1981   Walton J. Discussion of voluntary muscles. Ediburgh: Churchill Livingstone, 1981: 197–198.

Description of microscopic inflammatory changes observed in muscles following mild injuries, including the sternocleidomastoid and scalene muscles. The pattern includes overgrowth of connective tissue, giant and atrophic muscle fibers, and inflammatory cells.

1982   Carrol RE, Hurst LC. The relationship of thoracic outlet syndrome and carpal tunnel syndrome. Clin Orthop 1982; 164:149–153.

Review of 888 cases of carpal tunnel syndrome and 63 of TOS revealed no patients with both conditions, arguing against a "double crush syndrome." However, later studies disagree (see Wood 1990).

1982   Dale A. Thoracic outlet compression syndrome: critique in 1982. Arch Surg 1982; 117:1437–1445.

A national survey disclosed 273 brachial plexus injuries from transaxillary first rib resection among more than 100 surgeons. Complete recovery occurred in 80%, incomplete in 20%. Although the incidence of permanent nerve injuries is probably less than 1% of all such operations, the disabilities can be serious. The author stresses thorough diagnostic evaluation and a trial of nonoperative treatment before surgery is offered to these patients.

1982   Demeter SL, Pritchard JS, Piedad OH, Cordasco EM, Taherj S. Upper extremity thrombosis: etiology and prognosis. Angiology 1982; 33:743–755.

Review of 17 cases in 16 patients of axillosubclavian vein upper thrombosis. Treatment was heparin in most cases, surgery in four, and streptokinase in one. Surgery is only for patients with primary thrombosis who do not improve on conservative management. Secondary thrombosis is a benign form of the disease and is self-limiting.

1982   Ferguson TB. The crisis of excellence. J Thorac Cardiovasc Surg 1982; 84:161–171.

Between 1975 and 1978, 21% of all malpractice claims against thoracic surgeons involved operations for TOS.

1982   Roos DB. The place for scalenectomy and first rib resection in thoracic outlet syndrome. Surgery 1982; 92:1077–1085.

In a series of 1,332 transaxillary first rib resections for TOS, 92% resulted in good to excellent relief; 93 scalenectomies for upper plexus symptoms resulted in 100% relief. Length of follow-up is not stated. Clinical features of upper and lower plexus involvement are discussed; no laboratory tests were helpful in making a diagnosis; the indications for surgery are reviewed.

1982   Sallstrom J, Thulesius O. Noninvasive investigation of vascular compression in patients with thoracic outlet syndrome. Clin Physiol 1982; 2:117–125.

Doppler flowmetry in 377 patients with arm pain and 63 controls revealed a high correlation between arterial compression and brachial plexus compression. However, there was little significance to this correlation because of poor sensitivity (false negatives) and poor specificity (false positives). Correlation between clinical pulse palpation and Doppler flowmetry was very high, suggesting that Doppler flowmetry adds little to the diagnosis of TOS.

1982   Sessions RT. Recurrent thoracic outlet syndrome: causes and treatment. South Med J 1982; 75:453–461.

Reoperation for recurrence in 29 TOS patients who previously had undergone a variety of surgical procedures revealed scar tissue binding the nerves of the plexus in each case. Reoperations included scalenectomy, neurolysis, and resection of the first rib or a posterior stump when present. Three-quarters of the recurrences developed within six months of the first operation. Results were 79% good to excellent and 14% fair, with follow-ups from one month to seven years, averaging 23 months.

1982   Wiley E. Discussion in Roos DB: The place for scalenectomy and first rib resection in thoracic outlet syndrome. Surgery 1982; 92:1084.

Because of a substantial number of recurrences following transaxillary first rib resection, and because relief of symptoms was achieved by a later scalenectomy, the author changed his operation for TOS to a combined supraclavicular scalenectomy plus transaxillary first rib resection. Common observations were neck and shoulder pain, headaches, and a history of neck trauma immediately preceding the onset of symptoms.

1983   Batt M, Griffet J, Scotti L, LeBas P. Le syndrome de la traversee cervico-brachiale. A proposde 112 cas: vers une attitude tactique plus nuancee. J Chir Paris 1983; 120:687–691.

Following transaxillary first rib resection in 94 cases, there was a 19.5% failure rate and a 10% complication rate leading the authors to give up the transaxillary route in favor of the supraclavicular approach.

1983   Becker GJ, Holden RW, Rabe FE, Castaneda-Zuniga WR, Sears N, Dilley RS, Glover JL. Local thrombolytic therapy for subclavian and axillary vein thrombosis. Radiology 1983; 149:419–423.

Four patients with upper extremity venous thrombosis were initially treated with thrombolytic therapy using streptokinase or urokinase administered locally via a catheter buried in the clot. The procedure was monitored continuously and the catheter frequently advanced further into the clot as lysis occurred. Subsequently, one patient underwent venous bypass and another percutaneous balloon angioplasty.

1983   Daskalakis MK. Thoracic outlet compression syndrome: current concepts and surgical experience. Int Surg 1983; 68:337–344.

General review of the clinical features, etiology, diagnostic criteria, and treatment options for TOS. Of 45 patients, 40 had good improvement following transaxillary first rib resection.

1983   Fager CA. Evaluation of cervical spine surgery by postoperative myelography. Neurosurgery 1983; 12:416–421.

Following cervical nerve root decompression without entering a disc space, all 49 patients had both clinical and radiological improvement. Following surgery in 23 patients with disc disease, several noted worsening of their symptoms, which did not always correlate with postoperative myelograms.

1983   Grimby G, Saltin B: Mini-review: the ageing muscle. Clin Physiol 1983; 3:209–218.

General review of the influence of ageing on muscle characteristics, such as fiber size, number, strength, and fiber distribution. The main cause of reduction in muscle mass is loss of muscle fibers. There is no evidence that lifelong exercise retards this ageing process. However, exercise does keep those remaining muscle fibers fit. Several hypotheses to explain these changes are discussed.

1983   Kawaguti M, Hamano A. Numerical study on poststenotic dilatation. Biorheology 1983; 20:507–518.

A model was constructed to stimulate blood flow in a constricted artery. It was shown that one of the hydrodynamic causes of endothelial lesion of artery and poststenotic dilatation can be found in the large temporal variation of shear stress behind a constricted portion of artery.

1983   Ruckley CV. Thoracic outlet syndrome. Brit Med J 1983; 287:447–448.

Good, concise review of TOS. No new data.

1983   Sakellarides HT. The management of carpal tunnel compression syndrome: follow-up of 500 cases over a 25-year period. Orthop Rev 1983; 12:77–81.

In 500 cases, those operated upon within one year of the onset of symptoms had excellent recovery of motor function in 75%, moderate recovery in 25%; and 100% recovery of sensory function. Among those operated upon after 2 to 10 years of symptoms the results were not as good: moderate recovery of motor function in 30% and slight recovery in 70%; sensory function recovery was adequate in 60% and moderate in 40%. Surgery should not be delayed too long in the presence of muscle wasting.

1983   Sallstrom J, Gjores JE. Surgical treatment of the thoracic outlet syndrome. Acta Chir Scand 1983; 149:555–560.

Transaxillary first rib resection in 72 cases resulted in 81% good to excellent and 12% fair improvement. Follow-up was 15–69 months. Vascular tests and EMG studies were not helpful.

1983   Saltin B, Gollnick PD. Skeletal muscle adaptability: significance for metabolism and performance. In: Peachey LD, ed. Handbook of physiology, Sect 10: Skeletal Muscle. Bethesda, MD: Am Physiological Society, 1983:555–631.

Comprehensive review of the plasticity of skeletal muscle and discussion of all aspects of skeletal muscle anatomy, histology, chemistry, physiology, and adaptation.

1983   Siivola J, Pokela R, Sulg I. Somatosensory evoked responses as a diagnostic aid in thoracic outlet syndrome. Acta Chir Scand 1983; 140:147–150.

Sensory evoked responses were abnormal in 9 of 13 patients operated upon for TOS. Postoperatively, two of three who were tested reverted to normal.

1983   Thomas GI, Jones TW, Stavney LS, Manhas DR. The middle scalene muscle and its contribution to the TOS. Am J Surg 1983; 145:589–592.

Middle scalene muscle anatomical variations were observed in 58% of 33 cases of TOS. The commonest finding was anterior insertion of the middle scalene on the first rib, so it narrowed an already narrow space. Supraclavicular first rib resection with anterior and middle scalenectomy resulted in 91% good to excellent results.

1983   Travell JG, Simons DG. Myofascial pain and dysfunction: the trigger point manual. Baltimore. Williams & Wilkins, 1983: 331–476.

Handbook of fibromyositis and myofacial pain.

1983   Yiannikas C, Walsh JC. Somatosensory evoked responses in the diagnosis of thoracic outlet syndrome. J Neurol Neurosurg Psychiatry 1983; 46:234–240.

In 11 patients with cervical ribs, 5 had objective clinical signs of compression. Conventional EMG and conduction velocity studies were abnormal in three of the five, but sensory evoked responses were abnormal in all five.

1984   Bargar WL, Marcus RE, Ittleman FP. Late thoracic outlet syndrome secondary to pseudarthrosis of the clavicle. J Trauma 1984; 24:857–859.

Single case report of TOS due to pseudoarthrosis of the clavicle treated by claviculectomy with a successful result at two years.

1984   Carpenter S. Pathology of skeletal muscle. New York: Churchill Livingston, 1984; 20–22.

There are a variety of causes of type II fiber atrophy. These include inactivity, upper motor neuron deficit, starvation, steroids, Cushing's disease, primary hyperparathyroidism, many malignancies, and others. Females and people with sedentary occupations tend to have smaller caliber type II fibers than type I fibers. Type I atrophy occurs in a number of neuromuscular diseases of childhood and in rheumatoid arthritis. In muscles from which diagnostic biopsies are ordinarily obtained, fiber distribution is: type I fibers, 30–40%; type II fibers, 60–70%.

1984   Dunant JH. Subclavian vein obstruction in thoracic outlet syndrome. Inter Angio 1984; 3:157–159.

Venous pressures in 50 normals revealed 88% had a mean increase of 7.5 cm H_2O during shoulder bracing and 90-degree arm abduction. Venograms in 60 normals revealed 70% had venous obstruction under hyperabduction and shoulder retraction. Over a six-year period, 25 patients had acute primary subclavian vein thrombosis treated with fibrinolysis. In 80% of these, there was a history of subclinical intermittent venous compression prior to the onset of acute thrombosis. In all 25, transaxillary first rib resection was performed after fibrinolysis. Postoperatively, 68% were asymptomatic and 24% were improved. In addition, 15 of the 25 patients had venographic evidence of functional venous compression of the contralateral, unaffected side under mere abduction or slight shoulder bracing and a correlated marked increase in venous pressure in the same arm positions. In these 15 patients, rib resection was also performed prophyllactically to prevent possible thrombosis.

1984   Gilliat RW. Thoracic outlet syndrome. In Dyke PJ, Thomas PK, Lambert EH, Bunge R, eds. Peripheral neuropathy. London: WB Saunders, 1984: 1409–1424.

Good review and classifications of nerve compression syndromes associated with cervical ribs and resulting in muscle wasting.

1984   Gu Y, Wu M, Zheng Y, Gu YD, et al. Combined supra- and infraclavicular approach for excision of the first rib in the treatment of TOS. Chung Hua Wai Kotsa Chin, 1984; 22:692–693. (In Chinese).

Description of the combined approach for first rib resection.

1984   Gugenheim S, Sanders RJ. Axillary artery rupture caused by shoulder dislocation. Surgery 1984; 95:55–58.

Single case report of traumatic rupture of axillary artery treated by interposition prosthetic graft. Approach was combined infraclavicular and transaxillary. Graft is functioning well at six year follow-up.

1984   Heughan C. Thoracic outlet syndrome. Can J Surg 1984; 27:35–36.

Review of 44 cases of transaxillary first rib resection with a 75% success rate. Patients with hand and arm symptoms had better results than patients whose predominant symptoms are shoulder and neck pain.

1984   Jerret SA, Cuzzone LJ, Pasternak BM. Thoracic outlet syndrome: electrophysiologic reappraisal. Arch Neurol 1984; 41:960–963.

The combination of somatosensory evoked potentials (SSEP) and ulnar nerve F-wave determinations yielded abnormalities in 17 of 18 TOS patients.

1984   Lee BY, Thoden WR, Madden JL, McCann WJ. Subclavian artery aneurysm secondary to thoracic outlet syndrome. Contemp Surg 1984; 25:19–25.

Report of two cases of subclavian aneurysms due to arterial compression, one from a cervical rib, the other from an unstated cause. Repair via claviculectomy included aneurysm excision and vascular reconstruction with good improvement.

1984   Livingstone EF, DeLisa JA, Halar EM. Electrodiagnostic values through the thoracic outlet using C-8 root needle studies, F-waves, and cervical somatosensory evoked potentials. Arch Phys Med Rehabil 1984; 65:726–730.

Normal values in 20 subjects were established to help standardize techniques for C-8 nerve root needle studies, ulnar F-waves, and cervical somatosensory evoked potentials (SSEP).

1984   MacDougall J, Sale D, Alway S, Sutton J. Muscle fiber number in biceps brachii in bodybuilders and control subjects. J Appl Physiol 1984; 57:1399–1403.

The number of muscle fibers in the muscles of bodybuilders and normal controls was the same indicating that enlarged muscle mass comes from fiber enlargement rather than an increase in number of fibers. The amount of connective tissue in both groups was the same, 13%.

1984   Mahon M, Toman A, Willian P, Bagnall K. Variability of histochemical and morphometric data from needle biopsy specimens of human quadriceps femoris muscle. J Neurol Sci 1984; 63:85–100.

Multiple biopsies from different areas and depths in the same muscle of the same individual demonstrated significant differences in fiber size. Caution should be observed when interpreting apparent changes in such values derived from subsequent biopsies in the same individual.

1984   Noda EIF, Lopez S. Thoracic outlet syndrome: diagnosis and management with a new surgical technique. Herz 1984; 9:52–56.

In 71 patients, 119 scalenotomies were performed with 100% good results and no complications. The "new" technique uses a 4 cm incision, isolates the phrenic nerve or nerves, and divides the anterior scalene muscle with a cautery. This is the only reported study with 100% good results from scalenotomy!

1984   Qvarfordt PG, Ehrenfeld WK, Stoney RJ. Supraclavicular radical scalenectomy and transaxillary first rib resection for the thoracic outlet syndrome: a combined approach. Am J Surg 1984; 148:111–116.

Following transaxillary first rib resection in 97 patients, there were 21% failures. Combining transaxillary rib resection with supraclavicular scalenectomy in 94 cases resulted in only 1% failures. History of neck trauma was present in 44%; headache or facial pain in 29%. In 81% of those explored supraclavicularly, some type of anatomical scalene muscle anomaly or variation was observed.

1984   Roos DB. Recurrent thoracic outlet syndrome after first rib resection. Inter Angio 1984; 3:169–177.

There was an 82% improvement rate in 151 patients undergoing 207 operations for recurrent TOS. Upper plexus symptoms are best approached supraclavicularly with scalenectomy and neurolysis; lower plexus symptoms with neuroplasty through the axilla and removal of the posterior rib stump. Fat pads are used to cover nerves. Resting arm for at least a month postoperatively may help avoid the scar tissue formation that is always found as the cause in these cases.

1984   Sallstrom J, Schmidt H. Cervicobrachial disorders in certain occupations, with special reference to compression in the thoracic outlet. Am J Ind Med; 6:45–52.

Workers in occupations requiring the use of their arms in abducted positions, such as cash register and key board operators or assembly line workers, have an incidence as high as 76% of upper extremity symptoms, almost half of them being compatible with TOS.

1984   Scher LA, Veith FJ, Haimovici H, Samson RS, Ascer E, Sushil KG, Sprayregen S. Staging of arterial complications of cervical rib: guidelines for surgical management. Surgery 1984; 95:644–649.

A good, practical classification of managing cervical ribs with arterial complications is presented which employs four stages. Stage 0 represents a cervical rib without arterial involvement and requires no surgical treatment unless there are neurologic symptoms of TOS. Stage I lesions have only arterial stenosis with minimal poststenotic dilatation and are managed by cervical rib resection only. Stage II lesions have intrinsic arterial damage, often with aneurysm formation, and require rib resection, arterial resection, and arterial reconstruction. Stage III lesions present with distal embolic complications and require thromboembolectomy, thoracic outlet decompression, and arterial reconstruction. Sympathectomy was not utilized in their 15 cases.

1984   Stallworth JM, Horne JB. Diagnosis and management of thoracic outlet syndrome. Arch Surg 1984; 199:1149–1151.

Report of 194 operations for relief of TOS symptoms, 180 of which included division of the pectoralis minor tendon. The article does not provide the clinical symptoms and diagnostic criteria that were used to select patients for operation.

1984   Swift TR, Nichols FT. The droopy shoulder syndrome. Neurology (Cleveland) 1984; 34:212–215.

Symptoms of this condition are pain in the shoulder, neck, chest, and arm, and frequently paresthesia in the hand. The condition differs from TOS in that these symptoms develop with the arms hanging down while TOS symptoms usually develop with the arm elevated. Physical exam and diagnostic tests are usually normal. Physical therapy to strengthen shoulder suspension has been disappointing.

1984   Urschel HC. Evidence for conduction delay in thoracic outlet syndrome is challenged. N Engl J Med 1984; 310:1052–1053.

The author admits he falsified a figure in his article of 1972. However, he continues to defend measurement of ulnar nerve conduction velocity (UNCV) as the best objective test for TOS.

1984   Vo NM. Thoracic outlet syndrome: ten years later. Conn Med 1984; 48: 143–146.

A general review of the etiologies of TOS.

1984   Wilbourn AJ. Evidence for conduction delay in thoracic outlet syndrome is challenged. N Engl J Med 1984; 310:1052–1053.

The article published by Urschel and Razzuk in 1972 on ulnar nerve conduction velocities (UNCV) has a falsified drawing of a muscle response. The author subsequently admitted this falsification of data.

1985   Chodoroff G, Lee DW, Honet JC. Dynamic approach in the diagnosis of thoracic outlet syndrome using somatosensory evoked responses. Arch Phys Med Rehabil 1985; 66:3–6.

Six of 14 patients with clinical TOS had normal sensory evoked potentials (SEP) at rest but abnormal responses with the arm abducted to 90 degrees in external rotation. The values were normal in both positions in 14 controls.

1985   Costigan DA, Wilbourn AJ. The elevated arm stress test: specifically in the diagnosis of thoracic outlet syndrome. Neurology 1985; 35: (Suppl 1) 74–75.

Abducting the arms to 90 degrees in external rotation, the elevated arm stress test, was positive in 92% of patients with carpal tunnel syndrome and 74% of asymptomatic controls. A positive test in thoracic outlet syndrome is obviously nonspecific.

1985   DeWeese JA. Management of subclavian venous obstruction. In Bergen JJ, Yao JST, eds. Surgery of the veins. Orlando, FL: Grune & Stratton, 1985: 365–382.

Thorough review of thrombotic and nonthrombotic upper extremity venous obstruction, including pathogenesis, clinical features, diagnosis, treatment, and results of different treatments.

1985   Druy EM, Trout HH, Giordano JM, Hix WR. Lytic therapy in the treatment of axillary and subclavian vein thrombosis. J Vasc Surg 1985; 2:821–827.

Treatment of nine patients, five with primary and four with secondary axillosubclavian vein thrombosis, is reviewed. All received streptokinase or urokinase; the four with secondary thrombosis had good results and were required no further treatment. Three of the five with primary thrombosis became asymptomatic but two had rethrombosis and required rib resection (one case) and balloon angioplasty (one case).

1985   Dubowitz V. Muscle biopsy: a practical approach. Philadelphia: Bailliere Tindall, 1985.

Basic textbook describing techniques of skeletal muscle biopsy and histochemical staining. The microscopic picture of normal muscle and muscle from various pathological conditions are depicted. The book contains excellent photomicrographs demonstrating the features it describes.

1985   Horowitz SH. Brachial plexus injuries with causalgia resulting from transaxillary rib resection. Arch Surg 1985; 120:1189–1191.

Four case reports of patients suffering brachial plexus injuries following transaxillary first rib resection, the most severe sequela being causalgia.

1985   Jamieson WG, Mersly H. Representation of the thoracic outlet syndrome as a problem in chronic pain and psychiatric management. Pain 1985; 22:195–200.

Description of three patients with symptoms of TOS following auto accidents. There were no objective abnormalities; all were referred for psychiatric evaluation; all improved following first rib resection. This stresses the point that a number of people suffer prolonged discomfort because many physicians are reticent to diagnose and treat TOS surgically without positive objective tests.

1985   Larsson L, Ansved T. Effects of long-term physical training and detraining on enzyme histochemical and functional skeletal muscle characteristics in man. Muscle Nerve 1985; 8:714–722.

Detraining resulted in a 16% and 14% decrease in proportion of type 1 fibers of proximal arm and leg muscles, respectively. In a separate study by Tesch and Karlsson (1985), a comparable increase in proportion of type I fibers was noted in trained athletes.

1985   Layzer R. Complications of medical and surgical treatment: neuromuscular manifestations of systemic disease. Philadelphia: F. A. Davis, 1985:363–366.

Radiation therapy for breast cancer is one of the most common causes of brachial plexus neuropathy. This complication occurred 1–2 years following completion of therapy in 73% of a large series of patients.

1985   Melliere D, Becquemin JP, Etienne G. Les complications de la chirurgie des defiles thoraco-cervico-brachiaux. J Chir Paris 1985; 122:151–157.

In French, this is a comprehensive discussion of complications of thoracic outlet surgery. There are five groups of complications: arterial injury; nerve injury; complications from the surgical approach; inadequate operations; and recurrence.

1985   Newmark J, Levy S, Hochberg F. Somatosensory evoked potentials in thoracic outlet syndrome. Arch Neurol 1985; 42:1036.

Sensory evoked potentials (SEP) were abnormal in only one of five musicians with TOS. This test offers little advantage over clinical evaluation.

1985   Raskin NH, Howard MW, Ehrenfeld WK. Headache as the leading symptom of the thoracic outlet syndrome. Headache 1985; 25:208–210.

First rib resection was used to treat 30 TOS patients in whom intractable headache was a presenting complaint. The majority had significant relief of their headaches postoperatively.

1985   Ryding E, Ribbe E, Rosen I, Norgren L. A neurophysiologic investigation of thoracic outlet syndrome. Acta Chir Scand 1985; 151:327–331.

Electromyography (EMG), sensory and motor ulnar nerve conduction velocities (UNCV), and F-wave responses were measured. There were no statistically significant differences in the response to all tests between 41 TOS patients and controls. Conclusion: There is no clinically applicable neurophysiologic diagnostic test to reliably detect nerve compression in the thoracic outlet area.

1985   Sanders RJ, Raymer S. The supraclavicular approach to scalenectomy and first rib resection: description of technique. J Vasc Surg 1985; 2:751–756.

Graphic description of technique of anterior and middle scalenectomy and supraclavicular first rib resection. This method is similar to the description in Chapter 10 of this book.

1985   Sendzischew H, Hempel GK. Anterior approach for resection of the first rib and total scalenotomy. Surg Gynecol Obstet 1985; 160:275–276.

Description of the supraclavicular technique of first rib resection. No illustrations.

1985   Taylor LM Jr, McAllister WR, Dennis DL, Porter JM. Thrombolytic therapy followed by first rib resection for spontaneous ("effort") subclavian vein thrombosis. Am J Surg 1985; 149:644–647.

Report of two cases of acute subclavian vein thrombosis treated with systemic streptokinase. This was followed by improved symptoms and recanalization by x-ray. Heparin, followed by coumadin and first rib resection, led to good symptomatic improvement in both patients.

1985   Tesch P, Karlsson J. Muscle fiber types and size in trained and untrained muscles of elite athletes. J Appl Physiol 1985; 59:1716–1720.

An adaptive response to long-term endurance training was noted by an increase in specific muscles of the proportion of type I, slow twitch muscle fibers. In the vastus lateralis of runners, type I fibers increased from a mean of 45% to 67%; in kayakers, biceps muscle biopsies showed type I fibers increased from 55% to 70%.

1985   Vogel CM, Jensen JE. "Effort" Thrombosis of the subclavian vein in a competitive swimmer. Am J Sports Med 1985; 13:269–272.

Single case report of a swimmer with acute "effort" thrombosis who initially was treated with local infusion of low-dose streptokinase with good clot lysis. After four months of warfarin therapy, transaxillary first rib resection was done with good improvement.

1985   Wilbourn AJ. Thoracic outlet surgery causing severe brachial plexopathy: clinical and EMG features in five cases. Muscle Nerve 1985; 8:612–613.

Report of five patients with brachial plexus injuries secondary to first rib resection for TOS.

1986   Aziz S, Straehley CJ, Whelan TJ Jr. Effort-related axillosubclavian vein thrombosis: a new theory of pathogenesis and a plea for direct surgical intervention. Am J Surg 1986; 152:57–61.

Four case reports of primary axillosubclavian vein thrombosis treated surgically 1, 4, 23, and 90 days after the onset of symptoms. Treatment included medial claviculectomy; thrombectomy; excision of the chronic stricture in the proximal subclavian vein as well as the costoclavicular ligament in each patient; and venoplasty in two patients. Temporary arteriovenous fistulae to increase flow were used twice. Six months to 20 year follow-up revealed all four were asymptomatic.

1986   Beurger R. Transaxillary sympathectomy. Ann Vasc Surg 1986; 1:155–156.

Technique of transpleural dorsal sympathectomy via an axillary incision. Chest is entered through second interspace. The sympathetic chain is removed beginning just below the stellate to below the third ganglion.

1986   Capistrant TD. Thoracic outlet syndrome in cervical strain injury. Minn Med 1986; 69:13–17.

This is the second paper by this author (first, 1977) on the relationship of neck trauma to TOS. In 111 cases of cervical neck strain, whiplash flexion-extension neck injuries were the commonest cause; rear-end auto collisions were the most frequent event. TOS symptoms were present in 36%. Most patients improved on conservative treatment; 7% were operated upon for TOS.

1986   Cherington M, Machanic B, Harper I, Parry L. Surgery for thoracic outlet syndrome may be hazardous to your health. Muscle Nerve 1986; 9:632–634.

Report of five patients with complications of transaxillary first rib resection: two with reflex sympathetic dystrophy, two with brachial plexus injury, and one with hemorrhage from a subclavian artery tear. The incidence of these complications is not stated.

1986   Connolly JF, Dehne R. Delayed thoracic outlet syndrome from clavicular non-union: management by morseling. Neb Med J : 1986; 303–306.

Single case report of TOS from compression by the callous of a clavicular fracture. This was treated by resecting the clavicular callous and uniting the bone ends; good result at 18 months.

1986   Conte FA, Orzel JA. Superior vena cava syndrome and bilateral subclavian vein thrombosis: CT and radionuclide venography correlation. Clin Nuclear Med 1986; 11: 698–700.

Single case report of man with superior vena cava obstruction in whom radionuclide venography demonstrated the obstruction and collateral venous channels. This method was superior to CT scanning.

1986   De Silva M. The costoclavicular syndrome: a "new cause." Ann Rheum Dis 1986; 45:916–920.

Heavy breasts, pulling the clavicle downward and narrowing the costoclavicular space, are postulated as the cause of TOS symptoms in the upper extremities. No data are presented.

1986   Gloviczki P, Kazmier FJ, Hollier LH. Axillary subclavian venous occlusion: the morbidity of a nonlethal disease. J Vasc Surg 1986; 4:333–337.

Long-term follow-up of 95 patients with upper extremity venous thrombosis revealed 60% were asymptomatic or had mild symptoms; 27% had symptoms with moderate exercise; 13% had symptoms at rest. Seventy-two percent of patients receiving anticoagulants for at least three months had good results compared to only 35% good results in those not anticoagulated. Surgery in 15 extremities, 12 first rib resections, gave good results in seven cases, fair in five, and poor in three.

1986   Huffman JD. Electrodiagnostic techniques for and conservative treatment of thoracic outlet syndrome. Clin Orthop Rel Res 1986; 207:21–23.

General review of neuroelectric tests and different modalities used to diagnose and treat TOS.

1986   Kulick MI, Gordillo G, Javidi T, Kilgore ES Jr, Newmeyer WL. Long-term analysis of patients having surgical treatment for carpal tunnel syndrome. J Hand Surg 1986; 11A:59–66.

Of 130 carpal tunnel releases, relief of paresthesia occurred in 81% with an average followup of four years.

1986   Machleder HI, Moll F, Verity A. The anterior scalene muscle in thoracic outlet compression syndrome: histochemical and morphometric studies. Arch Surg 1986; 121:1141–1144.

Freezing and histochemical stains were used to evaluate scalene muscles in TOS patients. The authors found type I fiber predominance and type I fiber hypertrophy. However, the hypertrophy was based on a comparison to elderly control patients and these findings have not been confirmed (see Sanders, 1990).

1986   Mercier C. Transaxillary first rib resection: technique. Ann Vasc Surg 1:150–154.

Good graphic presentation of steps in performing transaxillary first rib resection.

1986   Moore M Jr. Thoracic outlet syndrome experience in a metropolitan hospital. Clin Orthop Rel Res 1986; 207:29–30.

This is an overview of the changing ideas about etiology, diagnosis, and treatment of TOS. There is now more attention to trauma, increased use of CAT scans and neurophysiologic testing, and less use of plethysmography and angiography.

1986   Narakas A, Bonnard C, Egloff DV. The cervico-thoracic outlet syndrome. Ann Chir Main 1986; 5:185–207.

Extensive analysis of 75 operated patients with TOS. Trauma was a cause in about one-half. Postoperative nerve complications occurred in 14%, including two cases of severe pain from injury to the second intercostal brachial cutaneous nerve. The current approach, based upon this review, is designed to reduce the risks of surgery. First, nonoperative therapy is tried; if unsuccessful, supraclavicular exploration with anterior and middle scalenectomy and excision of all bands and ligaments is performed. If there appears to be costoclavicular compression, a transaxillary first rib resection is added.

1986   Perler BA, Mitchell SE. Percutaneous transluminal angioplasty and transaxillary first rib resection: a multidisciplinary approach to the thoracic outlet syndrome. Am Surg 1986; 52:485–488.

Single case report of man who was twice anticoagulated for axillosubclavian vein thrombosis and pulmonary embolus and developed a postphlebetic symptomatic arm. Combined first rib resection followed by transluminal venous angioplasty was performed to release extrinsic and intrinsic obstructions. He was asymptomatic at 16 months follow-up.

1986   Pollak EW. Thoracic outlet syndrome: diagnosis and treatment. 1986. Mount Kisco, NY: Futura Publishing.

This is the first book to be published on the subject of TOS that provides complete coverage of the important areas of anatomy, clinical features, diagnostic studies, nonoperative and operative treatment, and results of treatment.

1986   Pratt NE. Neurovascular entrapment in the regions of the shoulder and posterior triangle of the neck. Phys Ther 1986; 66:1894–1900.

Good review of the differential diagnosis of nerve entrapment syndromes in the neck and shoulder.

1986   Riddell DH, Smith BM. Thoracic and vascular aspects of TOS. Clin Orthop Update 1986; 207:31–36.

Overview of neurogenic, arterial, and venous TOS. This includes etiology, anatomy, signs, symptoms, diagnostic tests, and treatment.

1986   Rutherford RB, Flanigan DP, Gupta SK, Johnston KW, Karmody A, Whittemore AD, Baker JD, Ernst CB. Suggested standards for reports dealing with lower extremity ischemia. J Vasc Surg 1986; 4:80-94.

Useful definitions and criteria for reporting the results of procedures to treat ischemic limbs.

1986   Schubart PJ, Haeberlin JR, Porter JM. Intermittent subclavian venous obstruction: utility of venous pressure gradients. Surgery 1986; 99:365–368.

Venous pressure gradient was obtained in a patient with intermittent right subclavian vein obstruction using transfemoral catheterization and electronic transducer. Both subclavian veins were measured and significant elevation found in the involved right arm. Following supraclavicular first rib resection, the pressure gradient was abolished and the symptoms gone.

1986   Shields RW, Wilbourn AJ. Headache and the thoracic outlet syndrome. Headache 1986; 26:209–210.

Critique of the article by Raskin (Headache 25: 208–210) in which the authors express their sarcastic opinion of "the ubiquitous, nebulous quagmire of TOS." In responding to this attack, Raskin points out that he was simply reporting the observations in his patients (many others can confirm Raskins findings).

1986   Smith-Behn J, Althar R, Katz W. Primary thrombosis of the axillary/subclavian vein. South Med J 1986; 79:1176–1178.

Single case report of 16-year-old athlete with axillosubclavian vein thrombosis and pulmonary embolus successfully treated with systemic streptokinase, heparin, and long-term warfarin. Post-treatment venogram confirmed venous patency.

1986   Snider H C, King GD. Minnesota multiphasic personality inventory as a predictor of operative results in thoracic outlet syndrome. South Med J 1986; 79:1527–1530.

The results of psychological personality tests correlated well with improvement following TOS surgery. Normal tests were associated with 10 good results in 11 patients; abnormal tests correlated with good results in only 5 of 14 patients.

1986   Statler KA, Stevens, GF, Sterling WA Jr. Late stenosis of the subclavian vein after hemodialysis catheter injury. Surgery 1986; 86:924–927.

Report of two cases and review of eight others of subclavian vein stenosis secondary to hemodialysis catheters. Arm is asymptomatic until arteriovenous fistula for dialysis is established in that arm. Severe pain and edema ensue. Early recognition and treatment of the stenosis may preserve the fistula.

1986   Steed DL, Teodori MF, Peitzman AB, McAuley CE, Kapoor WN, Webster MW. Streptokinase in the treatment of subclavian vein thrombosis. J Vasc Surg 1986; 4:28–32.

Of seven cases of axillary vein thrombosis treated with streptokinase, there was dissolution of the clot in only one. However, all seven showed clinical improvement. This stresses the importance of venography in evaluating results.

1986   Swensen WM, Vigesaa RE, Hieb RE, James EC. Thoracic outlet syndrome: the supraclavicular approach to first rib resection. Surg Rounds 1986; Sept, 73–79.

Graphic presentation of the supraclavicular technique of first rib resection.

1986   Synek V. Diagnostic importance of somatosensory evoked potentials in the diagnosis of thoracic outlet syndrome. Clin Electroencephalogr 1986; 17:112–116.

Sensory evoked potentials (SEP) in 14 patients with osseous abnormalities in the thoracic outlet area were abnormal in nine patients, all of whom improved following corrective TOS surgery. Other tests led to the conclusion that abnormal ulnar nerve SEP's in the presence of normal median nerve SEP's support the diagnosis of TOS.

1986   Urschel HC, Razzuk MA. The failed operation for thoracic outlet syndrome: the difficulty of diagnosis and management. Ann Thorac Surg 1986; 42:523–528.

Review of 225 cases of recurrent TOS reoperated upon through a posterior thoracoplasty approach with 79% good and 14% moderate improvement. True recurrence was noted in 182 patients while persistent symptoms, pseudorecurrence, was noted in 43. A posterior stump longer than 1 cm was present in 154 of the 182 true recurrent cases. The authors stress the importance of ulnar nerve conduction velocities (UNCV) as an important diagnostic test.

1987   Ameli FM, Minas T, Weiss M, Provan JL. Consequences of "conservative" conventional management of axillary vein thrombosis. Can J Surg 1987; 30:167–169.

In a follow-up study of sequelae of upper extremity thrombosis in 20 patients treated conservatively with heparin initially then three months of warfarin, 15 patients were asymptomatic; five had residual symptoms.

1987   Bandyk DF, Kaebnick HW, Stewart GW, Towne JB. Durability of the in situ saphenous vein arterial bypass: a comparison of primary and secondary patency. J Vasc Surg 1987; 5:256–268.

Primary patency of a vein graft is defined as functioning of the graft without revisions or interventions. Minor revisions, requiring incisions or invasions into the graft, such as lytic therapy, exclude the graft from primary patency. Secondary patency is defined as an open graft that required some intervention to maintain patency.

1987   Benoit BG, Preston DN, Atack DM, DaSilva VF. Neurolysis combined with the application of a silastic envelope for ulnar nerve entrapment at the elbow. Neurosurgery 1987; 20:594–598.

Sixty-six patients with ulnar nerve entrapment at the elbow were treated with neurolysis and application of a silastic sleeve to prevent postoperative scarring. Sixty-six percent improved, 36% failed with an average follow-up of 12 months.

1987   Berger AR, Busis NA, Logigian EL, Wierzbicka M, Shahani BT. Cervical root stimulation in the diagnosis of radiculopathy. Neurology 1987; 37:329–332.

Cervical root stimulation was performed on 34 patients with unilateral cervical radiculopathy. This was more sensitive than EMG.

1987   Dunant JH. Diagnosis of thoracic outlet syndrome and indications for surgery. VASA 1987; 16:345–348.

Good review of the author's 15 years of experience with more than 1,200 patients with TOS and 375 operations. The diagnostic criteria are stressed and strict indications for surgery are presented, which include the exclusion of every other differential diagnosis and prolonged conservative therapy.

1987   Hagberg M, Wegman DH. Prevalence rates and odds ratios of shoulder neck diseases in different occupational groups. Br J Indust Med 1987; 44:602–610.

Certain occupations characterized as "repetitive arm movement jobs" have a much higher rate of neck symptoms, arm symptoms, and TOS compared to other occupations. These include keyboard operators, assembly line workers, and cash register operators.

1987   Huey H, Morris DC, Nichols DM, Connell DG, Fry PD. Low-dose streptokinase thrombolysis of axillary-subclavian vein thrombosis. Cardiovasc Intervent Radiol 1987; 10:92–95.

Streptokinase infusion for upper extremity venous thrombosis resulted in recanalization in 70% of 10 extremities.

1987   Jamieson CW. Venous complications of the thoracic outlet syndrome. Eur J Vasc Surg 1987; 1:1–3.

First rib resection is appropriate for intermittent venous obstruction but its role for the postphlebetic arm is questionable.

1987   Landercasper J, Gall W, Fischer M, Boyd WC, Dahlberg PJ, Kisken WA, Boland T. Thrombolytic therapy of axillary-subclavian venous thrombosis. Arch Surg 1987; 122:1072–1075.

Systemic streptokinase infusion via the contralateral arm was successful in four patients. Two patients also underwent transaxillary first rib resection.

1987   Leffert RD, Graham G. The relationship between dead arm syndrome and thoracic outlet syndrome. Clin Orthop 1987; 223:20–31.

Anterior shoulder subluxation can present with TOS symptoms. On occasion, TOS may coexist. Treatment is directed first to the shoulder problem.

1987   Leivseth G, Tindall A, Myklebust R. Changes in guinea pig muscle histology in response to reduced mobility. Muscle Nerve 1987; 10:410–414.

In guinea pigs, immobilization of one limb resulted in significant atrophy of type I and type II fibers in both gastrocnemius and soleus muscles.

1987   Machleder HJ, Moll F, Nuwer M, Jordan S. Somatosensory evoked potentials in the assessment of thoracic outlet compression syndrome. J Vasc Surg 1987; 6:177–184.

Transaxillary first rib resection in 59 patients with abnormal SEP's resulted in improvement in 86%; 21 patients with normal SEP's experiences 76% good results following surgery, although this group underwent operation on the basis of positive vascular compression on physical exam. Postoperative SEP's reverted to normal values in 91% of 40 patients who had good results from surgery.

1987   Mandel S. Neurologic syndromes from repetitive trauma at work. Postgrad Med 1987; 82:87–92.

Overuse and repetitive activities can cause repeated trauma to the upper extremities and produce a variety of compression syndromes, one of which is TOS. There is a good discussion of the mechanisms.

1987   O'Leary MR, Smith MS, Druy EM. Diagnostic and therapeutic approach to axillary-subclavian vein thrombosis. Ann Emer Med 1987; 16:889–893.

Report of four cases of upper extremity venous thrombosis managed by a variety of modalities including streptokinase, first rib resection, and transvenous angioplasty. Results were mixed.

1987   Pittam MR, Drake SG. The place of first rib resection in the management of axillary-subclavian vein thrombosis. Eur J Vasc Surg 1987; 1:5–10.

Venography in eight patients with symptomatic upper extremity venous thrombosis, three acute and five chronic, demonstrated complete venous occlusion in seven and marked narrowing in the eighth. Acute patients were anticoagulated: two slowly improved; one did not. Seven transaxillary first rib resections were performed, five with success. The two failures underwent axillary-internal jugular vein bypass with saphenous vein graft; both occluded. Venography in the contra-lateral arms of the eight patients revealed six with narrowing or occlusion. One became symptomatic within two years and required surgery.

1987   Roos D. Thoracic outlet syndromes: update 1987. Am J Surg 1987; 154:568–573.

Good overview of the subject of TOS including its history, etiology, vascular and neurogenic forms, clinical features, diagnosis, and treatment options.

1987   Sanders RJ, Rosales C, Pearce WH. Creation and closure of temporary arteriovenous fistulas for venous reconstruction or thrombectomy: description of technique. J Vasc Surg 1987; 6:504–505.

Technique is described for preparation of an arteriovenous fistula with Teflon reinforced polytetrafluoroethylene (PTFE). The graft is looped superficially, where it is buried subcutaneously, near the skin. This permits closure under local anesthesia several weeks later.

1987   Shuttleworth RD, Van der Merve DM, Mitchell WL. Subclavian vein stenosis and axillary vein "effort thrombosis": age and the first rib bypass collateral, thrombolytic therapy and first rib resection. S Afr Med J 1987; 71:564–566.

Report of three patients with upper extremity venous thrombosis treated first with streptokinase, then heparin for 10 days, followed by transaxillary first rib resection in two. Early results were good.

1987   Smith T, Trojaborg W. Diagnosis of thoracic outlet syndrome: value of sensory and motor conduction studies and quantitative electromyography. Arch Neurol 1987; 44: 1161–1163.

Ten patients with wasted hands and sensory symptoms were operated upon for TOS with improvement in sensory symptoms in all. Sensory and motor conduction velocities were normal in all and of no help. However, abnormal electomyographic

(EMG) studies of ulnar and median innervated small hand muscles and reduced amplitudes in sensory action potentials (SAP) from digit 5 were compatible with compression of C-8 and T-1 roots or the lower cord of the brachial plexus.

1987   Swenson WM, Rennich D, Capp KA, James EC. Axillary vein thrombosis due to thoracic outlet syndrome: correction via the supraclavicular approach. AORN J 1987; 46:878.

Description of technique of supraclavicular venous thrombectomy and first rib resection.

1987   Takagi K, Yamaga M, Morisawa K, Kitagawa T. Management of thoracic outlet syndrome. Arch Orthop Trauma Surg 1987; 106:78–81.

Report of 60 cases of TOS, 45 treated by transaxillary first rib resection and 15 by scalenotomy with a success rate of 78% and 80% respectively. Follow-up time was 12–96 months. No specific tests were helpful; diagnosis was made by exclusion and history.

1987   Warrens A, Heaton JM. Thoracic outlet compression syndrome: the lack of reliability of its clinical assessment. Ann R Coll Surg Engl 1987; 69:203–204.

Four maneuvers for assessment of thoracic outlet compression in 64 randomly chosen volunteers revealed 58% had a positive result in at least one of the maneuvers. The maneuvers and percentage positive were: Adson's, 15%; costoclavicular, 27%; erect hyperabduction, 14%; and lying hyperabduction, 5%. These results did not correlate with the findings of digital plethysmography.

1987   Wiles PG, Birtwell JA, Davies JA, Chennells P. Subclavian vein notch: a phlebographic abnormality associated with subclavian-axillary vein thrombosis. Brit J Hosp Med 1987; 37:349-50.

Four patients with axillosubclavian vein thrombosis were treated with streptokinase. Following lysis, they were placed on heparin for a few days and continued on warfarin for a few months. Two cases were successful, the other two rethrombosed. Following lysis, venography demonstrated a consistent filling defect in the subclavian vein with overlying thrombus. The implications of this notch-like defect are discussed with regard to additional treatment by rib resection to avoid rethrombosis.

1987   Zarins CK, Zatina MA, Giddens DP, Ku DN, Glagov S. Shear stress regulation of artery lumen diameter in experimental atherogenesis. J Vasc Surg 1987; 5:413–420.

Response of the arterial wall and intima to increased blood flow was studied in an atherogenic monkey model. Blood flow in one iliac artery was increased sixfold with an arteriovenous fistula. The arterial caliber doubled in size to accommodate the flow; wall shear stress remained unchanged suggesting that shear stress may be the factor regulating artery lumen diameter. There was no change in wall thickness or composition.

1988   Al-Hassan HK, Sattar MA, Eklof B. Embolic brain infarction: a rare complication of thoracic outlet syndrome. A report of two cases. J Cardiovasc Surg 1988; 29:322–325.

Report of two patients with cervical ribs, right subclavian artery thrombosis, and retrograde cerebral emboli. Treatment was by medial claviculectomy and resection and graft (vein and PTFE). One patient died from the stroke.

1988   Aminoff MJ, Olney RK, Parry GJ, Raskin NH. Relative utility of different electrophysiologic techniques in the evaluation of brachial plexopathies. Neurology 1988; 38:546–549

Standard conduction studies are helpful primarily to exclude lesions distal to the plexus. Supraclavicular nerve stimulation is not helpful as the results were normal in most TOS patients. Needle electromyography (EMG) is the most helpful test for TOS.

1988   Araujo JO, Azenha F, Barros ET, Marconi A. Reciprocal compression between the axillary artery and brachial plexus. J Cardiovasc Surg 1988; 29:172–176.

It was noted on arteriography in 10 of 60 TOS patients that there was total compression of the axillary artery under the head of the humerus, which the authors interpreted as being due to compression by a branch of the lower trunk of the brachial plexus. Treatment was by division and reanastomosis of the axillary artery on the other side of the nerve branch. Three of the 10 patients developed arterial stenosis at the suture line requiring reoperation. [Editorial comment: The existence of this condition is questionable. The authors may be misinterpreting compression by the humoral head for compression by a nerve branch. Arterial resection and reanastomosis carries serious risks and should not be undertaken lightly.]

1988   Blair SJ. Avoiding complications of surgery for nerve compression syndromes. Orthop Clin North Am 1988; 19:125–130.

Description of technical precautions designed to avoid nerve injuries in several upper extremity operations.

1988   Brown SC, Charlesworth D. Results of excision of a cervical rib in patients with the thoracic outlet syndrome. Br J Surg 1988; 75:431–433.

Review of 23 cervical rib excisions. Neurologic symptoms were present in 15, nine of whom were cured, five improved, and one failed. Among eight with vascular symptoms, one was cured and six improved. Conclusion was that rib resection alone may be insufficient for patients with vascular involvement and cervical ribs.

1988   Campbell PT, Simel DL. Left arm pain isn't always angina. NC Med J 1988; 49:564–567.

Chest pain simulating angina may be due to other causes. Two such cases are reported, one with left subclavian artery compression and a vertebral steal, the other with neurogenic TOS. Carotid-subclavian bypass in the first case and first rib resection in the second relieved symptoms in each patient.

1988   Colon E, Westdrop R. Vascular compression in the thoracic outlet: age dependent normative values in noninvasive testing. J Cardiovasc Surg 1988; 29:166–171.

Finger plethysmography revealed that 120 degree arm abduction reduced blood flow to zero in 44% of normals while no flow with the military position (costoclavicular compression) or the Adson maneuver produced zero blood flow in less than 10% of normals.

1988   Davies AL, Messerschmidt W. Thoracic outlet syndrome: a therapeutic approach based on 115 consecutive cases. Del Med J 1988; 60:307–330.

Trauma was present in the history of 65% and headaches a symptom in 26% of 115 patients undergoing 122 transaxillary first rib resections. Follow-up by questionnaire, with 85% followed for over two years, revealed relief of headaches in 20 of 30 patients; 20% had residual symptoms; 90% felt the operation helped them.

1988   Fredericks EJ. Brachial plexopathy complicating thoracic outlet syndrome surgery. Letter Musc Nerve 1988; 11:1090.

Short report of four cases of brachial plexopathy following transaxillary first rib resection. There is no mention of the incidence.

1988   Grant DS, Adiseshia M, Shaw PJ. Vascular compression in thoracic outlet syndrome—a potentially missed diagnosis. J R Soc Med 1988: 81.

Case report of positional arteriography being helpful in the diagnosis of TOS in a patient with symptoms of paresthesia and discoloration that occurred only in the erect position with the shoulders braced.

1988   Gu YD, Zhang GM, Chen DS, Yan JG, Cheng XM. Thoracic outlet syndrome. Chin Med J 1988; 101:689–694.

A variety of operations were used in 60 cases of TOS followed for 2–15 years with 82% good to excellent results. Anterior scalenotomy has been replaced by combined anterior and middle scalenectomy with improved results. When first rib resection is indicated, the approach of choice is a combining supra- and infraclavicular incisions.

1988   Horattas MC, Wright DJ, Fenton AH, Evans DM, Oddi MA, Kamienski RW, Shields EF. Changing concepts of deep venous thrombosis of the upper extremity—report of a series and review of the literature. Surgery 1988; 104:561–567.

Prospective study of subclavian venous catheterizations revealed 28% had venous thrombosis, often subclinical. Such catheters caused 39% of the 33 cases of axillary and subclavian vein thrombosis seen over six years. Pulmonary emboli occurred in 12%.

1988   Jain KM, Smejkal R. Use of spiral vein graft to bypass occluded subclavian vein. J Cardiovasc Surg 1988; 29:572–573.

Single case report of successful axillary-internal jugular vein bypass using a spiral vein graft fashioned over a size 32 French chest tube.

1988   Jackson CGR, Dickinson AL. Adaptations of skeletal muscle to strength or endurance training. In: Granna WA, ed. Advances in sports medicine and fitness. Vol 1. Chicago: Year Book Medical Publishers, 1988:45–60.

The cellular response of human skeletal muscle covers a wide spectrum of changes from strength training on the one hand to endurance conditioning on the other.

1988   Johnson EW. Practical electromyography. Second Edition. Baltimore: Williams & Wilkins, 1988.

Handbook of electromyography describing techniques and interpretations.

1988   Kritzer RO, Rose JE. Diffuse idiopathic skeletal hyperostosis presenting with thoracic outlet syndrome and dysphagia. Neurosurgery 1988; 22:1071–1074.

Case report of an unusual entity, diffuse idiopathic skeletal hyperostosis, which produced TOS and was successfully treated by infraclavicular first rib resection.

1988   Lalka SG, Cosentino C, Malone JM, Reinert RL, Bernhard VM. Hemodynamics of revascularization for iliofemoral venous occlusion: a short-term canine model. J Vasc Surg 1988; 8:592–599.

Acute animal study of venous hemodynamics that suggests large vein conduits may not need arteriovenous fistulae to maintain patency, but small conduits do need them. Precise location of the fistula is also discussed.

1988   Liebenson CS. Thoracic outlet syndrome: diagnosis and management. J Manipulative Physiol Ther 1988; 11:493–499.

Good general review of etiology, diagnostic criteria, and treatment of TOS. No data.

1988 Lindgren KA, Leino E. Subluxation of the first rib: a possible thoracic outlet syndrome mechanism. Arch Phys Med Rehabil 1988; 68:692–695.

Describes 22 patients with TOS and reflex sympathetic dystrophy, each with a hypomobile first rib, detected by reduced motion of the first rib on expiration and inspiration. As possible explanations, it is hypothesized that this action irritates the stellate ganglion causing symptoms, or that scalene muscle spasm reduces motion of the first rib.

1988 Lord JW Jr, Urschel HC Jr. Total claviculectomy. Surgical Rounds 1988; 11:17–27.

Technique of claviculectomy is graphically described and the indications and results in 37 cases are discussed.

1988 Machleder HI. Veno-occlusive disorders of the upper extremity. Curr Probl Surg 1988; 25:44–67.

Comprehensive review of the etiology, diagnosis, medical therapy, and surgical management of venous obstruction of the axillosubclavian vein.

1988 Manabe S, Tateishi A, Ohno T. Anterolateral uncoforaminotomy for cervical spondylotic myeloradiculopathy. Acta Orthop Scand 1988: 59:669–674.

Thirty-four of 35 patients with cervical spondylotic radiculopathy and abnormal myelograms had good response to surgical decompression. Follow-up time was not stated.

1988 Mandel S. Thoracic outlet syndrome (Editorial). Muscle Nerve 1988; 11:1090–1091.

A neurologist's approach to neurogenic TOS without objective findings. After thorough workup and unsuccessful trial of conservative therapy, over 100 patients were operated upon, with no permanent nerve complications and a 1-year improvement rate of 80%.

1988 Molina JE. Thrombolytic therapy of axillary-subclavian venous thrombosis: Letter to editor. Arch Surg 1988; 123:662–663.

There is no data to support the use of thrombolytic therapy alone, without another follow-up procedure. Lysis does not relieve extrinsic pressure nor internal venous webs, thickenings, and scar.

1988 Pang D, Wessel HB. Thoracic outlet syndrome. Neurosurgery 1988; 22:105–121.

Good, extensive review article of etiology, diagnosis, and treatment options for TOS.

1988 Rayan GM. Lower trunk brachial plexus compression neuropathy due to cervical rib in young athletes. Am J Sports Med 1988; 16:77–79.

Two case reports of TOS in athletes with cervical ribs. Transaxillary first rib and cervical rib resection gave good symptomatic relief in both.

1988 Rauwerda JA, Bakker FC, van der Broek TAA, Dwars BJ. Spontaneous subclavian vein thrombosis: a successful combined approach of local thrombolytic therapy followed by first rib resection. Surgery 1988; 103:477–80.

Five patients were treated for upper extremity venous thrombosis with local fibrinolysis followed in 3–12 weeks by transaxillary first rib resection. Postop venography revealed all five veins were open.

1988 Reilly LM, Stoney RJ. Supraclavicular approach for thoracic outlet decompression. J Vasc Surg 1988; 8:329–334.

Supraclavicular anterior and middle scalenectomy with first rib resection in 40 patients resulted in 58% good and 33% fair improvement. Postoperative complications included temporary brachial plexus palsy in 12% and temporary phrenic nerve palsy in 10%. There was one case of winged scapula, one with a self-limited chylothorax, and one patient had a subclavian vein repaired. At surgery, a variety of scalene muscle variants and anomalies were noted.

1988   Salo JA, Varstela, E, Ketonen P, Ala-Kulja K, Luosto R. Management of vascular complications in thoracic outlet syndrome. Acta Chir Scand 1988; 154:349–352.

Review of 12 cases of arterial TOS and six of venous TOS. Treatment of arterial cases required arterial reconstruction in three instances and mechanical decompression in nine. Early diagnosis and treatment reduces the need for major arterial reconstruction. Treatment of venous obstruction was transaxillary first rib resection in five and scalenotomy in one. No venous thrombectomies were done. All but one of the arterial cases were improved. Of the venous cases, three were asymptomatic and three had some symptoms.

1988   Sellke FW, Kelly TR. Thoracic outlet syndrome. Amer J Surg 1988; 156:54–57.

Transaxillary first rib resection in 473 cases resulted in a 79% complete and 14% partial relief of symptoms. Arterial symptoms were rare; 97% of symptoms were neurological, including coldness, which was most likely due to sympathetic nerve irritation or peripheral neuropathy and not arterial compression. EMG and UNCV studies were done in 182 cases and were mostly normal; yet the large majority of these patients experienced good results from surgery. Similarly, positional obliteration of the radial pulse was not found to be helpful. On physical examination, four positive findings were common: 90-degree AER stress test; supraclavicular tenderness and reproduction of symptoms with pressure over the scalene muscles; hypesthesia to touch and light pinprick over the ulnar nerve distribution of the arm and forearm; and weakness of the triceps or interosseous muscles of the hand. Thirteen patients had venous thrombosis; six had thrombectomy performed through the axilla.

1988   Stanton PE Jr, Vo NM, Haley T, Shannon J, Evans J. Thoracic outlet syndrome: a comprehensive evaluation. Am Surg 1988; 54:129–133.

Of 480 patients evaluated for TOS, the diagnosis was established in 300, 83 of whom underwent transaxillary first rib resection, four scalenotomy, and three pectoralis minor tenotomy. Nerve conduction studies and Doppler testing were positive in 75% and 60%, respectively. Both tests had high positive correlation with clinical results of surgery. Overall results were 81% good and 7% fair.

1988   Sullivan KL, Minken SL, White RI. Treatment of a case of thromboembolism resulting from thoracic outlet syndrome with intra-arterial urokinase infusion. J Vasc Surg 1988; 7:568–571.

Urokinase lysed a totally occluding thrombus in the subclavian artery and partially cleared peripheral emboli in a patient with recent ischemic hand symptoms. An open-ended guide wire was used for infusion rather than a catheter to minimize pericatheter thrombus formation. Angioplasty partially improved a stenosis in the subclavian artery in this patient who demonstrated no osseous abnormality.

1988   Veilleux M, Stevens JC, Campbell JK. Somatosensory evoked potential: lack of value for diagnosis of thoracic outlet syndrome. Muscle Nerve 1988; 11:571–575.

Analysis of neuroelectric diagnostic studies in 20 TOS patients noted sensory evoked potentials (SEP) were of little value; nerve conduction studies (NCS) and electromyography (EMG) were most helpful in excluding nerve compression at more distal sites in the arm than the thoracic outlet.

1988   White BE. Diagnosis of thoracic outlet syndrome. Del Med J 1988; 60:606–607.

Editorial comment critical of those who diagnose TOS on the basis of clinical criteria alone; the clinical criteria are all nonspecific. The author claims the diagnosis is quite rare if one uses as criteria hypothenar atrophy, C-8 sensory dysfunction, positionally related symptoms, and accurately performed neurophysiological studies.

1988   Wilbourn AJ. Thoracic outlet syndrome surgery causing severe brachial plexopathy. Muscle Nerve 1988; 11:66–74.

Description of symptomatic pattern from brachial plexus injuries in eight patients following first rib resection, six via the axilla.

1988   Wilbourn AJ. Thoracic outlet surgery: a reply (editorial). Muscle Nerve 1988; 11:1092.

The author responds to a criticism by a fellow neurologist of his position regarding "disputed TOS." He attempts to justify his stance by repeating his skepticism but provides no substantial data.

1988   Wood VE, Twito R, Verska JM. Thoracic outlet syndrome: the results of first rib resection in 100 patients. Orthop Clin North Am 1988; 19:131–146.

One hundred twenty transaxillary first rib resections in 100 patients resulted in improvement in 90%. The nine types of congenital bands identified by Roos are described in detail. Nine patients previously had cervical spine surgery; 44% had histories of trauma; many had a second nerve compression syndrome ("double crush syndrome"), the commonest being 25 patients with carpal tunnel syndrome. Postoperative complications included long thoracic nerve paralysis, 12%; snapping scapula, 11%; and persistent ICB nerve pain. Neurophysiological studies were of little help in diagnosing TOS; they were better for carpal tunnel or cubital tunnel compression. The most reliable diagnostic maneuvers on physical exam were duplication of symptoms with the arms at 90 degrees in AER and pain on direct pressure over the brachial plexus.

1988   Young MC, Richards RR, Hudson AR. Thoracic outlet syndrome with congenital pseudarthrosis of the clavicle: treatment by brachial plexus decompression, plate fixation, and bone grafting. Can J Surg 1988; 31:131–133.

One case report of a 20-year-old with TOS symptoms due to a constricting band running from the distal clavicular fragment to the first rib. Dividing the band relieved the symptoms.

1989   Barker WF. An historical look at the thoracic outlet compression syndrome. Ann Vasc Surg 1989; 3:293–298.

An excellent overview of the history of TOS covering the salient features of the eighteenth and nineteenth centuries, the cervical rib, scalenotomy, and first rib eras.

1989   Baumgartner F, Nelson RJ, Robertson JM. The rudimentary first rib: a cause of thoracic outlet syndrome with arterial compromise. Arch Surg 1989; 124:1090–1092.

Two case reports of arterial TOS due to rudimentary first ribs with poststenotic dilatation. First and second rib resection were performed to remove the osseous exostoses; arterial repair was not needed.

1989   Bilbey JH, Muller NL, Connell DG, Luoma AA, Nelems B. Thoracic outlet syndrome: evaluation with CT. Radiology 1989; 171:381–384.

Eight of 12 TOS patients with normal plain x-rays had abnormal findings on CT scan. These consisted of impingement of the C-7 transverse process on the scalene triangle or the middle scalene muscle.

1989   Cherington M. A conservative point of view of the thoracic outlet syndrome. Am J Surg 1989; 158:394–395.

This editorial presents the arguments against the existence of neurogenic TOS in the absence of electrodiagnostic abnormalities. All patients suspected of having TOS should undergo neurophysiologic testing even though it is rare for these tests to make a diagnosis of TOS by themselves; clinical interpretation is necessary. The author's reservations against surgery for TOS include the fact that serious complications have occurred from operations to remove first ribs and some patients do not improve postoperatively.

1989   Cikrit DF, Haefner R, Nichols WK, Silver D. Transaxillary or supraclavicular decompression for the thoracic outlet syndrome: a comparison of the risks and benefits. Am Surg 1989; 55:347–352.

Comparison of 30 transaxillary first rib resections with 15 supraclavicular anterior and middle scalenectomies revealed an early success rate of 81% for transaxillary rib resection versus 93% for scalenectomy. Seven cervical ribs were removed in the transaxillary first rib group; four cervical ribs and one first rib were removed in the supraclavicular group. Long term follow-up, with a mean of three years, found five recurrences in the rib resection group, reducing the success rate to 67%; there were no recurrences in the scalenectomy group, continuing at 93% success. Several complications occurred following rib resection, none following scalenectomy.

1989   Connolly JF, Dehne R. Nonunion of the clavicle and thoracic outlet syndrome. J Trauma 1989; 29:1127–1133.

Of 15 adult patients with nonunion of clavicular fractures treated with figure-of-eight bandages, seven developed symptoms of intermittent brachial plexus compression. Two of these resulted from resection of the mid-portion of the clavicle and impingement by the hypertrophied lateral stump. Nonunions of the clavicle respond well to reduction and adequate fixation making excision of the midclavicle unnecessary. If the mid-portion of the clavicle is removed to facilitate subclavian vascular exposure, it should be reimplanted and held with plate fixation to protect the neurovascular structures.

1989   Cormier JM, Amrane M, Ward A, Laurian C, Gigou F. Arterial complications of the thoracic outlet syndrome: fifty-five operative cases. J Vasc Surg 1989; 9:778–787.

To date, this is by far the largest single report of arterial TOS cases from one institution. Etiology in 55 cases was cervical rib in 31, abnormal first rib in 15, fracture in 3, and soft tissue compression in 8. Treatment was surgical through a combined supra-and infraclavicular route. Decompression was achieved by excision of the cervical and first ribs. Vascular reconstruction was by excision and end-to-end anastomosis in 23 and replacement vein graft in 11. Emboli were present in 35 cases and were extracted if possible. Of 39 patients available for follow-up, 35 were asymptomatic; four had claudication.

1989   Cormier JM, Tabet G. Resultats du traitement des complications arterielles des syndrome de la traversee thoroco-brachialle. In Kieffer E., ed. Les syndromes de la traversee thoraco-brachialle; Paris: AERCV, 1989:169–179.

1989   Cuetter AC, David MB: The thoracic outlet syndrome: controversies, overdiagnosis, overtreatment, and recommendations for management. Muscle Nerve 1989; 12:410–419.

In 14 patients, diagnoses other than TOS were found to explain patients' symptoms following unsuccessful first rib resection. These diagnoses could have been made preoperatively. First rib resection for TOS should be considered only after other diagnoses have been excluded and patients have not responded to conservative treatment.

1989   DeMaesemeer M, De Hert S, Van Schil P, Vanmaele R, Schoofs E. Deep venous thrombosis of the upper extremity: case reports and review of the literature. Acta Chir Beig 1989; 89:253–261.

Good discussion of etiology and treatment with report of three cases.

1989   Dobrusin R. An osteopathic approach to conservative management of thoracic outlet syndromes. J Am Osteo Ass 1989; 89:1046–1057.

General review of the etiology, diagnosis, and treatment of TOS. This includes a good description of osteopathic manipulative treatment.

1989   Goldberg BJ, Light TR, Blair SJ. Ulnar neuropathy at the elbow: results of medial epicondylectomy. J Hand Surg 1989; 14A:182–188.

Forty-eight cases of ulnar neuropathy treated by epicondylectomy had an overall improvement rate of 77%. Degree of postoperative improvement was directly related to amount of preoperative neurologic deficit. Sensory loss had the best results, motor loss the worst.

1989   Kaar G, Broe PJ, Bouchier-Hayes DJ. Upper limb emboli: a review of 55 patients managed surgically. J Cardiovasc Surg 1989; 30:165–168.

Causes of emboli in 55 patients were atrial fibrillation (33), myocardial infarction (5), subclavian artery aneurysm (20), atrial myxoma (2), unknown (14). Treatment was embolectomy (51) and primary amputation (2). The two aneurysms were not operated upon. There were no cases of TOS.

1989   Kieffer E, Ruotolo C. Arterial complications of thoracic outlet compression. In: Rutherford RB, ed. Vascular surgery, 3rd ed. Philadelphia: WB Saunders Co., 1989: 875–882.

Good review of the causes, diagnostic tests, and treatment of arterial TOS.

1989   Kolodinsky SD, Brandschwei FH. Axillary vein thrombosis in a female backpacker: Paget-Schroetter syndrome.

One case report of an unusual complication of backpacking.

1989   Kunkel JM, Machleder HI. Letter: Subclavian vein thrombosis. Surgery 1989; 106:114.

Following successful fibrinolytic therapy of upper extremity venous thrombosis, there is often a persistent focal stenosis at the point where the vein crossed the first rib. This should be managed by first rib resection as the initial procedure, as this is frequently due to perivenous fibrosis or extrinsic venous compression. If the defect persists postoperatively, percutaneous balloon angioplasty is tried.

1989   Kunkel JM, Machleder HI. Treatment of Paget-Schroetter syndrome: a staged, multidisciplinary approach. Arch Surg 1090; 124:1153–1158.

Excellent description of the management of 25 patients with axillary-subclavian vein thrombosis. Lytic therapy followed by anticoagulation was uniformly used and evaluated with venography. First rib resection was performed in 17 of the 25 patients because of residual symptoms after three months of warfarin therapy. After encountering three patients with separate thrombotic events in both upper extremities, bilateral venography was performed in the subsequent 15 cases, 12 of whom demonstrated venous compression on the contralateral side. Four of these patients underwent prophylactic first rib resection.

1989   Lepantalo M, Lindgren K-A, Leino E, Lindfors O, vonSmitten K, Nuutinen E, Totterman S. Long term outcome after resection of the first rib for thoracic outlet syndrome. Br J Surg 1989; 76:1255–1256.

Report of 112 transaxillary first rib resections for TOS with one month excellent results in 52%, fair in 25%. Follow-up after a minimum of 30 months, revealed only 37% excellent results, but no comment on number of fair results. Poorer results were in patients with work related etiology, neck pain, or symptoms worse at night. One instance of permanent plexus damage occurred.

1989   Lindgren SHS, Ribbe EB, Norgren LEH. Two year follow-up of patients operated on for thoracic outlet syndrome. Effects on sick-leave incidence. Eur J Vasc Surg 1989; 3:411–5.

One hundred seventy-five cases of TOS with two-year good or fair success in 59%. Of 110 TOS patients with anomalies, ribs or bands, 75(68%) had success. Prolonged sick-leave postoperatively correlated well with poor results from surgery.

1989   Loh CS, Wu AVO, Stevenson IM: Surgical decompression for thoracic outlet syndrome. J R Coll Surg Edin 1989; 34:66-8.

Fifty operations for TOS were performed, 40 through the supraclavicular route and 10 with an additional incision: Better access to the first rib was obtained by dividing the clavicle in three cases and adding an infraclavicular incision in seven. In 14 cases, fibrous or constricting bands were divided; cervical ribs were removed in another 14. In the remaining 22 cases, the first rib was removed as no specific compressing structure was identified. There was complete relief of symptoms in 74% and partial relief in 20%. The majority of patients noticed improvement on the day following surgery. Postoperatively, temporary phrenic nerve paresis occurred in six patients (12%).

1989   Lord JW Jr. Critical reappraisal of diagnostic and therapeutic modalities for thoracic outlet syndromes. Surg Gynecol Obstet 1989; 168:337-40.

This article emphasizes the serious complications of first rib resection and stresses that surgery should be limited to patients with positive objective findings after other diagnoses have been eliminated and conservative therapy has failed. It criticizes the large number of TOS operations performed in the United States between 1965 and 1985 on the basis of the fact that only 91 first rib resections were performed in seven New York hospitals between 1979 and 1986. The author implies that since so few were done in a big city like New York, surgeons in the rest of the country must be operating too often.

1989   McAllister RMR, Watkin G, Adiseshiah M. Unusual cause of thoracic outlet syndrome. Br J Surg 1989; 76:1257–1258.

Case report of TOS symptoms produced by a benign schwannoma arising from within a nerve root of the brachial plexus. There is a discussion of plexus tumors, their rarity, and their incidence.

1989   McCarthy WJ, Yao JS, Schafer MF, Nuber G, Flinn WR, Blackburn D, Suker Jr. Upper extremity arterial injury in athletes. J Vasc Surg 1989; 9:317–327.

Eleven athletes had TOS symptoms related to vigorous use of their arms. Arteriography revealed arterial compression of the subclavian artery or its branches in all, often during positional maneuvers only. Two patients with cervical ribs and subclavian aneurysms had the ribs resected and interposition vein grafts inserted. Eight patients had muscle resections: anterior scalene alone in five; pectoralis minor alone in one; and both muscles in two. Postoperative noninvasive studies demonstrated relief of arterial compression in the playing position of each patient and all had resumed their playing careers. One player with distal emboli was treated conservatively.

1989   Nelson DA. TOS = TMJ: True of false? Del Med J 1989; 61:339-40.

Editorial comment linking together TOS and TMJ syndrome as conditions often diagnosed by subjective clinical pictures in the absence of positive objective testing.

1989   Ojha M, Johnston KW, Cobbold RSC. Evidence of a possible link between post-stenotic dilatation and wall shear stress. Abs Int Soc Cardiovasc Surg Scientific Meeting 1989; 37:52.

1989   Pavot AP, Ignacio DR, Gargour GW. Assessment of conduction from C-8 nerve root exit to supraclavicular fossa—its value in the diagnosis of thoracic outlet syndrome. Electromyogr Clin Neurophysiol 1989; 29:445–451.

Description of a method of measuring nerve conduction time across the thoracic outlet. With a recording electrode over the abductor digiti quinti, measurements note the difference in latencies of stimulation at the C-8 nerve root and in the supraclavicular fossa. Normals had values of 0.4–1.2 msec while TOS patients had values of 1.0–2.6 msec.

1989   Pretre R, Spiliopoulos A, Megevand R. Transthoracic approach in the thoracic outlet syndrome: an alternate operative route for removal of the first rib. Surgery 1989; 106:856–860.

Description of first rib resection via an anterolateral thoracotomy through the second or third interspace. Success in 87% at one year in 18 cases compared to 84% in 13 cases of transaxillary rib resection. This approach avoids damage to the brachial plexus.

1989   Roos DB. Thoracic outlet nerve compression. In: Rutherford RB, ed. Vascular surgery, 3rd ed. Philadelphia: WB Saunders Co, 1989:858–875.

Good discussion of the etiology, clinical features, diagnosis, and surgical treatment of neurogenic TOS.

1989   Rutherford RB, Piotrowski JJ. Axillary-subclavian vein thrombosis. In: Rutherford RB, ed. Vascular surgery, 3rd ed. Philadelphia: WB Saunders Co, 1989:883–889.

Good review of etiology, signs, symptoms, diagnosis, and management of upper extremity vein thrombosis.

1989   Sanders RJ, Roos DB. The surgical anatomy of the scalene triangle. Contemp Surg 1989; 35:11–16.

Anatomical studies of 117 scalene triangles in cadavers established a number of anatomical variations in the normal relationship of muscles and nerves of the brachial plexus. Similar observations in 116 triangles in TOS patients demonstrated that TOS patients had a narrower triangle and anatomical predisposition to develop symptoms if a neck injury were to disturb the scalene muscles.

1989   Sanders RJ, Pearce WH. The treatment of thoracic outlet syndrome: a comparison of different operations. J Vasc Surg 1989; 10:626–634.

Life-table comparison of transaxillary first rib resection (111 cases), anterior and middle scalenectomy (279 cases), and combined supraclavicular first rib resection with scalenectomy (278 cases) revealed almost identical results to 15 years: 91–93% initial improvement, 70–73% at 3–5 years, and 64–65% at 10–15 years. There was less morbidity following scalenectomy alone.

1989   Sessions RT. Reoperation for thoracic outlet syndrome. J Cardiovasc Surg 1989; 30: 434–444.

Causes and treatment of recurrent TOS are thoroughly discussed. Sixty cases were treated with a variety of operations, but anterior scalenectomy and neurolysis were the most common. Most recurrences developed within a few months of the primary operation. Results were 79% good to excellent; 12% fair. Clinical features of upper and lower plexus involvement are reviewed. Removal of the posterior rib stump and covering the plexus with fat or a piece of PTFE may help prevent another recurrence.

1989   Strange-Vognsen HH, Hauch O, Andersen J, Struckmann J. Resection of the first rib following deep arm vein thrombolysis in patients with thoracic outlet syndrome. J Cardiovasc Surg 1989; 30:430–433.

Following successful fibrinolytic recanalization of thrombosed axillosubclavian veins, venograms revealed partial compression of the vein in the costoclavicular space in 11 of 20 cases at rest and in another six with the arms elevated. First rib resection was performed to prevent rethrombosis in 12 of these cases and none had developed rethrombosis during the one to six year follow-up. Two patients who did not have rib resection did experience rethrombosis.

1989   Winsor T, Winsor D, Mikail A, Sibley AE. Thoracic outlet syndromes: application of microcirculation techniques and clinical review. Angiology 1989; 40:773–782.

Quantitative measurements of fingertip blood flow using a laser instrument were performed with shoulders, arms, and head in various positions used to diagnose different compression points in TOS. The technique was highly successful in separating normals from patients with costoclavicular or scalenus anticus vascular compression.

1989   Wood VE, Verska JM: The snapping scapula in association with the thoracic outlet syndrome. Arch Surg 1989; 124:1335–1337.

Following 120 first rib resections, 15 instances of pain and "snapping" of the medial border of the scapula developed. Symptoms improved in 11 patient-sides following resection of the superior angle of the scapula. The technique is described.

1990   Dobrin PB. Arterial poststenotic dilatation. Surg Gynecol Obstet 1991.

Poststenotic dilatation is produced by flow disturbances sufficient to produce an audible bruit and a palpable thrill. Moderate arterial stenosis fulfills this requirement, while very mild or very severe stenosis do not. Although the exact flow disturbance is uncertain, abnormal shear stresses, eddy currents, jets, and turbulence all have been suggested as the cause. To produce poststenotic dilatation, the flow disturbance must cause the vessel wall to vibrate; the vibrations are thought to alter the elastin in the wall. Mild dilatation is often reversible within hours of removing the stenosis while dilatation to twice normal diameter may result in permanent aneurysm formation and require resection. Arterial dilatation as little as one-third greater than normal may contain ulceration with overlying thrombus. These vessels also require resection.

1990   Roos D. The thoracic outlet syndrome is underrated. Arch Neurol 1990; 47:327–328.

Editorial comment stressing the large number of patients with clinical symptoms of TOS who undergo prolonged conservative treatment for many months with no improvement, receive excessive worthless diagnostic tests, and are never offered a chance for symptomatic relief by surgical decompression. [See Wilbourn, Arch Neurol 1990; 47:228–230.]

1990   Roos DB. Transaxillary thoracic outlet decompression and sympathectomy. In: Bergan JJ, Yao JST, eds. Techniques in arterial surgery 1990; Philadelphia: WB Saunders Co., 1990: 305–316.

Description of the transaxillary technique of first rib resection and dorsal sympathectomy as performed by the author.

1990   Sanders RJ. Supraclavicular scalenectomy, first rib resection, and dorsal sympathectomy. In: Bergan JJ, Yao JST, eds. Techniques in arterial surgery 1990; Philadelphia: WB Saunders Co., 1990: 317–323.

Technical description of the supraclavicular approach for anterior and middle scalenectomy, dorsal sympathectomy, and first rib resection as performed by the author.

1990   Sanders RJ, Jackson CGR, Banchero N, Pearce WH. Scalene muscle abnormalities in traumatic thoracic outlet syndrome. Am J Surg 1990; 159:231–236.

Description of histologic changes in the scalene muscles of 45 traumatic TOS patients, all of whom had histories of neck injury. The microscopic features are type I fiber predominance, type II fiber atrophy, and an increase in connective tissue (from under 15% in normals to an average of 36% in TOS patients). A classification of TOS bases upon osseous abnormalities and a history of trauma is presented.

1990   Sanders RJ, Haug C, Pearce WH. Recurrent thoracic outlet syndrome. J Vasc Surg 1990; 12:390–400.

Recurrent or persistent TOS in 134 cases is presented. Postoperative scarring is the most common cause. Treatment depends upon what operation was done first: Scalenectomy and neuroplasty is performed for recurrence if the first operation was rib resection; first rib resection is done for recurrence if the first operation was scalenectomy. Using life-table methods, there was good to excellent improvement initially in 84%; this fell to 50% at the 3–5 year level and to 41% at 10-15 years. Patients with fair improvement were not included in these results and represent another 10%.

1990   Wilbourn AJ. The thoracic outlet syndrome is overdiagnosed. Arch Neurol 1990; 47:228–330.

Editorial comment stressing the lack of objective findings in "disputed" neurogenic TOS; the lack of consensus among its advocates regarding etiology and diagnostic criteria; and the failure to routinely use neuroelectric diagnostic testing. Iatrogenic nerve injury is pointed out as an unfortunate consequence of an operation done for what may have been inadequate indications. (See Roos, Arch Neurol 1990; 47:227–228).

1990   Wilson JJ, Zahn CA, Newman H. Fibrinolytic therapy for idiopathic subclavian-axillary vein thrombosis. Am J Med 1990; 159:208–211.

Of eight cases of axillary vein thrombosis treated with streptokinase, five developed total and two partial recanalization. Although all five of the total recanalized veins revealed residual narrowing at the upper margin of the first rib, none of the patients developed postphlebitic symptoms during the five-year follow-up. This supports the view that first rib resection is unnecessary in these patients.

1990   Wood VE, Biondi J. Double-crush nerve compression in thoracic outlet syndrome. J Bone Joint Surg 72A:85–87.

Compression of a nerve distal to the thoracic outlet was demonstrated by neurophysiologic studies in 44% of 165 patients undergoing transaxillary first rib resection for TOS. Carpal tunnel compression was the commonest. In 13 cases, operation at three sites was needed to relieve symptoms.

1991   Jackson CGR, Banchero N, Sanders RJ. The histochemistry of traumatic thoracic outlet syndrome. In Preparation.

Description of the techniques used by muscle physiologists to examine skeletal muscle and the findings in normal and in TOS scalene muscle. (See Sanders, Jackson, Banchero, Pearce, 1990)

Index